LIFE CYCLE
GROUP WORK
IN NURSING

LIFE CYCLE GROUP WORK IN NURSING

Ellen Hastings Janosik, R.N., M.S.

Alfred University, Alfred, New York.

Lenore Bolling Phipps, R.N., M.S.

Western Monroe Mental Health Center, Rochester, New York.

Jones and Bartlett Publishers, Inc.

Boston   Monterey

Printed in the United States of America

10 9 8 7 6 5 4

ISBN 0-86720-388-9

Editorial office: Jones and Bartlett Publishers, Inc., 23720 Spectacular Bid, Monterey, CA 93940
Sales and customer service offices: Jones and Bartlett Publishers, Inc., 20 Park Plaza, Boston, MA 02116

Subject Editor: Judy Joseph
Production Editor: Maggie Schwarz
Interior Design: Meryl Levavi
Cover Design: Fred Charles
Illustrations: L.E.P.I. Graphics, Albany, N.Y.
Typesetting: L.E.P.I. Graphics, Albany, N.Y.

Dedicated
to
Ed Janosik
and
Art Phipps

PREFACE

"No man [or woman] is an island entire of itself; every man is a piece of the continent, a part of the main . . ."

John Donne
1573–1631

Life Cycle Group Work in Nursing combines theory and clinical application of theory in a unique way. The book has a strong theoretical foundation, and examples from clinical practice that illustrate the theoretical concepts are included in every chapter. Part 1 begins with a discussion of alternative models for group work and presents the recurrent life cycle model as the most effective approach for undertaking and understanding groups. Intrapsychic and interpersonal groups are explained by comparing psychoanalytic concepts with gestalt-experiential concepts. Application of crisis theory in a group setting is described fully. Stages and levels of group development are contrasted and compared. Process and content are defined operationally through communication theory, conflict issues, and curative group factors.

Part 2 builds on the theories presented in the first part. The activities needed to organize groups are discussed in detail. Selection criteria, preparation of members, and the group contract are included in the guidelines. Adaptive and maladaptive behaviors of group leaders and group members are treated extensively, with clinical examples firmly based on group theory.

Part 3 deals with special population groups and their purposes. Chapter 10 on health-care teams contains original material that is based on clinical observation and research and explores such group aspects as collegiality as it affects the functioning of health teams. Chapter 15 on group work with substance abusers presents original research findings that have implications for selecting alcoholics for certain types of group treatment. The recurrent life cycle model is used in this section to link group work to the resolution of developmental and situational tasks. Group work with children and adolescents, couples and families, the elderly and chronically ill is presented in Chapters 11–14. Chapter 16 describes the wide range of group psychotherapy and concludes this comprehensive section. Here, as elsewhere in the book, clinical examples based on preceding theoretical constructs are included. Principles for assessing needs, planning the group, and implementing interventions are given for each special population under discussion.

Part 4 is concerned with evaluation of group work and the analysis of evaluative data. Chapter 17 discusses some research strategies used to evaluate groups. The advisability of combining intrasubject/intersubject studies with intragroup/intergroup investigation is considered. In Chapter 18, there are brief descriptions of behavioral, physiological, and psychological measures of group effects. A few useful analytic procedures for data are outlined. Numerous sources of measurement tools are cited in the chapters. For purposes of evaluation, the dimensions of group research are delineated as structure, process, and outcome.

This book is an integration of group theory and practice. Theory is not treated as abstract knowledge but as an integral component of group work. Readers need not struggle to translate theoretical concepts into clinical realities. That has been our intention and constitutes the primary strength of the book. It is our hope that *Life Cycle Group Work in Nursing* will answer the requirements of nursing practitioners and students seeking to engage in group work from an ethical and enlightened vantage point.

Ellen Hastings Janosik
Lenore Bolling Phipps

ACKNOWLEDGMENTS

We wish to recognize the contributions of the following colleagues: Betty Evans, whose encompassing knowledge of psychodynamics and the human experience enriched our theoretical and clinical foundation; Gertrude E. Flynn, whose devoted efforts to expand the scope of nursing have enhanced the profession; Linda Carter-Jessep, Elaine Hubbard, and Gerri Lamb, whose discussions contributed to the development of ideas in Chapter 10; and Eva McLaughlin of the Neurology Department of Hospital for Sick Children in Toronto, Canada, for sharing her experience in working with a group program organized for young people with epilepsy.

We also thank the following people for their reviews and suggestions during the early stages of *Life Cycle Group Work in Nursing:* Barbara Backer, Herbert H. Lehman College, CUNY; Roberta Brown, University of California, Los Angeles; Patricia Campion O'Neill, SUNY, Stony Brook; Rose Constantino, University of Pittsburgh; Caroline Pendzick, SUNY, Stony Brook; Karen Sewall, George Mason University;

Moira Shine, George Mason University; Penny Starkey, Arizona State University; and Jane White, George Mason University.

We also wish to acknowledge the many individuals and families whose participation contributed to our understanding of the complexities of group work.

Finally, we extend appreciation to the following individuals and publishers for permission to use selected materials from their copyrighted works:

Bales, R.F. *Interaction Process Analysis: A Method for the Study of Small Groups*. Midway Reprint Series, Chicago: University of Chicago Press, 1951. Used by permission of the University of Chicago Press.

Bellak, L. *The Best Years of Your Life*. N.Y.: Atheneum Publishers, 1975, pages 12, 13. Used by permission of Dr. Bellak to whom the copyright reverted.

Murray, R., Huelskoetter, M., and O'Driscoll, M.S. *The Nursing Process in Later Maturity*. Englewood Cliffs, N.J.: Prentice Hall, Inc., 1980.

Sampson, E., and Marthas, M. *Group Process for the Health Professions*. N.Y.: John C. Wiley and Sons, 1977.

Wurmser, L. "Drug Abuse: Nemesis of Psychiatry," *American Scholar* 41(3), 1972. Copyright by the United Chapters of Phi Beta Kappa; adapted by permission of the publishers.

CONTRIBUTORS

JOAN E. BOWERS, ED.D., R.N., Assistant Professor and Coordinator, Department of Psychosocial Nursing, Family and Child Pathway, University of Washington, Seattle, Washington.

VEDA BOWLER BOYER, M.S., R.N., Assistant Professor, Indiana University Hospitals, Psychiatric Nurse Clinician, Indianapolis.

RICHARD S. DEFRANK, PH.D., M.A., Post-Doctoral Fellow in Social Psychology, Prevention of Cardiovascular Disease Program, University of Houston, Houston, Texas.

LYNN WEST GRIFFITH, M.S., R.N., Assistant Professor of Nursing and Chairperson, College of Nursing, Alfred University, Alfred, New York.

ELLEN HASTINGS JANOSIK, M.S., R.N., Psychiatric Nurse Clinician, Assistant Professor of Nursing, Afred University, Alfred, New York.

LOIS KOCH MARVIN, M.S., R.N., Assistant Professor of Nursing, Roberts Wesleyan College, Rochester, New York.

JEAN R. MILLER, PH.D., R.N., Associate Dean of Research and Development, College of Nursing, University of Utah, Salt Lake City, Utah.

LENORE BOLLING PHIPPS, M.S., R.N., Psychiatric Nurse Clinician. Consultant in psychiatric-mental health nursing, Western Monroe Mental Health Center, Rochester, New York.

MADELINE H. SCHMITT, PH.D., R.N., Associate Professor of Nursing and Sociology, University of Rochester, Rochester, New York.

THOMAS R. ZASTOWNY, PH.D., M.A., Research Associate in Pediatrics, University of Rochester, Rochester, New York.

CONTENTS

LIFE CYCLE
GROUP WORK
IN NURSING

PART ONE

Group Theory

1

Group Work: History and Overview

Lenore Bolling Phipps

Individuals are social beings. Since the beginning of time human beings have shaped and been shaped by the groups to which they have belonged. All individuals are born into an original, or primary, group known as the family. This is the group that helps to mold identity and transmit cultural patterns of behavior. The original group continues to serve as the foundation from which individuals relate to other groups and to the larger community.

The word "group" may have different meanings for people, depending on experiences and perceptions. The term "group" as it is used in this text refers to an interdependent association of two or more persons united by a common interest, whose actions are interrelated so that each person influences and is influenced by each other person (Sampson, 1977).

Human beings live and work in groups that influence them in multiple ways. Groups provide interactional experience which alters behavior, attitudes, and ideas. Whether through affiliations with education, religion, industry, medicine, politics, or mental health, interdependence and interrelatedness within groups are the mechanisms by which individuals develop and extend their innate potential. Groups constitute essential social systems which organize, shape, and enrich our lives.

HISTORY OF GROUP WORK

Attention to the study and understanding of how and why groups work has followed an erratic course during the twentieth century. At times this understanding of groups has been the result of serendipitous discovery; at other times understanding has been the result of controlled scientific experimentation.

The Early Years

The use of groups within the health-care system was first introduced in 1907 by a Boston internist, Dr. Joseph Pratt, in the treatment of despondent tuberculosis patients. Pratt met regularly with groups of patients and, in an atmosphere of support and reassurance, taught them about diet and hygiene (Freedman, 1972). While the primary task of these groups was educational, Pratt may have been aware of other therapeutic ingredients at work within these groups, such as a mutual sharing of concerns in a supportive environment. He continued to use auxiliary-group treatment at his Boston clinic for many years (Wilson, 1979).

Other physicians began to employ Pratt's lecture format with patient groups, using the premise that education is inherent in treatment. Marsh and Lazell, among others, utilized didactic lectures in attempts to treat groups of mental patients. Lazell believed that improvement occurred in these populations not only because of the educational material presented but also because of increased social interaction and diminished levels of fear in the group (Freedman, 1972).

The Twenties and Thirties

During the 1920s and 1930s psychiatrists began to study group social interaction, including the way in which group members related to each other and to the group as a whole. Therapy groups were thought to possess characteristics which recreated the climate of the family of origin. Expanding on this theme, group therapists believed that the individual member related to other members and to the group leader in ways reminiscent of patterns that had existed in the original family (Freedman, 1972). Freud would have endorsed the idea that it was essential to understand one individual in relation to significant others, since the basic mechanisms in any group replicate identification, empathy, and sharing present in the original family. This idea was later extended to include the concept that any group may become a social microcosm. The social microcosm concept suggests that the group provides the medium in which members' styles of relationships parallel their lives outside the group. These interactional styles are spontaneously and unconsciously expressed, both verbally and nonverbally (Loomis, 1979). The significance of this phenomenon for psychotherapy groups lies in the belief that a corrective change in the group will be transposed to external relationships and an opportunity will be provided for understanding the customary roles or behavior patterns of group members.

Important contributions to the advancement of group work were provided by Trignant Burrow in 1927. A precursor of the encounter movement, Burrow stressed the importance of "here and now" events and encouraged the spontaneous expression of current physical and emotional experiences. He believed many of these experiences were universal, which when shared with other group members, lessened feelings of isolation and increased feelings of belonging. His approach was innovative in method and in the concept that members were not considered "sick" patients being treated by a "well" physician but rather that together they were participants sharing the human experience (Anthony, 1971).

Jacob Moreno, another pioneer in group work, devised his "theater of spontaneous man" using drama and role playing to enact problem situations. This role playing enabled group members to seek and practice alternative behaviors and to increase their cognitive and emotional self-awareness (Freedman, 1972).

The Northfield Experiment

The study of group work probably received its greatest impetus from the stresses and demands of World War II. Because of the scarcity of psychiatrists available to treat the vast numbers of battle-fatigued, emotional casualties of the war, development of a group approach was hastened, and it became economical and effective to use group work as a method of treatment. European and American psychiatrists working together at military centers helped nurture and develop one another's ideas on group treatment. In Northfield, England, doctors suspended army protocol and treated military patients in small groups like civilians. It was here that Foulkes, a psychiatrist, developed the concept of a community "network." Foulkes's idea was that the patient's network of personal relationships with friends and family at the time of illness had a profound effect on recovery (Anthony, 1971). The Northfield experiment not only provided rich training in the applied theory of group work but also furnished the creative impetus for much of its development in the watershed years which followed World War II.

Kurt Lewin

Our current understanding of group characteristics comes mainly from the work of Kurt Lewin, who expanded the horizons of applied group theory. Lewin was a proponent of using the experimental method in social science to test leadership styles, communication patterns, and social pressures which influence behavior (Mills, 1967). He proposed that any group works as a unit to determine its goals and standards, and that these standards, or norms, are maintained by group social pressures which insure individual member conformity. Individuals' attitudes and habits are greatly influenced by the group to which they belong or in which they desire membership. A sense of acceptance and belonging are the rewards for behavior which corresponds to the group's expectations. Altering an individual's group-approved behavior requires an *unfreezing* of those behaviors, either reducing the person's dependence on the group or changing the standards of the group as a whole. *Refreezing* is the process of retaining the new behavior through interaction with a group whose standards support and reinforce it (Sampson, 1977).

One example of group pressure and the refreezing process may be seen in some contemporary weight-reduction groups. An individual raised in a family in which food was equated with love and finishing one's dinner was rewarded with praise, continues to practice overeating because it is a family-approved behavior, even at the price of obesity in later years. The decision to join a weight-reduction group enables this person to identify with a new group, and to receive approval from this group in return for an alteration in eating habits. The person shifting from one set of group values to that of another group may feel conflict for a time.

According to Lewin, conflict is innate and essential to any group. Conflict is not detrimental in itself but it carries the potential for the group's growth or its destruction. Conflict usually arises between the conformity demanded by the group and the individual support it provides to its members. Lewin identifies possible conflicts arising among the individual's wish to merge and yet to be separate, the needs of one member versus the needs of the group as a whole, and the forces which contribute to group survival or group destruction. If the group is to survive, its subtask is to negotiate successfully any of these inherent conflict issues (Anthony, 1971).

The Postwar Years

Between 1945 and 1970 the applied theory of group work began to interest many disciplines. Group theory was introduced into the university curricula of sociology, psychiatry, education, nursing, and psychology. Industry and government saw the advantages of understanding the ways in which groups function and thus supplied financial support for the development of applied theory. In 1947 the National Training Laboratory for Applied Behavioral Science (NTL) was established in Bethel, Maine, with the objective of teaching group dynamics to government and industrial managers. Understanding that human relations skills were vital in contemporary society, NTL used training groups, *T-groups*, as an educational method. The objectives of these groups were to increase the member's awareness of his or her influence and interaction within the group, increase the member's understanding of group dynamics, increase the member's competency in handling difficult situations, and relate these ideas to job performance effectiveness (Anthony, 1971). In 1973, at the University of Chicago, the noted theorist and clinician Carl Rogers described a group program to help Veterans Administration counselors increase their effectiveness in guiding veterans in postwar adjustment.

The postwar years brought marked socioeconomic changes in American society which contributed to the development of the encounter group movement of the 1960s. A booming economy carried the double-edged sword of affluence and alienation. On the one hand the economy provided sufficient income to meet most physical needs, and on the other it imposed computerized technologies which increased the impersonal aspects of contemporary society. The primary group, or the family, is highly mobile and dispersed geographically, while the numbers of single-parent families are markedly increasing. Groups focusing on growth, awareness, and relatedness have been aimed at decreasing that alienation. Carl Rogers, in 1973, commented that physical affluence has contributed to our sometimes desperate search to meet psychological needs. Individuals hunger for close and genuine relationships in which feelings are expressed spontaneously, experiences are shared, and new behaviors are tested.

Abraham Maslow Abraham Maslow, in 1968, formulated a vigorous humanistic psychology which stated that physiological and psychological health are obtainable through the gratification of basic hierarchical needs. For most people, basic needs are satisfied neither through ascetic self-denial nor hedonistic self-indulgence. Instead, human needs tend to follow an ordered pattern of urgency. Maslow's hierarchy of needs is 1) food, shelter, and physical survival; 2) protection, safety, and security, 3) belongingness, friendship, affection, and love; 4) respect, self-esteem, approval, and dignity; and 5) self-actualization or the freedom to develop one's full potential. Maslow regarded the lowest level of needs to be most urgent, but also considered high level, nonmaterial needs important.

Powers of self-actualization must be exercised if they are to remain functional, just as muscles must be used if they are to remain strong. In the affluent years following World War II, when lower level needs could be satisfied easily, popular clamor arose for opportunities to experience the need levels of personal fulfillment and self-actualization. Because material needs were easily satisfied, people turned to the pursuit of "peak" experiences, which were considered a form of psychological growth. Although Maslow did not think that self-actualization was a "peak" experience, these two terms were sometimes used interchangeably by the public. The popular idea of self-actualization and "peak" experiences incited enormous demand for groups in which self-growth was a major goal. A widespread result of the clinical and experimental projects of Maslow and Rogers, among others, was to support group work among persons without conspicuous psychiatric disorders. The work of growth-oriented social psychologists provided further impetus by presenting theory on self-actualizing group experiences.

The Encounter Movement The need for personal growth, or self-actualization, was the catalyst for the subsequent development of the encounter group movement of the 1960s. While diverse groups fell under the category of "encounter movement," they all recognized the basic needs an individual has to feel competent, worthwhile, and loveable, and they held as their goal the improvement of interpersonal relationships through the expression of genuine feelings. Heightened perception of emotion, living in the present, and qualities of openness and honesty were emphasized (Sayre, 1979).

The encounter movement, which was initially regarded as a panacea, was evaluated by a Stanford research team in 1973. Their data suggest that while these groups may provide opportunities to increase self-awareness and self-expression, encounter groups leave no lasting positive change in most people (Lieberman, 1973).

STUDYING GROUP BEHAVIOR

The challenge of studying group behavior has taken two major routes: these are the NTL (National Training Laboratory for Applied

Behavioral Science) model and its English counterpart, the Tavistock model. Advocates of the latter model study group process and development by focusing on the relationship between the group and the leader. The NTL model examines member-to-member relationships (Stafford, 1978).

There has been increasing interest in data-collecting techniques to measure group variables. Moreno devised the *sociogram,* a simple instrument which shows the pattern of emotional relations in a group by identifying the most liked or disliked group members. Sociologist Robert Bales saw the group as a miniature social system or problem-solving unit and developed a scoring technique to quantify group interaction. Bales' scoring has become a standard research method for the evaluation of small groups. His technique is described in Chapter 17 of this text. At Harvard University, experiments were conducted in small self-study groups in which members studied their own reactions and behaviors in order to learn about group development and process. The current trend in the study of group behavior is the use of mathematical measurements to analyze the complex process of group dynamics.

The use of therapeutic small groups has grown in sophistication and applicability since Dr. Pratt's first formal lectures to tuberculosis patients in 1907. Theodore Mills, a sociologist, noted in 1967 that certain trends were becoming evident:

1. The small group functions as an interface between the individual and the community.
2. The current focus of study is on the internal dynamics, or process.
3. Groups are being created to test specific hypotheses for experimental research purposes.
4. Self-analytical groups in which members simultaneously act as participants and observers provide an exchange of objective and subjective information.
5. Mathematical models are being developed to analyze group process in conjunction with general systems theory.

GROUP WORK IN NURSING

The therapeutic value of group work is evident in many ways. Groups provide opportunities to share similar problems in a supportive and responsive atmosphere, and to learn and test new behaviors. Group work is a therapeutic tool which the skillful and knowledgeable nurse can use in his or her repertoire of practices. It is the nurse's task to assimilate the theory and practice of group work. This will require understanding and knowledge of:

- personal behavior in the group
- group development
- theoretical frameworks
- leadership skills
- membership roles (Marram 1973).

While nurses have traditionally worked with large groups of patients in wards or clinics, their role as formal leaders of small groups has emerged only recently. There are several factors which have contributed to this role expansion during the past two decades.

Contemporary society has been described as an age of alienation, characterized by geographic mobility and the breakdown of traditional family, neighborhood, religious, and social-support systems. Nurses have often viewed illness in a social context, providing care while understanding the ramifications of illness to family and community. As traditional support systems have become unavailable, nurses have expanded their practice to meet this need. This role expansion frequently has taken the form of leadership of small supportive and educational groups such as those for preoperative patients, postpartum mothers, and diabetics.

Perhaps the most influential of the factors contributing to the role expansion of nurses as leaders of small groups is the changing pattern of health care. The current trend is toward community rather than hospital health care, and toward distributive rather than episodic care. Prevention has introduced new approaches and new terminology. Gerald Caplan (1970), a mental health theoretician, spoke of primary prevention, which diminishes the incidence of illness; secondary prevention, which decreases the prevalence of illness; and tertiary prevention, which maintains the patient at an optimal level of functioning. Group work is applicable at any and all levels of prevention, serving both patients and nonpatients. For example, neonatal classes prepare young families at the primary prevention level. Parents Anonymous groups enable child-abusing parents to learn more positive and less destructive parenting behaviors at the secondary prevention level. At the tertiary prevention level, remotivation groups assist recently discharged mentally ill patients to re-enter the community. Today's health care system provides challenges and opportunities for nurses to assist groups, families, and communities to prevent illness and to treat and restore health.

Another factor in the promotion of group work in nursing has been the impressive number of articles on the subject. An informal survey of articles in nursing journals reflects the scope of the group approach, with its applicability to all nursing specialties. There are articles relevant to direct and indirect nursing practice, to supervisory and interdisciplinary roles, and to consultation.

A third factor, related to the second, has been the inclusion of group dynamics into the nursing curricula at the undergraduate and graduate levels. The earliest efforts to include group therapy in a university began at Wellesley College in 1952 with the introduction of group experiences to ease the adjustment of freshmen students into the nursing role. Later, sensitivity training was included in many graduate curricula in psychiatric nursing to enhance self-awareness and clinical effectiveness. In these groups students were participant-observers. Using an unstructured format, members focused on their feelings and reactions as well as on the process of group dynamics. The reaction to these group experiences was generally favorable and the result was a more knowledgeable and accepting attitude toward human relationships on the part of participants (Adams, 1971).

In the future the nursing profession may expect additional and continued pressure to work with groups. With the soaring costs of health care and the focus on primary prevention, it has become necessary to incorporate this tool into nursing practice (Gardner, 1979).

THE NEED FOR A THEORETICAL FRAMEWORK

How do nurses work with groups? What are the guidelines for group interventions? A theoretical framework provides a basis for direction and decision making in therapeutic interventions (Armstrong, 1963). A theoretical framework is composed of interrelated concepts and principles which predict and explain certain phenomena. It standardizes practice and promotes greater objectivity. Using a theoretical framework provides a frame of reference for intervention, a systematic process which guides the leader's assessment and approach. A theoretical foundation insures a sound, logical approach and contributes the knowledge and expertise so essential to any profession (Marram, 1973). Numerous theoretical frameworks have evolved out of psychiatry, psychology, and sociology. Among these are psychoanalytic, gestalt-existential, communication, interactional, and crisis groups. A detailed discussion of these frameworks is presented in the following chapters.

Some controversy surrounds the use of a single theoretical frame-work versus an eclectic approach. There are arguments that using a solitary theory impedes the leader's spontaneity or natural style by forcing an artificial subjection of the group to the theory. An eclectic orientation provides greater flexibility and freedom in that it enables the leader to select concepts and principles from multiple theories according to their suitability for a particular group or situa-tion, thus expanding the options to predict and to explain more group phenomena than is possible using a single framework. Eclecticism may also provide greater flexibility and freedom in the selection of goals and interventions which may be tailored to individual or group needs.

The disadvantages of eclecticism lie in the depth of approach and the breadth of leader experience. Group work which utilizes multiple theories may lack completeness and yield broader but more super-ficial results. Eclecticism may prove a burden for the beginning prac-titioner trying to master a solid theoretical foundation. The inexper-ienced leader quite often relies on an intuitive rather than a deliberative approach. For the newcomer to group work a solitary theoretical framework often provides a necessary measure of security (Marram, 1973).

MEMBERSHIP AND CATEGORIES OF GROUPS

There are three major categories of groups: primary, secondary, and reference. Everyone belongs to each of these groups in a lifetime, though membership in any specific group may change over time. Mem-bership may be inherited, as in a family group, or acquired, as in an occupational group.

Membership defines who is and who is not included in the sphere of influence of the group. Members of a group are expected to con-form to certain attitudes and behaviors, which may be clearly defined or vaguely implied, depending on the group. Membership is contingent on the eligibility and attraction which the group has for the potential member. It is one thing to be acceptable to a group and quite another to wish to join the group. Therefore, membership is determined by eligibility or noneligibility and by negative or positive attractiveness.

Nonmembership has interesting ramifications. The nonmember who is independent and eligible but who refuses to join a group may threaten group integrity by refusing to acknowledge the group. This phenomenon was exemplified in the actions of certain political leaders who refused to join social clubs that excluded ethnic and racial minorities.

Another uncertain and difficult situation involves the marginal nonmember who wishes to be accepted but is currently ineligible. This position often precipitates anxiety, which may be expressed in excessive conformity or in rebellion, confusion, anger, or despair. For example, the adolescent is often psychologically a marginal, nonmember of the family. Though technically a family member, psychologically he or she may be an outsider, lacking full adult status with its privileges and responsibilities (Sampson, 1977).

Categories of Groups

The Primary Group   The *primary group* wields important influence in a person's life. This is the significant face-to-face group which confirms identity, influences social values, behavior, and provides support (MacLennan, 1968). People have a lifelong need for primary-group affiliation, with the close and informal ties which bind them together and help satisfy emotional needs. The family, as the patient's primary-group network, has profound implications in patient care. Because family members have marked influence on each other, illness in one member has great impact on the others. Consequently, prevention and treatment require family participation (Phipps, 1980).

The Secondary Group   *Secondary groups* play less of a role in self-definition than primary groups. These are also small, face-to-face groups but they are less intimate and more impersonal. Secondary groups are limited to a specialized purpose or function which is task- or work-oriented. These groups may be informally or formally structured in terms of leadership, rules, or tasks, and they occur in occupational, educational, or recreational spheres of activity (Sampson, 1977).

Both primary and secondary groups have two major functions: maintaining the members' interpersonal needs and accomplishing the group's task. The importance of these two functions may vary though both functions are vital to the life of the group and are influenced by the leader. For example, the family, as a primary group, must meet the socioemotional as well as the material needs of its members. These two types of needs may be provided by one or both parents. The health team, as a secondary group, may have a major physical role in the management of a patient's illness but it also must provide internal respect and cooperation to insure the morale of its members.

The Reference Group *Reference groups*, the third category
of groups, are groups in which individual membership may not be apparent, but which nevertheless influence attitudes, values, and behaviors. Reference groups provide an implied standard of behavior. A
person may have many reference groups and may change, discard, or
acquire groups over time, but usually one reference group is most
influential at any one time. Membership in a reference group is often
characterized by a vague but enveloping identification with other group
members, so that the self is evaluated in terms of group values, standards, and goals (Marram, 1973). What constitutes a reference group
for one person may be a secondary group for another. Conversely,
an all-encompassing membership may transform a secondary group
into a reference group. Nurses whose identity is shaped by professional activities regard their professional organization as a reference
group rather than a secondary group. Reference groups are characterized by powerful racial, religious, ethnic, or occupational affiliations. A minority with negative self-image and powerlessness may
use reference-group affiliation as a form of affirmative action. Recently, minority memberships have gained reference-group strength with
slogans such as "Black Is Beautiful" and "Women Are Equal." One
can accept or deny minority group membership. Denial of reference-
group allegiance causes one to identify with what the reference group
is not. Interracial and interreligious marriages often represent a
repudiation of inherited reference-group affiliation.

Adopting a new reference group carries the potential for redefining
oneself, creating conflict between one's personal values and group
values, or dividing oneself between the old and new reference groups.
In short, changing reference groups can be constructive or destructive
in terms of self-definition, role adjustment, and self-esteem. Reference groups that are constructive increase self-esteem, provide a sense
of belonging without a loss of identity, and minimize conflict with
other reference-group affiliations.

A lack of reference-group membership may have a detrimental
effect. Any individual without reference-group affiliation lives at
the fringes of society, alienated and uncertain regarding identity
and values (Marram, 1973).

SUMMARY

This chapter introduced group work with a historical review of groups
both within and beyond the health-care system. The significance of
group work as it relates to nursing practice was discussed, and the
basic concepts and categories of group membership were presented.

REFERENCES

Adams, J. "Student Evaluations of an Interactional Group Experience," *Journal of Psychiatric Nursing and Mental Health Services* Vol. 9, No. 4, 1971, pages 28–36.

American Psychiatric Association Services Division. *A Psychiatric Glossary.* 3rd ed. Washington, DC, 1969.

Anthony, E.J. "The History of Group Psychotherapy." In *Comprehensive Group Psychotherapy*, H.I. Kaplan and B.J. Sadock, Eds. Baltimore: Williams and Wilkens, 1971.

Armstrong, S., and S. Roulin. *Group Psychotherapy in Nursing Practice.* New York: Macmillan, 1963.

Caplan, G. *The Theory and Practice of Mental Health Consultation.* New York: Basic Books, 1970.

Cartwright, D., and A. Zander. *Group Dynamics, Research and Theory.* New York: Harper & Row, 1968.

Freedman, A.; H. Kaplan; and B. Sadock. *Modern Synopsis of Psychiatry.* Baltimore: Williams and Wilkins, 1972.

Gardner, K. "Small Groups and Their Therapeutic Force," *Principles and Practice of Psychiatric Nursing.* St. Louis: C.V. Mosby, 1979.

Lieberman, M.A.; I.D. Yalom; and M.B. Miles. "Encounter: The Leader Makes the Difference," *Psychology Today* Vol. 6, No. 10, March 1973, pages 69–76.

Loomis, M. *Group Process for Nurses*, St. Louis: C.V. Mosby, 1979.

Luft, J. *Group Processes: An Introduction to Group Dynamics.* 2nd ed. Palo Alto, CA.: National Press Books, 1970.

MacLennan, B., and N. Feldsenfeld. *Group Counseling and Psychotherapy with Adolescents.* New York: Columbia University Press, 1968.

Marram, G. *The Group Approach in Nursing Practice.* St. Louis: C.V. Mosby, 1973.

Mills, T.M. *The Sociology of Small Groups.* Englewood Cliffs, N.J.: Prentice-Hall, 1967.

Phipps, L. "Theoretical Frameworks Applicable to Family Care," *Family-Focused Care.* New York: McGraw-Hill, 1980.

Rogers, C. *Carl Rogers on Encounter Groups.* New York: Harper and Row, 1973.

Sampson, E., and M. Marthas. *Group Process for the Health Professions.* New York: Wiley, 1977.

Sayre, J. "Alternative Healing Therapies," *Psychiatric Nursing*, H.S. Wilson and C.R. Kneisl, Eds. Menlo Park, CA: Addison-Wesley, 1979.

Stafford, L. "Two Methods for Study of Group Behavior," *Journal of Psychiatric Nursing and Mental Health Services* Vol. 16, No. 4, 1978, pages 32–34.

Wilson, H.S., and C.R. Kneisl, Eds. *Psychiatric Nursing.* Menlo Park, CA: Addison-Wesley, 1979.

Yalom, I. *The Theory and Practice of Group Psychotherapy.* New York: Basic Books, 1975.

2

Models of Groups: Rationale and Typology

Ellen Hastings Janosik

A model may be described as a set of related ideas applied to groups in order to explain what is being observed or investigated, and to organize the data. Models are interpretative or selective approaches to the study of groups which influence the observer's viewpoint.

RATIONALE FOR GROUP MODELS

The search for meaning in group events may prove overwhelming to the nurse who is functioning as a group leader or participant-observer. Complex relationships among such variables as group goals, composition, process, and outcomes make it difficult to understand group phenomena in a coherent way. When one's understanding of the group is based only on random clinical observation, definite conclusions are seldom reached. This is true even when observations are made on a regular basis. Clinical observation of the group carried out over time does, however, permit assumptions about group phenomena and hypotheses about what interventions worked and why. For most group leaders, planning for future sessions depends largely on data obtained through observations. Despite its limitations, sustained clinical observation is essential to the search for meaning in group dynamics.

The only common characteristic of all groups is that they are composed of individuals engaged in a process which has meaning (Loomis, 1979). A nurse involved with group work cannot turn to technical instruments such as stethoscopes or microscopes to define what is being observed. The application of a group model attempts to do this, although it is less precise.

Three basic requirements which have been advocated for theory building may be adapted by the nurse attempting to assess group dynamics (Henderson, 1955). They are intimate contact and familiarity with the phenomena; collection and organization of data; and effective cognitive approaches to the observed phenomena. In this paradigm a search for meaning must begin with sustained observation, communication, or other involvement with the group whose dynamics are being assessed.

Group Interaction

Group interaction takes place between individuals protected by psychological boundaries which are more or less penetrable. Such boundaries tend to inhibit full comprehension by observers of what is taking place. Individual boundaries encircle each person in the group, while larger boundaries surround the group itself. The nurse who is a leader or participant-observer must transcend protective individual boundaries to some extent. An outside observer must transcend both group and individual boundaries in order to assess group phenomena.

The term *boundaries* is subject to interpretations which concern the extent of individual involvement with others and the extent of group involvement with the environment. Individual boundaries may be described as outer limits within which selfhood is contained. In group terminology, boundaries consist of rules and role expectations which define which persons belong to the group and how they function as group members. Boundaries facilitate group development by separating the group from external systems in order to promote task accomplishment. At the same time the boundaries of individual members function to prevent excessive loss of self as group forces begin to emerge. Usually there is more interaction or energy exchange inside individual or group boundaries than across these boundaries.

Protective boundaries can only be bridged or transcended through sustained observation, which validates or refutes what has been seen previously. Unfortunately, independent observation and assessment may be threatened by the same close contact which is required. Therefore, any group observer wishing to be objective has a technical problem which has been articulated as follows (Mills, 1967).

- The group observer must transcend boundaries to permit adequate examination of group phenomena.
- The group observer must also maintain boundaries, remaining separate in order to avoid being psychologically incorporated by the group.
- The group observer must progress from random observation to structured assessment of group phenomena.

Clinical observation of group phenomena may inadvertently be affected by the biases or predilections of observers. Prolonged contact with spontaneous interactional processes often causes confusion in the group observer. Because group interaction takes place at several levels, cognitive understanding may be jeopardized. In addition, objectivity may be impaired by the feelings aroused in the observer witnessing the interactions of the group. Some members stir feelings of hostility while others arouse sympathy. The actions of a leader may be viewed with admiration or distaste. This hazard is particularly formidable for a participant-observer, whether a group leader or a group member. Using a model helps avoid this by changing random observations into structured observations, which moderate the affective responses of observers.

Because every group is unique, it is dangerous to use one group to typify many. Yet the nurse who observes, leads, or participates in groups needs a unifying model which recognizes complexities but also introduces a degree of order among variables. Using a model increases the perceptiveness of the observer by providing a focus.

A group model helps the observer to discern patterns, and offers analytic tools to deal with the data. Application of a model to the data encourages categorization and generalization, two processes which assist inductive thinking. Models of groups are usually two-dimensional in that they trace spatial and temporal developments and thereby help clarify abstract ideas (Anthony, 1971). They are not all-inclusive nor are they a substitute for systematic research. If an appropriate group model has been selected, data collection and organization are facilitated and there is more likelihood of achieving adequate cognitive understanding of the data.

SYSTEMS MODEL OF GROUPS

There is a wide selection of group models, none of which is superior in all respects. General systems theory is sometimes applied to the assessment of group dynamics with good results. The properties of a system include boundaries, structure, function, interdependence, and feedback processes, all of which are evident in groups. Because groups are made up of individuals rather than components, they are considered social systems in which all participants are interacting units relating directly or indirectly to each other. As social entities or systems, groups can be distinguished by their properties from the environment, which constitutes a larger system or systems.

Although a group is composed of individual members, it displays characteristics which are different from the total characteristics of its members. The group may be less or more than the sum of its parts, for the experience of being in a group alters the participants in negative as well as positive ways. As a result, groups possess a distinct wholeness different from the sum of their parts. This is a consequence of interdependent activities occurring in the group.

Three group models were contrasted and designated as the member to leader model, the group to leader model, and the systems model. In the first two models relationships show linearity, but not in the third. In the systems-group model the leader is described as a regulatory agent whose interventions produce circular rather than linear effects (Astrachan, 1970). This is the result of feedback loops which maintain reciprocal interactions among all participants in the system. Systems theory considers group organization and participant behavior to be inextricably linked. Groups cannot be understood except by examining participant behavior in the context of boundaries, structure, function, and interrelatedness which are major characteristics of groups as social systems (Olsen, 1968).

One drawback in applying a systems model to groups is that there is a developmental or maturational aspect to group life which a systems model overlooks. Group development is an emerging process, and the nurse assessing group dynamics should select a model which accounts for changes over time. There are three important models of groups which direct attention to developmental changes: the *linear-progressive* model, the *life cycle* model, and the *recurrent or pendular life cycle model.* Each model considers developmental changes in a different way. The interpretation which the observer makes is influenced by the group model being used. It is the model and the theoretical orientation of the observer which determines what is being observed and how it is being assessed (Watzlawick, 1976).

Linear-Progressive Models of Groups

Linear-progressive models see change in the group as an evolutionary, forward movement. Various group theorists have imposed their own developmental stages on this progression. One simple formulation of the linear-progressive model divides group dynamics into an initial stage, a working stage, and a final stage. Certain behaviors are thought to be characteristic of the various stages, but the duration of each stage may vary greatly. For example, a time-limited group scheduled to last twelve weeks may, because of time pressures, move quickly from the initial to the working stage, especially if motivation is high. On the other hand, a long-term group with a life expectancy of several years and low motivation might spend twelve weeks in the initial stage. Chronology alone is not reliable in determining the stage of group development. It is important to analyze the linear-progressive model and other developmental group models in behavioral rather than temporal terms.

Behavior Patterns Investigation supports the idea that stages in group development are characterized by prevailing behaviors. In a study of encounter groups Carl Rogers (1970) identified ten patterns or stages based on the clustering of events and behaviors. In these stages, which were named *process patterns*, group behavior moved from early conditions of testing and resistance to trustfulness and the development of a *healing capacity* in the group. Following the appearance of a healing capacity, resistance to change seems to weaken and the group begins to move toward therapeutic growth (Anderson and Carter, 1978; pages 94-95). Other investigators (Kaplan and Roman, 1963) noted the clustering of behaviors during group development and identified three sequential stages in which prevailing behaviors indicate feelings of dependency, power, or intimacy. In some respects these stages of group behavior are analogous to the stages of psychosexual behavior formulated by Freud (Burgess and Lazare, 1976). Behaviorally and experientially, the dynamic conflicts of an immature group resemble the dynamic conflicts of a child moving from one psychosexual developmental stage to the next. This analogy is illustrated in Table 2-1.

Table 2–1   INTEGRATION OF GROUP AND INDIVIDUAL DYNAMIC
CONFLICTS

Phases of Group Development (Kaplan and Roman, 1963)		Phases of Individual Psychosexual Development (Burgess and Lazare, 1976)
Phase 1.	Dependency		Oral Phase: To be cared for and protected
Phase 2.	Power	Early Period	Anal Phase: To be in control and secure
			Phallic Phase: To achieve; To be strong and powerful
		Later Period	Latency Phase: To collaborate and cooperate
Phase 3.	Intimacy		Genital Phase: To be intimate; To be mature

This three-stage model of groups delineates behaviors likely to appear before the task of the group can be undertaken. Frequently a new group or new members joining an established group will manifest behaviors which reveal wishes for dependency, striving for power, or overtures toward intimacy. The nurse observing a group where such behaviors are dominant should assess the group or some of its members as unready to confront the task, whatever the task of the group may be.

The group model just presented approaches but does not include a working phase. A more complete linear model, still based on behavior, is that of Tuckman (1965) who found that groups in general, regardless of their goals, undergo the following developmental changes:

- Forming: a group stage of testing and dependency.
- Storming: a group stage of conflict and emotional expression.
- Norming: a group stage of establishing norms and cohesion.
- Performing: a group stage of task accomplishment and role relatedness.

In Tuckman's scheme, as in most forms of the linear-progressive model, group movement is considered to move toward efficiency and to remain there. A maturing group moves from unproductive behavior into competent performance. It is assumed in Tuckman's model that productivity remains at a high level until the group separates.

Just as Freud's psychosexual phases of individual development end with puberty, so the linear-progressive model stops short of examining the group in its period of decline and separation. No attention is paid here to the possibility of developmental lag, regression, or even premature demise, although these events occur with some frequency. Since the last phases of group life are as consequential as the first, there are strong arguments for preferring a life cycle model over the linear-progressive model for understanding groups.

Life Cycle Models of Groups

The linear-progressive model suggests that group development resembles the movement of individuals from infantile dependence to mature interdependence. This model implies that productivity is lasting once maturity is reached and that there is no period of decline. The same curious omission is evident in Freud's psychosexual stages, but is remedied in the work of Erikson (1963) whose eight-stage developmental model encompasses the entire life cycle. Groups, like individuals, seldom maintain maximum productivity to the end of their existence. The life cycle model takes for granted the diminution of productivity, the dissipation of energy, and the eventual dissolution of the group.

Few theorists have presented life cycle developmental frameworks as inclusive as Erikson's eight stages of man, but there have been some noteworthy attempts to deal with the declining aspects of group life. Mills (1964) described five periods of group development which are similar to those of Tuckman except for the addition of a last phase called *separation*. During the separation phase members deal with the approaching death of the group by reviewing the impact of the group experience and coping with their feelings about separating. According to Mills, this period is accompanied by behaviors which symbolize a search for a "benediction" before the group ceases to exist. Members may reminisce about the history of the group or evaluate its successes and failures. Although the formulation of Mills is less extensive than that of Erikson, similarities between the two are shown in Table 2-2 on the following page.

Another group theorist who made notable contributions to the life cycle model was Shutz (1960), whose framework was interpersonal, rather than psychosexual (Freudian) or psychosocial (Eriksonian). Three basic interpersonal needs common to everyone are a need for inclusion, a need for control, and a need for affection. Sequential needs for inclusion, control, and affection are stages which groups experience in that order (I-C-A). Only after resolving questions of

Table 2–2   INTEGRATION OF GROUP AND INDIVIDUAL PSYCHOSOCIAL
STAGES

Periods of Group Development (Mills, 1964)		Stages of Individual Psychosocial Development (Erikson, 1963)
Period 1.	Encountering	Stage 1. Oral/Sensory: Basic Trust versus Mistrust
Period 2.	Boundary Testing and Role Modeling	Stage 2. Anal/Muscular: Autonomy versus Shame and Doubt
		Stage 3. Locomotor/Genital: Initiative versus Guilt
		Stage 4. Latency: Industry versus Inferiority
Period 3.	Establishing Norms	Stage 5. Puberty/Adolescence: Identity versus Role Confusion
Period 4.	Working and Producing	Stage 6. Young Adulthood: Intimacy versus Isolation
		Stage 7. Adulthood: Generativity versus Stagnation
Period 5.	Separating	Stage 8. Maturity: Ego Integrity versus Despair

who is committed to being in the group and who dominates whom in the group can the members relate easily to one another. As termination approaches, the group begins to relinquish established ties of affection. Problems about control resurface. The final phase of the group finds members again preoccupied with issues of inclusion (A-C-I) (Sampson and Marthas, 1977).

Pendular or Recurrent Life Cycle Model of Groups

The life cycle model is more comprehensive than the linear-progressive model but not much more complex. In both, the constraints of a simple developmental framework may cause recurrent conflicts in a group to seem inexplicable. This is a cogent argument for looking further for a satisfactory group model.

It is significant that Erikson expresses individual developmental progression in bipolar terms which bring an "either-or" quality to the resolution of critical life tasks. He implies the presence of positive and negative influences which cause recurrent movement between two poles representing success or failure in overcoming stage critical tasks. The bipolarity found in the Eriksonian stages of man is a possible explanation for recurrent or pendular swings which are discernible in the lives of many individuals whose behaviors swing uneasily between the polarities of success and failure.

Among other group theorists, Wilfred Bion (1959) noted the pendular or recurrent nature of group issues. Bion identified *basic-assumption* activities which groups adopt as alternatives to productive work. The basic-assumption activities described by Bion consist of dependency, fight-flight, and pairing behaviors. Although dependency activities are likely to prevail in early stages of group life and pairing in later stages, Bion did not consider basic-assumption activities in a developmental context. The behaviors shown by basic-assumption groups distinguish them from work groups, but groups are not thought to advance sequentially from one basic-assumption activity to the next, ultimately becoming a work group. Instead, group activities move in a recurrent fashion among the three kinds of basic-assumption activities until the group is ready to confront and surmount the impediments to work. Even then there is no assurance that a work group will not revert from time to time to basic-assumption activities. Although the underlying feelings in the group may be covert, overt group interactions can be very revealing. It is the observable activities of the members which justify assessment of the group as being engaged in basic-assumption activities or as functioning as a work group.

CHOOSING A MODEL OF GROUPS

The linear-progressive model offers the nurse-observer a fairly uncomplicated view of groups. A disadvantage of this model is that not all groups forge onward and upward, directing themselves to goal attainment and high productivity until they end. The life cycle model recognizes the fact that groups may become less effective and less task-oriented as their end nears. The pendular or recurrent life cycle model follows a developmental pattern but has the potential to explain group deviation from maximum productivity. Since this model helps account for regression and digression in groups, it has undeniable advantages. The pendular or recurrent life cycle model resembles the universal human condition: problems are not solved once and for all but must be faced repeatedly as the life of the group continues.

A nurse attempting to assess group phenomena may select the life cycle model because it includes a terminal phase but is less complicated than the recurrent model. The life cycle model has the advantage of being complete, yet it is within the grasp of an inexperienced observer who is relatively unfamiliar with group concepts. If the more sophisticated pendular or recurrent life cycle model is used, impasses, recurring problems, and diversionary activities within the group may be easier to explain. Pendular movement in groups may be related to conflict regarding goal attainment as opposed to emotional satisfaction. If this is happening, the observer will find that the group oscillates between two poles — emotional expressiveness and instrumental productivity.

Sometimes tasks can be accomplished without sacrificing group expressiveness, but more often task accomplishment must take precedence over emotional satisfaction. The pendular or recurrent life cycle model explains movement in the group between expressiveness, which is given up reluctantly, and productivity, which is taken up reluctantly. The polarity seen in pendular or recurrent life cycle groups may be compared to individual movement between Freud's pleasure and reality principles — the first governed by the id and the second by the ego — or to individual alternatives between Erikson's bipolarization of crucial tasks in stages of the life cycle (Anderson and Carter, 1978; Mills, 1967). Included in Erikson's psychosocial theory is the concept that incomplete resolution of early critical tasks affects the resolution of later tasks. This is true of group development as well as individual development. Bipolarization and epigenetic development are inherent in the recurrent or pendular life cycle model. These concepts adapted from the work of Erikson enhance our understanding of group development which proceeds with relative, though seldom absolute, predictability.

CLINICAL EXAMPLE: APPLICATION OF GROUP MODELS TO A SCHOOL COMMITTEE

The outmoded health suite of an urban high school was scheduled for renovation, subject to restrictions based on safety and budgetary limitations. A seven-member committee was organized to plan the renovation and forward detailed recommendations to the school board. The committee was composed of an architect, an engineer, a draftsman, the school principal, the school nurse, and two parents representing the Home and School Association. All committee members except the parents were employees of the school board. The committee was charged with meeting biweekly to discuss the remodeling and to arrive at decisions within guidelines formulated by the school board. Group members agreed that the facilities of the health suite were antiquated; however, each member entered the committee with a hidden agenda based on personal priorities. Any group model illuminates some aspects of group behavior; and the specific model affects the selection and organization of salient data. This can be shown by applying various group models to the same situation and contrasting the data obtained.

Systems Model of Groups

The committee met as a social system committed to a group task which rendered the members accountable to a larger system in the form of the school board. The school board was an external system which wielded great power, especially over committee members who were employees. In general the committee members perceived the school board as a bureaucracy whose chief function was the control of forces wishing drastic change. Also operating within the committee were complex relationships based on status, roles, and vested interests.

Status within the committee depended upon prestige related to the high school and on prestige related to the bureaucracy which was the school board. Roles derived from the status of individual members, and shaped the attitudes and behaviors of committee members holding a certain status.

The school board was one important system affecting the status of committee members, another was the high school. For the architect, the engineer, and the draftsman it was the school board which significantly affected their actions. The two parents on the committee believed their major responsibility was to the high school; the principal and the nurse felt an allegiance both to the school board, which employed them, and to the high school, where they were employed. Complicating the issue of allegiance were the vested interests brought by the committee members into group transactions. The following table illustrates complexities of status, allegiance, and vested interests operating during committee meetings (Table 2-3).

Table 2–3 STATUS, VESTED INTERESTS, AND ALLEGIANCE OF COMMITTEE MEMBERS

Committee Member	High School Status Rank	School Board Status Rank	Vested Interest	Allegiance
Principal	1	3	Efficiency Appearance	School Board High School
Nurse	2	6	Convenience Practicality	High School School Board
Parents	3	5	Comfort Privacy	High School
Architect	4	1	Economy Feasibility	School Board
Engineer	5	2	Safety Economy	School Board
Draftsman	6	4	Design Accuracy	School Board

During the meetings leadership was shared between the principal and the architect, each of whom enjoyed superior status with one of the important external systems. Opinions of the principal concerning the needs of high school students and staff were countered by the architect, who stressed cost and feasibility. Other committee members were more or less active depending on the issue being discussed and the relevance of the issue to their vested interests. All the members were relatively committed to the group task, but also sought to achieve private goals. Since the private goals were interrelated but conflicting, compromise was necessary. Ultimately, the private goals of the members became subordinate to the group task.

Linear-Progressive Group Model Two subgroups formed under the leadership of the architect and the school principal. Members who considered themselves accountable only to the school board acknowledged the dominance of the architect. The school nurse and the parents aligned themselves with the principal. As the committee continued to meet, intimacy increased within the subgroups but not between them. Only after the two leaders showed willingness to compromise were the subgroups able to overcome their differences. Genuine trust did not develop between the subgroups but differences were resolved in order to complete the task. By setting aside personal interests and reconciling the values of the members, the committee was able to perform competently. Productivity remained high until the necessary recommendations were sent to the school board, at which time the committee was dissolved. Table 2-4 shows the progression of group and individual dynamic issues as committee members addressed themselves to the group task.

Life Cycle Model of Groups Having progressed through phases of dependency, conflict, and intimacy to task performance, several committee members experienced feelings of dissatisfaction as termination neared. Imminent dissolution of the committee reminded them that personal interests had been compromised. The cost of the renovations recommended to the school board were disquieting to the cost-conscious architect, while the engineer feared that safety features had been sacrificed to expediency. The school nurse regretted compromising on new equipment and improved working conditions. These unspoken reservations caused the members to renew acrimonious discussion of issues which had already been settled. The architect and the school principal responded to the rising dissension

Table 2–4 GROUP AND INDIVIDUAL DYNAMIC CONFLICTS OF THE
COMMITTEE MEMBERS

Phases of Group Development (Kaplan and Roman, 1963)			*Phases of Individual Development (Burgess and Lazare, 1976)*
Phase 1.	Dependency		Oral Phase: Members wish to be protected and directed by group leaders
			Subgroups form and align with each leader
Phase 2.	Power	Early Period	Anal Phase: Leaders vie for dominance
			Subgroups compete by supporting their respective leaders
			Phallic Phase: Competition continues
			Vested interests of some members become apparent
		Later Period	Latency Phase: Leaders reconcile divergent goals in order to accomplish the task
			Subgroups begin to cooperate with each other
Phase 3.	Intimacy		Genital Phase: Common efforts are devoted to finishing the group task
			Mature role performance is enacted by the members

by expressing satisfaction with the decisions and by praising the entire group for its efforts. Recognition from the leaders counteracted the disaffection of individual members and strengthened group agreement. The leaders used their influence to persuade the other committee members to deal realistically with termination.

Pendular or Recurrent Life Cycle Model The committee members accepted the group task but were also motivated by personal interests which impeded progress. Discrepancy between self-interest and group interests established polarized values representing conflict between personal interests and group interests. Divergence between individual desires for gratification and group orientation to the task prolonged the negotiation process. During negotiations conflict developed between expressive and instrumental behaviors of the members. Expressive behaviors were those which met the emotional needs of members while instrumental behaviors were those which focused on the group task.

The expressive behaviors performed integrative functions which helped maintain the group; the instrumental behaviors performed adaptive functions which enabled the group to complete the task. The formation of subgroups was an example of integrative behavior and the eventual collaboration between the subgroups was an example of adaptive behavior. In some respects the subgroups fulfilled narcissistic or egocentric needs of members who were unready for generative efforts. Status was an important factor in the committee, as shown by the leadership roles. An additional polarity might be identified as the ability of members to relinquish hierarchical or vertical role enactment in favor of equalitarian or horizontal role enactment.

The pendular life cycle model identified recurrent movement between positive and negative poles (Table 2-5). Contending behaviors of the two subgroups could be identified as aspects of recurrent changes. Behaviors of individual members could be measured against prevailing group behaviors, and shifts in prevailing group behaviors could be studied over time. Since the committee successfully reached

Table 2-5 PENDULAR OR RECURRENT POLARIZATION
AMONG COMMITTEE MEMBERS

Negative Polarization	Positive Polarization
Personal Goals ↕ Motivated by Self-Interest	Group Goals ↕ Motivated by Group Interests
Expressive (Socio-Emotional) Behaviors ↕ Promoted Group Integration	Instrumental (Task) Behaviors ↕ Promoted Group Adaptation
Egocentric (Narcissistic) Operations ↕ Gratified Individual Needs	Generative Operations ↕ Gratified Group Needs
Vertical Interactions ↕ Hierarchical Role Enactment	Horizontal Interactions ↕ Equalitarian Role Enactment

agreement, it discharged its responsibility despite recurrent pendular swings. Adequate task performance was achieved because movement was in the direction of positive poles, which encouraged productivity.

SUMMARY

In this chapter, models were described as selective approaches to the study of groups which are helpful in the systematic observation of group phenomena. Group models are particularly important for observers who must note and organize data without being incorporated into the group. The characteristics of various models of groups were presented; among these were the systems model, the linear-progressive model, and the life cycle model. The pendular or recurrent life cycle model was described as the most adaptable, encompassing the polarities of Erikson's psychosocial framework and the basic-assumption activities of Bion. Each model presented was considered to have inherent strengths and limitations, but the pendular or recurrent life cycle model was identifed as the most useful in understanding the regressive and progressive forces present throughout the development of groups.

REFERENCES

Anderson, R.E., and I. Carter. *Human Behavior in the Social Environment.* 2nd ed. Chicago: Aldine, 1978.

Anthony, E.J. "Comparison Between Individual and Group Psychotherapy." In *Comprehensive Group Psychotherapy*, H.I. Kaplan and B.J. Sadock, Eds. Baltimore: Williams and Wilkins, 1971.

Astrachan, B.M. "Towards Social Systems Model of Therapeutic Groups," *Social Psychiatry* Vol. 5, No. 2, 1970, pages 110–119.

Bion, W.R. *Experiences in Groups.* New York: Basic Books, 1959.

Burgess, A.W., and A. Lazare. *Psychiatric Nursing in the Hospital and Community.* Englewood Cliffs, N.J.: Prentice-Hall, 1976.

Erikson, E. *Childhood and Society.* New York: Norton, 1963.

Gibbard, G.S.; J.J. Hartman; and R.D. Mann. *Analysis of Groups.* San Francisco: Jossey-Bass, 1974.

Henderson, L.J. "Procedure in a Science." *Human Relations: Concepts and Cases in Concrete Social Science* Vol. I. Cambridge: Harvard University Press, 1953, pages 24–39.

Kaplan, S.R., and M. Roman. "Phases of Development in an Adult Therapy Group." *International Journal of Group Psychotherapy*, 1963, pages 10–26.

Loomis, M.E. *Group Process for Nurses.* St. Louis: C.V. Mosby, 1979.

Mills, T.M. *Group Transformation: An Analysis of a Learning Group.* Englewood Cliffs, N.J.: Prentice-Hall, 1964.

————. *The Sociology of Small Groups.* Englewood Cliffs, N.J.: Prentice-Hall, 1967, pages 25–35.

Olsen, M. *The Process of Social Organization.* New York: Holt Rinehart & Winston, 1968.

Rogers, C. *Carl Rogers on Encounter Groups.* New York: Harper & Row, 1970.

Schutz, W.C. *FIRO: A Three Dimensional Theory of Interpersonal Behavior.* New York: Holt Rinehart & Winston, 1960.

Tuckman, B.W. "Developmental Sequence in Small Groups." *Psychological Bulletin* 63, 1965, pages 384–399.

Watzlawick, P. *How Real Is Real?* New York: Random House, 1976.

3

Theoretical Frameworks: Intrapsychic Groups

Ellen Hastings Janosik

A theoretical framework is a set of related concepts which may or may not have been validated systematically. Unlike a model, a theoretical framework is not superimposed on a group in order to make group events more comprehensible. Instead, a theoretical framework is the foundation for group organization and leadership strategy. Theoretical frameworks used in group work are often eclectic in that they draw upon more than one school of thought.

TYPOLOGY OF GROUPS

There are two major categories of groups — regardless of whether they are organized for primary, secondary, or tertiary health care — those that produce intrapsychic or intrapersonal changes in members and those that promote interpersonal or social changes for members. From these divergent goals, many differences in leadership strategy and membership outcomes follow.

The first category includes, among others, psychoanalytic and gestalt-existentialist groups. Traditional psychoanalytic groups usually deal with members by excluding or ignoring contemporary forces, except when they reflect the past. The current problems of group members are considered to have originated in early life; psycho-analytic groups, therefore, are preoccupied with past events. Gestalt-existentialist groups are present-oriented, dealing with current behaviors and events. There is little emphasis on the origin and meaning of what is happening; instead, the emphasis is on the experiential state of members at that moment. In the gestalt-existential framework, members and their social field are inextricably related.

Simply stated, then, gestalt-existential groups are engaged in a process of integration and synthesis; psychoanalytic groups are engaged in a process of interpretation and analysis. Both are concerned with the inner psychological life of their members, but use different methods. Psychoanalytic and gestalt-existential groups attempt to alter the internal psychological experience of their members, since both assume that behavioral and social alterations follow intrapsychic change.

The second major category of groups includes those concerned with interpersonal changes or changes in the social environment of members: communication-interactional groups, which have been influenced by the work of Sullivan (1953), and crisis groups, which have been influenced by the work of Caplan (1963). Interpersonal groups are based on the assumption that behavioral or social change can ameliorate intrapsychic distress.

PSYCHOANALYTIC FRAMEWORK

Nurses do not often lead psychoanalytic groups as such but utilize concepts contributed by psychoanalytic theorists, sometimes without being aware of the source. Persons who are engaged in a group experience often seem different from people who are engaged in singular or dyadic transactions. A popular but plausible explanation is that group members are responsive to a mysterious influence called *group pressure*. Slavson, a psychoanalytic theorist (1974), described human beings as battlegrounds for conflicts between instinctual urges and restrictions imposed by established social groups. Social inclusion and the survival of the group to which one belongs may become a more imperative need than individual survival.

Individuals who are part of a group may find themselves merged or submerged in the group, feeling that neither the group nor its members can survive separately. This merging of individual identity in the matrix of the group means that considerable power is exerted over members. Mature and highly organized groups can restrain and harness the impulses of individual members in order to reach the objectives of the group. Less mature groups may permit or encourage unrestrained aggressive or erotic behavior on the part of individual members, which thus perverts the objectives of the group as a whole.

Under the influence of the group, individuals are capable of heroic actions which place the welfare of the group before their own. In such instances a sense of being part of the group supersedes the individuality of the members. Psychoanalytic theory uses the term *ego ideal* to describe an idealized image of what one wants to be. *Esprit de corps* seems to make the ego ideal of the group and the ego ideal of the hero become one. The outcome may, on the one hand, be a deed of courage. On the other hand, group pressure and the merging of the individual with the group may sometimes provoke questionable actions, at least when an immature, disorganized group acts in a manner which suggests the absence of group responsibility (*group superego constraints*). When a group gives free rein to aggressive behavior, merging with the group may threaten an individual member's mature ego integration. A decrease in feelings of autonomy and personal responsibility may, for example, incite group members to such violent acts as looting, rape, or assault. Although psychoanalytic concepts grew out of work with individuals, many group theorists apply Freudian topographic (*conscious* and *unconscious mental activity*) and structural (*id, ego, superego,* and *ego ideal*) formulations to the study of groups.

Sometimes membership in durable, established groups mitigates the impact of primitive groups. Primary and reference groups may effectively counter an individual's wish to merge with a secondary group. An exchange student from Britain reported being able to resist the regressive tendencies of an unauthorized encounter group on a college campus by reminding himself that "Englishmen do not behave in that fashion."

The Kennedy Airport Snow-In   At times a group experience may arouse neither heroism nor antisocial behavior but rather apathy or aimlessness. In an account of a blizzard which immobilized Kennedy Airport, stranded passengers relapsed into listless dependency (Hammerschlag and Astrachan, 1971). No cohesiveness developed between persons suffering the same predicament, except within certain nuclear families. Even though there was no actual danger, hoarding behaviors appeared among those marooned together. There were fantasies of an unknown, omnipotent rescuer who would appear and lead everyone to safety. Neither panic (*flight*) nor effective mobilization for action (*fight*) was exhibited. Breakdown of the organizational system at the airport and the absence of outside resources created social immobility. The travelers were too numerous to constitute a small group, although it is possible that within the crowd smaller constellations were formed whose members engaged in sharing behaviors. The general mood of dependency and helplessness, however, precluded the formation of group measures to decrease discomfort or find rescue.

The previous examples indicate some possible effects of group pressure: 1) heroism and self-sacrifice on behalf of the group; 2) guilt-producing (ego-alien) acts committed in collusion with the group; and 3) apathy and helplessness which prevent interdependence and utilization of group resources. A number of group theorists have attempted to explain these and similar phenomena in psychoanalytic terms.

Dual Nature of Groups

A consistent theme in psychoanalytic group theory is the dual nature of group life. The recurrent life cycle model contrasts progressive and regressive elements in group life, and accepts the inevitability of recurrent conflicts during its existence. This is comparable to the experiences of individuals as they move through developmental life stages. The Freudian psychosexual progression and the Eriksonian psychosocial progression allow the possibility of recurrent conflict or crisis throughout the individual's life span, and help explain the duality in group life. Some theorists in the psychoanalytic mold (Bion, 1959; Slater, 1966; Gibbard and Hartman, 1973) compare the total group to a preoedipal mother toward whom members feel regressive wishes for *symbiosis* (merging) and progressive pulls toward *individuation* (separating), not unlike the opposing needs of individuals to relate and to differentiate in the family of origin. Duality is inherent in the preoedipal conflict between the regressive influence of the group as a maternal entity and the opposing wish of members to maintain boundaries between themselves and the group.

Lewin The field theorist Kurt Lewin (1951) observed progressive and regressive forces in groups and considered these attributable to conflicts arising as members vie for territory or life space. The duality in this explanation refers to the balance which must be preserved between the sacrifice of individual freedom and the security which the group provides. Because this is a delicate balance, with members weighing their choices, group tension results. In a poorly organized group — where leadership is inadequate — tension may mount to disruptive heights. In well-organized groups tension is disseminated or distributed among the members. With group tension regulated, the group can direct its energy toward work and growth. Channels of communication can be established and the group task can be undertaken.

Bion   An important proponent of the dual nature of groups was Wilfred Bion (1959), who discerned primitive elements of groups which he called *psychotic,* or out of touch with reality. Bion used a number of descriptive phrases to refer to aspects of group experience which are not within the conscious awareness of members. The term *basic assumption* was applied to the experiential condition of a group and the mechanisms used by the group to express that condition. It is the prevailing basic assumption of a group which affects all group interactions and expresses commonalities among members which establish the group culture at a particular point in time.

According to Bion, groups exist on two levels, conscious and unconscious. The unconscious level contains processes which are latent and covert, but are always operative. This is the level of group life which Bion considered psychotic or irrational. These psychotic elements can only be controlled by strong organization and leadership. Through organization and leadership a basic-assumption group can be transformed into a work group. Without a leader, a work group may continue to function for a while but will soon falter. A group search for a new leader will then ensue. One strong member may become the leader, or the group may adopt creeds or rituals which symbolize the lost leader. In Alcoholics Anonymous or Recovery Inc. (for discharged psychiatric patients), a doctrine or creed provides leadership. Such groups adhere to a fairly rigid dogma in which common terminology and goals are accepted by the members. Groups which are unsuccessful in finding a new leader, or an embodiment of the lost leader, may regress to irrational, unproductive levels and eventually disband.

On the conscious level group members are initially brought together by the task to be undertaken. A legitimate task and meaningful communication concerning it control the unconscious aspects of group life, but cannot banish them altogether. Unconscious processes within the group contend with desires to accomplish the task and are rooted in the members' instinctual impulses for immediate gratification. The instinctual, unconscious processes in the group cause basic assumptions. Bion found that there are three kinds of basic-assumption group cultures in which unconscious needs are expressed: 1) basic-assumption dependency groups, 2) basic-assumption fight-flight groups, and 3) basic-assumption pairing groups.

The alternative to displaying a form of basic-assumption group culture is to become a group with a work orientation. It is necessary to add that the basic-assumption and work-group hypotheses of Bion are not developmental. Basic-assumption groups are not sequential, moving from dependency through fight-flight to pairing assumptions until a working phase is reached. Instead there is recurrent movement which may be regressive or progressive (Table 3-1). A work group may regress to basic-assumption activities because of changes in leadership, membership, or the perceived nature of the task. Loss of a valued member or leader may generate panic (flight) or rage (fight) in the group. The introduction of new members may arouse siblinglike competition. Here the result may be attenuation of group cohesion and a return to group pairing behavior when members were not workers but lovers or enemies. Belated recognition or acknowledgment of barriers to completing the task may cause a work group to revert to a basic-assumption culture.

Because members of a group forfeit their individuality they become susceptible to the *contagion* of neighboring minds (Anthony, 1971a). Since the group is illogical, it will conform to any dominant force or influence; it is capable of responding to positive as well as

Table 3-1   BASIC-ASSUMPTION AND WORK-GROUP
                      FORMULATION

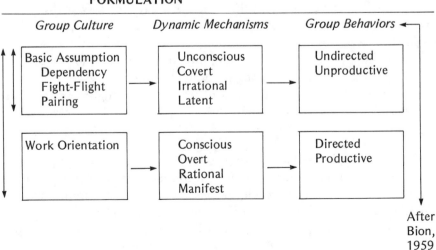

Group Culture	Dynamic Mechanisms	Group Behaviors
Basic Assumption Dependency Fight-Flight Pairing	Unconscious Covert Irrational Latent	Undirected Unproductive
Work Orientation	Conscious Overt Rational Manifest	Directed Productive

After Bion, 1959

negative influences, and thus is capable of either succeeding or failing. The group must be controlled by effective organization so that the collective experience can be one of achievement. Another duality is that members inhabit both the past and the present (Anthony 1971 b). In the group, members are offered the opportunity to relive the conflicts of childhood and family in a remedial way by connecting the historic past to present realities.

The consensus of psychoanalytic group theorists is that effective organization requires continuity and consistency; patterned group relationships; regulated stimulation of *intergroup* competition; development of group traditions; and distribution, differentiation, and specialization of functions, and effective leadership strategy. The competition advocated is between groups rather than within groups, where intense rivalry among members can be destructive.

Freud   Freud's professional interest was directed toward the psychoanalysis of the individual, but some of his insights into group dynamics are worthy of mention. He valued the idealization of the leader, identification among fellow members, and group empathy through which members could appreciate each other's feelings. Among the positive group influences admired by Freud were imitation, relatedness, sympathy, common purpose, and mutual interests. In his opinion members projected their own narcissistic or egocentric qualities onto the group, making it special and important. There is a reciprocal quality to this use of the mechanism of projection. If I am important and the group is important to me, then the group must be important. Conversely, if the group is important and I am a member, then I must be important as well. Like other psychoanalytic theorists, Freud believed that strong organization safeguarded groups and that leadership was essential. He thought that leader-centered groups fostered dependency and regression, but that regression in the service of the ego was desirable. During individual psychoanalysis, regression is fostered so that developmental conflicts can be brought to conscious awareness, analyzed, and worked through (Freud, 1957).

Revolt in the Group

Psychoanalytic theorists are interested in how and why groups come into existence. One explanation is that human beings are *herd* animals whose evolutionary cellular development is from the simple to the complex, and from the unit to the aggregate. In this explanation humans are thought to feel incomplete unless they are members of groups, which represent the next advance in the evolutionary hierarchy.

Freud (1950) disagreed with the concept of an innate social instinct, believing that humans are not herd but *horde* animals who gather round a strong leader. In essence the group is a primal horde or band ruled by a leader whose strength protects the group. The leader of the horde is despotic and demanding. In return for his protection his sons must slavishly obey him. As a result the leader is resented as well as venerated. Resenting the father, the sons are temporarily immobilized by fear of reprisal if they revolt. They fear retaliation from the father-leader if they fail, and they fear being attacked by jealous brothers if they assume the mantle of leadership. Eventually the sons move into a state of trustfulness in which they can join together to overthrow the leader. The revolt against the leader has a catalytic effect on the group. It is comparable to an oedipal struggle after which the group becomes cohesive, mature, and ready to confront the task (Mills, 1967).

A great deal of psychoanalytic theory is expressed in the language of literature and mythology. This sometimes causes the psychological value of the concepts to be discounted. Comparing a group to a primal horde may seem fanciful, but immature groups are often extremely dependent on a leader and entertain unrealistic expectations of the leader's power. As groups mature, confidence in their own ability and disappointment in the leader produces rebellion, which builds cohesion among members, after which productive work usually starts. Theorists who support the herd theory tend to emphasize leadership which emanates from the group rather than from a designated leader.

Struggles within the Group In general, the psychoanalytic theorists conceptualize the presence of two struggles in the group. A group begins with a collection of separate persons who soon begin to experience the group as a symbiotic mother. In addition the group replicates family conditions so that the leader becomes a father figure. Because expectations of the leader are unrealistic, most of the members become disillusioned, which in turn produces anxiety with the result that members move toward each other and against the leader. The symbolic revolt against the authority of the leader resolves the group oedipal struggle. It also counteracts the preoedipal wishes of members to merge with the group, since rebelling against the leader signifies differentiation rather than symbiosis. Feelings of guilt and the appearance of a group superego are thought to follow the revolt. Having united to overthrow the father-leader, the group becomes a community in which members have equal rights and share equal responsibility for patricide (*revolt*).

A variation of the collective revolt is one in which only a single member attacks the leader. The member who heads the revolt may be looked upon either as a hero or a threat, since this member may become the new leader. Freud thought that emotional ties between members could not be established until reliance on the leader weakened, either through collective revolt or the emergence of a hero to challenge the leader. In group terminology, intimacy between members is likely to develop only after authority issues have been faced.

The consequence of the revolt is that members must take responsibility for the group. Regardless of the developmental stage of any member, there is ongoing conflict between group needs and personal needs. While the group lasts, members experience anew the transition from symbiosis to differentiation. As the group matures, becomes cohesive, and learns to work together, boundaries between self and group become less troublesome.

Transference

Transference has been called one of the most important psychological mechanisms of life (Anthony, 1971b). Freud, at first, regarded transference as a form of resistance toward the therapist transmitted from the patient's early experience with significant persons. Later in his work Freud regarded transference as a therapeutic tool rather than a form of resistance. In the context of the relationship with the therapist the patient is able to relive childhood attitudes toward significant persons. Since transference is a useful tool, the psychoanalytic therapist encourages its appearance. This is done by having the therapist adopt a strict neutrality which conceals his or her personality. The therapist becomes a *tabula rasa* on which distortions can be projected. As a result of positive transferences in the group the leader is thought to have unlimited power and knowledge. At the same time the paradoxical nature of group life causes negative transference to the leader. The leader is idealized as loving and wise, but is also feared and distrusted as the enemy. Like the parent from the past, the leader is seen as giving and punishing, gratifying and withholding. The ultimate effect of this confusing distortion is ambivalence toward the leader.

Techniques of individual analysis show that the more passive a therapist becomes, the more powerful the transference. Some definitions of transference include only displacements from patient to therapist of attitudes derived from childhood experiences. More liberal definitions expand transference to include any distortion or irrationality involving displaced feelings regardless of the target. This definition of transference applies to group situations. Yalom (1975) believes that transference is always present in groups and considers it essential for leaders to recognize this. Transference can exist between members and the leader, and among fellow members.

Ambivalence toward the leader creates problems for the group. Members want the leader to reveal human qualities, but also to be larger than life. The leader is imbued by the group with superhuman powers so that all the needs of members can be met. Dependent members exalt the leader and minimize their own abilities. Other members feel helpless and want to be cared for, but resent the feeling. These are counterdependent or counterphobic members who react to feeling helpless by showing distrust or defiance of the leader. Positive transferences are usually the pattern of dependent members; negative transferences are usually the pattern of counterdependent members.

Handling Transferences Two specific techniques have been recommended in dealing with transferences in groups (Yalom, 1975). The recommended techniques are 1) to turn to the whole group for consensual validation in order to correct transference distortion; and 2) to engage in careful self-disclosure in order to make the leader known (*transparent*) to the group. Consensual validation of transference distortion means that the leader solicits from members their impressions of what is happening in the group, particularly with respect to how the leader is perceived. Agreement among the majority of group members may not mean that their perceptions are necessarily accurate, but merely show that members are functioning at the same affective or cognitive level. Since transference is usually idiosyncratic, the inclination of the group majority would not be to support the distortions of any one member.

The second way of dealing with transference is for the leader to disclose information of a personal nature. The leader disclaims the exceptional powers which the group has bestowed and tries to shrink to human proportions. This gradual self-disclosure makes it harder for the group to continue transference distortion. Passivity and neutrality from the leader preserve transferences; self-disclosure allows the leader to relinquish the central position and confer power on the group. One tactic suggested by Yalom as a way of handling transference is to tell the group how its displaced attitudes are affecting the leader. A statement is suggested such as, "I feel uncomfortable when Lisa expects me to tell her what to do. There are members of the group who are more able to help. Why not ask one of them, Lisa?"

The leader using self-disclosure to reduce transference should not mistake transparency for the abdication of leadership responsibility. Timing is important, and a mature, confident group can tolerate more self-disclosure from a leader than an immature group made up of needy members. The obligation of the leader is to serve the group, and this obligation must not be discarded along with self-concealment. It is not only members who are conflicted about boundary management in groups. Occasionally a leader may engage in reckless self-disclosure, using the group as a vehicle for personal catharsis. Even when fostering transparency, the leader should be mindful of role, never merging but remaining apart from the group in order to observe, reflect, and generalize so that the corrective experiences in the group can be applied in everyday life. Marram (1978) states that a leader may share functions with group members but never responsibility.

Countertransference

The reverse side of transference is countertransference. In this phenomenon the group leader experiences an emotional response to a group member or members which is subjective and has its origin in some previous experience of the leader. Countertransference, which is unconscious, represents a threat to the group and must be brought to conscious awareness by the introspection of the leader, with help from a coleader, or the observations of qualified group supervisors.

Regressive-Reconstructive and Repressive-Inspirational Groups

A continuum depicting the personality change achieved in different types of groups demonstrates the relative effects of leader concealment and leader transparency (Table 3-2). The leader who is passive and neutral has the potential to produce the most personality change in members. This is done by encouraging transferences which induce dependency and regression. Leadership of this sort is appropriate for long-term analytic groups, known as regressive-reconstructive groups, in which personality change is a primary goal.

At the opposite end of the continuum are the repressive-inspirational groups. Here transference is negated by active leaders because adjustments in daily living are sought, rather than personality change. Other groups on the continuum show degrees of personality change ranging from considerable to negligible. There are intervening variables, but a very influential one is thought to be leadership functions (Mullan and Rosenbaum, 1962).

Table 3–2 GROUP TYPOLOGY BASED ON PERSONALITY CHANGE

Groups are placed on a continuum which represents the extent of personality change being sought. The regressive-reconstructive groups attempt to achieve the greatest personality change. The repressive-inspirational groups do not attempt personality change.

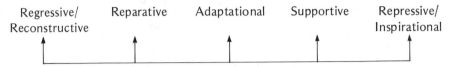

| Regressive/
Reconstructive | Reparative | Adaptational | Supportive | Repressive/
Inspirational |

Comparison of Regressive-Reconstructive and Repressive-Inspirational Groups

Regressive-Reconstructive

Group Organization: Members are prepared in individual sessions for an indefinite time based on their needs.

Group life is long-term, often from 3 to 5 years.

Group selection is based on capacity for insight and change. Group may be open to new members and is therefore described as open-ended.

Group Techniques: Leader allows members to experience whatever unfolds, accepting the irrational and unconscious, including dreams and fantasies.

Leader uses therapeutic skills to analyze the group experience, relating latent and manifest behavior to early family experiences.

Group Leadership: Leader is passive and neutral, does not engage in self-disclosure.

Goals: Leader desires that each member develop responsibility for setting personal goals, and that personality change be accomplished by dealing with historical antecedents to present behaviors.

Termination: The decision to leave the group belongs with the member. Members are aware of the meaning of the decision to terminate, which once made is considered final.

Repressive-Inspirational

Group Organization: Members are prepared in an arbitrary number of sessions, usually minimal in number.

Group life is usually short-term, from 2 months to 1 year.

Group is often closed to new members. Group selection centers on a particular need, problem, or population.

Group Techniques: Leader actively controls content and process by directing, teaching, inspiring members. Task accomplishment and conscious processes are stressed, especially in current relationships. Leader advises, supports, and counsels.

Group Leadership: Leader engages in gradual self-disclosure and shares leadership with the members.

Goals: Goals are group goals. The group is considered effective if members adjust better to their environment. Symptom relief is sought without necessarily relating symptoms to historical antecedents.

Termination: Termination is a decision made by the leader and members as part of the group contract. Termination usually occurs as a group unit.

Beginning leaders tend to favor the activism of repressive-inspirational groups, but most groups belong at points somewhere between the extremes of the continuum. Supportive groups raise self-esteem through encouragement from the leader and fellow members. Little intrapsychic change takes place, but the group represents a caring environment in which empathy and identification are present. Adaptational groups are directed toward functional behavioral or transactional changes. Intrapsychic change per se is not a goal except as a concomitant of conscious improvement. Reparative groups are concerned with building stronger psychological defenses and relinquishing inadequate defenses in favor of better ways of coping.

Nurses are frequently called upon to lead reparative, adaptational, supportive, and repressive-inspirational groups. In most groups led by nurses leadership style is active, flexible, and democratic. Leaders of groups may be active without being authoritarian. It is the passive, neutral leader who easily becomes an authority figure, since this leader is perceived unrealistically. Except in the most traditional regressive-reconstructive groups, transference to the leader is eroded by self-disclosure and consensual validation. These erosions are deliberate, calculated adjustments based on group needs, goals, and the therapeutic contract. Here, as elsewhere, assessment is the basis of adjustments which affect group transferences.

CLINICAL EXAMPLE: PSYCHOANALYTIC CONCEPT IN A SUPPORTIVE MOTHER'S GROUP

A supportive group for mothers of preschool children was organized by an elementary school principal and led by Debbie, a community health nurse, and Jane, a psychiatric mental-health nurse. The school was located in a stable, working-class neighborhood, and the group was sponsored by the adult education division of the local school board. Preschool children accompanied their mothers to the school and engaged in supervised play in the next room while their mothers met. The group met weekly for a period of five months and there were two group objectives. Didactic information was presented on the developmental tasks of young children, and the mothers were encouraged to express their feelings about themselves and their roles in the family. Both nurses were experienced group leaders, but Jane was an older, married woman with grown children, while Debbie was single and childless. During the first meetings the members showed deference toward Jane (*idealization of the leader*) and indifference or distrust toward Debbie (*negative transference*). Jane's contributions to the meetings were warmly received while Debbie's were ignored, except when a member would refer sarcastically to Debbie's free and childless state. It was apparent that Jane represented a mother figure to the group, while Debbie was treated like a schoolgirl.

Jane and Debbie responded to the problem by allocating the tasks of the group between the two of them. Debbie was described to the group as the undisputed authority on all child-rearing subjects. When a question on this topic was directed to Jane, she pleaded ignorance, asserting that she couldn't remember the time when her own children were toddlers, but that Debbie would know the answer (*leader transparency*). After a while the status denial practiced by Jane had an effect. Debbie began to be asked questions and to be heard. After one helpful response by Debbie a mother commented, "You remind me of my sister. She doesn't have any kids either, but she teaches school and thinks a lot. Sometimes she can help me figure things out."

Altering the negative transference to Debbie did not altogether lessen the positive feelings members had for Jane, but did make them more realistic. With the expertise of Debbie established, Jane was able to use her leadership role to elicit interactions among the members themselves and reduce her own centrality. The group became cohesive as the mothers began to share ideas, recipes, and life experiences. One of the members gave birth to a baby during the months that the group met. The baby became a great source of excitement and interest (*empathy*). As a group, the members collected money for a gift and visited the new baby. Both leaders were excluded from these activities, and the group spokesperson explained, "We didn't ask Jane and Debbie to join in. They're both so busy and it's not like they're really part of the gang" (*revolt*).

After this shared activity there was less reliance on the leaders for guidance and greater spontaneity among the members. During the first group meetings the mothers repeatedly left the group to see how their children were. As the mothers became more comfortable with each other, this behavior decreased. Eventually the mothers became so engrossed in the group discussions that when children tapped on the door to see their mommy, they would be told impatiently not to bother mommy when she was busy (*egocentric* or *narcissistic projection*).

As termination neared, one session was devoted to evaluating the group experience. The group was pronounced a success, so much so that the members planned to meet in each other's homes. The judgment was that "Jane and Debbie helped us some, but they haven't answered all our questions. And since all of us are in the same boat maybe we can help each other" (*identification*).

GESTALT-EXISTENTIAL FRAMEWORK

Gestalt psychology and existential psychology began as separate traditions but have much in common. Existentialists assert that individuals do not exist as separate beings in the world but that the world exists only because individuals inhabit it. Individuals exist, therefore, only because they experience the world they inhabit. Behavior is not construed as a result of environment acting on the individual but is a complex response to a situation as interpreted by the individual. Thought, learning, perception, and interpretation all contribute to one's experience of reality (Gendlin, 1968).

Individuals are free to choose what they will be and do, and it is up to the individual to make decisions. Freedom to choose means that some choices may not be good. Existentialists do not accept the Freudian concept of psychic determinism except in the sense of self-determination. Few persons reach their full potential, but most of them make progress toward a real or authentic life experience. In any case human beings and the world depend on each other for existence (Hall and Lindzey, 1970).

Gestalt psychologists define the individual and the environment as a configuration or organization which gives meaning to one's experience. Intrinsic to gestalt psychology is the statement that human nature can only be understood in its relation to the environment. When individuals and the environment are seen in their entirety, the result is a gestalt or shape (Downing, 1976). Completeness and unity are essential to gestalt psychology, which rejects *linear causality*. Human beings are considered rational and emotional simultaneously; *psyche* and *soma* are not merely joined but are one.

The gestaltists object to behaviorism, particularly to the stimulus-response formula. For behaviorists, S means the sum of stimuli affecting the sensory apparatus at a given point and R means the motor response. It is the direct, simple connection of the two which the gestaltists reject. Their emphasis is on the organism's ability to respond to a pattern of stimuli rather than discrete components. The ability to organize patterns out of sensory stimuli leads naturally to the ability to organize one's experience into a coherent form (Wertheimer and Kohler, 1968).

Dominant Needs   The gestalt group leader is unconcerned with antecedents of behavior. Dwelling on the past is not encouraged; immediate events have their own significance (O'Hearne, 1976). Human instincts are not rigid structures but are constantly modified by the experiences of the individual. Gestalt psychologists explain the presence of a dominant need in an individual's experience which takes over the foreground of the gestalt, as other needs recede into the background. An alcoholic drinking at a tavern experiences ingesting alcohol as his or her most pressing need. Conviviality, food, and other aspects of the gestalt are secondary to the dominant need to drink. For the bartender, working hard to serve customers constitutes the most urgent need. A woman entering the tavern in search of her husband experiences a need different from that of a woman looking for any man who will buy her a drink. Each individual produces a different gestalt, yet the environment of the tavern has not changed except in the inner experience of the persons involved (Perls, 1976).

The hierarchy of needs presented by Maslow (1968) helps explain the relative importance of dominant and recessive needs in the gestalt created by the relationship between the individual and the environment. The gestalt theorist does not use the labels health and illness, but prefers instead the term *self-actualization,* which means becoming fully human in the sense that one's abilities, energies, and experiences are integrated. Since human beings differ, self-actualization differs for everyone. Satisfying a dominant need may not necessarily contribute to positive self-actualization, as in the example of the alcoholic, but all persons have freedom of choice.

Supplies obtained from the environment are used in ways chosen by the individual, so that development is directed more by internal than by external forces. Maslow stated that change is not merely the acquisition of new habits but involves a total shifting of the organism. The most important impetus for change comes from life events such as catastrophes, births, deaths, and peak experiences which drastically affect the individual.

Phenomenology To a gestaltist, self-actualization means expressing one's experiential state, whatever it is, rather than acquiring coping skills. Gestalt and existential psychology are concerned with *phenomenology,* which is a method of understanding immediate experience. Phenomenology is used to investigate perceiving, learning, remembering, thinking, and feeling, which constitute one's total experience. The gestalt-existentialist uses personal subjective experience as the beginning of knowledge, and the purpose of the group is to make members aware of what they are experiencing at any point in time. Gwen Marram, a nurse theorist (1978), found that gestaltists and existentialists share these beliefs: 1) within certain limits every individual has great freedom to reach full human potential; 2) awareness of present reality affects what one may become and facilitates ability to change; and 3) for an individual to deal with problems it is necessary only to know what they are, and not why they exist.

The lack of conceptual structure which marks gestalt and existential theory may be disconcerting for nurses trying to see the relevance of concepts such as self-actualization to group work. Nevertheless, gestalt-existential principles may be readily adapted to health-care groups led by nurses. Many individuals tend to hold on to maladaptive behaviors, attempting to manipulate their environment in adverse ways. Gestalt-existential group leaders encourage their members to experience their feelings, and express the fears and frustrations of current reality in order to mobilize their potential for change.

Gestalt Production and Destruction   Proponents of gestalt-existential theory have extended their work to populations which are not considered clinically ill. Counseling of college students, sensitivity training of professionals, and assertiveness programs for the timid are only a few areas where these theories are being used to advantage. The concept of hierarchical levels of needs as defined by Maslow (1968) is already familiar to nurses. All that remains is to envisage needs as dynamic forces which organize gestalts representing the way one experiences the world. Needs develop, are satisfied, and recede, to be replaced by other needs. This continuous process is referred to as *gestalt production* (needs appear and become compelling) and *gestalt destruction* (needs are satisfied, recede, and are replaced by other needs). When this process is not impaired, the world experienced by the individual is orderly and gratifying. The individual is able to obtain selectively what he or she needs from the environment. When need fulfillment fails, the result is confusion, indecision, and incoherence in the gestalt, which represents the individual's relation to the environment.

The gestalt-existential group framework is action-oriented, deals with the here and now, and stresses responsibility and free choice. The group leader works with what is going on in the group. Improvement begins when the individual recognizes and acknowledges all aspects of the self. Willingness to change helps prepare individuals to live in this changing world (Fagan and Shepherd, 1970). The next question is: What methods and techniques can be used by the gestalt-existential group leader to facilitate need fulfillment and change in the members?

Change through Self-Awareness

The goal of the gestalt-existential group leader is to help members identify desirable changes, to recognize self-defeating behaviors, and to encourage experimentation and choice. Gestalt theory can be condensed into three precepts: living in the present; reaching for self-awareness; and assuming personal responsibility.

Striving for self-awareness may be eased through judicious use of the following questions by the group leader (Perls, 1978). The questions, any or all of which may be asked of group members, are:

- What are you doing?
- What are you feeling?
- What do you want?
- What are you avoiding?
- What do you expect?

The Hot Seat

The verbal answers to these questions may be cognitive, but non-verbal responses help reveal the total person. There may follow "a confusion, a hesitation, a knitting of the brow, a shrug of the shoulders . . . a bit of embarrassment . . . an eager leaning forward . . . ." (Perls, 1976, p. 75). Leaders of gestalt groups are attentive to incongruence in communication. The verbally seductive member who sits with legs tightly crossed and arms folded protectively reveals incongruence between words and body language. The observed incongruence may be brought to the attention of the group member who then becomes the occupant of the *hot seat*. The objective of this technique is to make the occupant aware of the nature of the inner experience. Since taking the hot seat is the fate of every member at different times, it is important that group members be able to handle this. Anxiety levels in gestalt groups may become quite high. Members must be carefully selected who can withstand anxiety, and the leader must monitor proceedings so that anxiety does not reach unbearable levels.

Self-disclosure by the leader is an accepted part of the proceedings. The group is an encounter in which the leader is permitted to communicate openly, with members free to accept or reject interventions as they decide. In the gestalt-existential group the myth of the omnipotent leader is less pervasive than in psychoanalytic groups, for the leader is presented as a helping person very much like the group members. Magical expectations rarely persist, nor is transference important since the leader cultivates transparency. The leader is presumed to be the healthiest person in the group. Unhampered by rigid, repetitive behavior the leader may intrude or withdraw, participate or abstain. By means of role modeling the leader tries to release the walled-off expressiveness of members. Because the leader is seen exercising choices, hope is born that perhaps everyone has choices or options. Experiences within the group form a new reality in which members begin to trust and take risks.

Psychodramatization

There are times when a gestalt leader will bring past events into the group but in a special way. The mother of a retarded child may be encouraged to relive the experience of discovering that her child will not develop normally. This is done by enabling the mother to return *psychodramatically* to the experience by role-playing scenes of talking to her husband, her parents, or even to her retarded child. Talking about an experience is considered relatively ineffective. Talking as though the experience were happening immediately helps the individual assimilate the feelings. For example, a son might reconstruct the deathbed scene of his mother, or a father might act out in fantasy the expected death of a leukemic child. Leaders respond to what is happening in the group as members reveal their unmet needs through gestures, movements, and inflections as much as through words. Opportunities are available in the accepting group climate to complete unfinished business through active re-enactment and re-experience.

Congruence

Many gestalt techniques are nonverbal, although some attention is paid to language. Psychoanalysts have often taken action words and transformed them into nouns. "I deny" became the defense mechanism of denial. "I have borrowed some of your characteristics which I admire" became identification. To a gestaltist this structuralization of verbs increases distance between the individual and the experience. Gestaltists try to reconnect individuals to their experience by insisting on action verbs and the use of personal pronouns.

Questions asked by the leader are really observations directed to members. The leader disguises observations as questions to which members must respond. The question, "Are you aware of what you are doing in the group?" directed to the seductive but conflicted female member is really a comment on incongruent communication, and could be translated as, "You flirt verbally and give a come-on message to the men in the group but your body language says you are scared to get involved. What are you really trying to tell us?"

Homework

Members of gestalt groups are sometimes asked to imagine themselves back in a group session and to go over it in memory. It is unusual for an entire session to be recalled easily. If there are blank segments, the individual is asked to remember what he was feeling at that time. Did he freely express feelings? Were feelings held back or falsified? Could the feelings be expressed now? This exploration reinforces self-awareness and indicates whether group members are able to say what they feel and genuinely feel what they are saying.

The gift the gestalt leader hopes group members will accept is self-awareness, which helps people see how they contribute to their own problems, what the problems are, and how they might be solved. If the group is successful, unresolved issues from the past may disappear even though they are not faced directly. Dissociations, tensions, and discontents from the past become less burdensome as the present becomes more satisfying.

Expressiveness

Language is used to increase personal responsibility. By using action words and the pronoun "I," the statement that a valuable book has been lost must be restated as "I lost a valuable book." Evasions and omissions are not accepted, even though authentic expressiveness does not come immediately. In trying to reconnect individuals to their experience, gestaltists have resorted to categorization (Perls, 1976). There are four stages of expressiveness: *blocked, inhibited, exhibitionistic,* and *spontaneous* (see chart below).

To reach the goal of spontaneous expressiveness the gestalt leader encourages members to communicate through all avenues appropriate in the group. All the senses — taste, touch, smell, sound, and sight — are

Stage of Expressiveness	*Behavioral Manifestation*
• Blocked Stage	Individuals are nonexpressive, not knowing what they want to express.
• Inhibited Stage	Individuals are nonexpressive but know what they want to say even though they won't say it.
• Exhibitionistic Stage	Individuals can express what they want to say but are not wholly comfortable because expressiveness has not been integrated into their experiences.
• Spontaneous Stage	Individuals can express what they want fully and easily; expressiveness is compatible, assimilated, and integrated.

used to establish meaningful communication among members and to help members contact their own inner experience. Verbal techniques and exercises involving sensory and motor apparatus may be employed by activist leaders (Polster and Polster, 1974).

CLINICAL EXAMPLE: GESTALT–EXISTENTIAL CONCEPTS IN AN ADOLESCENT GROUP

The gestalt group leader is willing to take risks in order to destroy rigid behavioral patterns. A group of five adolescents referred because of school-related problems met weekly under the leadership of a nurse practitioner. One of the members, Sam, was depressed and had little interaction with others in the group. The most verbal member was Cherie, a black girl with a disorganized family life and a record of truancy. Laurie was a happy-go-lucky underachiever who seemed not to take the group or herself very seriously. Tim was a gifted musician who had become involved in drug use. The fifth member was Mary, a withdrawn, nonverbal girl who looked younger than her fifteen years. Group members ranged in age from fourteen to eighteen years. On a behavioral level an impasse developed quickly as the members consistently sat in the same chairs. The two males, Sam and Tim, sat side by side but did not interact with each other (*repetitive behaviors*).

After several weeks the leader literally pushed apart the chairs Sam and Tim were sitting in, saying that she chose to sit between them. This caused much moving and shifting of chairs as members were freed from habit by the action of the leader. Sam, who usually sat at a distance from Laurie, left his chair and sat beside her. This was recognized and reinforced by Cherie who moved into the seat next to the leader which had been vacated by Sam. Since they no longer sat side by side, Tim and Sam began to eye each other warily. The intrusive move of the leader was planned and implemented to create spatial and social mobility and to demonstrate to the group that alternatives were available.

In a group setting where the leader hopes to encourage expressiveness and meaningful dialogue, it is necessary to indicate that negative feelings may be expressed. The leader of the adolescent group became aware that some behaviors in the group made her feel angry. In touch with her own anger, the leader considered it likely that other members were experiencing similar feelings. The leader's anger had been aroused by Mary, the most silent member, who consistently monopolized the group's attention. An unfailing way for Mary to attract attention from other members was to begin to cry quietly. When this happened Cherie would take Mary's hand while Laurie murmured sympathetically (*blocked expressiveness*). Deciding to risk the disapproval of the group, the leader remarked that in her opinion Mary's crying spells were boring.

Laurie immediately accused the leader of being heartless, but Cherie began to giggle (*inhibited expressiveness*). Sam supported the leader by remarking that Mary cried in front of everyone, but there were lots of ways to cry — like privately. Tim indirectly supported Sam and the leader by singing "Laughing on the outside, crying on the inside" (*exhibitionistic expressiveness*). On hearing this the group members began to laugh and the tension dropped. When this happened the leader commented that perhaps it was easier for Mary to cry than talk about her problems, and asked the group how Mary could be helped to participate in a different way. The members then became able to express anger at Mary's tears, telling Mary they couldn't help her unless she told them what was going on. It was evident that the members actually considered the tears a nuisance and an impediment to helping Mary. The negative reaction of the leader to Mary's behavior was an accurate barometer of the group's feelings.

Although Mary wept on other occasions it was not necessary for the leader to voice annoyance a second time. The group members had learned from the leader that it was permissible to express true feelings rather than the stereotyped gestures which they thought were required (*spontaneous expressiveness*).

In this example a gestalt-existential group leader risked the anger of the group in order to release authentic emotion which was being blocked. At the same time the group was persuaded not to abandon Mary. If this had happened, Mary would have felt rejected and the group would have felt guilty for expressing negative feelings. The intervention enabled the leader to criticize the protracted weeping on behalf of the group, and at the same time confirm the importance of Mary to the group.

SUMMARY

A dichotomy was used to differentiate groups designed to produce intrapsychic change in members from groups designed to produce interpersonal or social change for members. The intrapsychic groups were further dichotomized as psychoanalytic and gestalt-existential. Contrasts were made between the historic or antecedal emphasis of psychoanalytic groups and the here-and-now emphasis of gestalt-existential theory. Various psychoanalytic concepts such as regression, symbiosis, differentiation, transference, and countertransference were described and illustrated. Basic premises of Bion regarding work groups and basic-assumption groups were cited. A continuum based on the extent of personality change showed the range between regressive-reconstructive groups, which seek personality change, and repressive-inspirational groups, which do not. Leader behaviors such as status denial and self-disclosure were recommended as methods which effectively reduce transference and unrealistic expectations of the leader.

In describing gestalt-existential groups, relevant concepts of need hierarchy and self-actualization were addressed. Among the various techniques of the gestalt-existential group leader, the "hot seat," psychodramatization, and "homework" were presented. Stages of expressiveness were identified, and features of each stage were described. Activism, directiveness, and risk-taking were advocated for the leaders of gestalt-existential groups.

REFERENCES

Anthony, E.J. "The History of Group Psychotherapy." In *Comprehensive Group Psychotherapy*, H.I. Kaplan and B.J. Sadock, Eds. Baltimore: Williams and Wilkins, 1971 a, pages 5–31.

_____. "Comparison Between Individual and Group Psychotherapy." In *Comprehensive Group Psychotherapy*, H.I. Kaplan and B.J. Sadock, Eds. Baltimore: Williams and Wilkins, 1971b, pages 104–117.

Bion, W.R. *Experiences in Groups.* New York: Basic Books, 1959.

Downing, J., Ed. *Gestalt Awareness.* New York: Harper & Row, 1976.

Erikson, E.H. *Identity, Youth, and Crisis.* New York: W.W. Norton, 1968.

Fagan, J., and I. Shepherd. *Gestalt Therapy Now.* Palo Alto, CA.: Science and Behavior Books, 1970.

Freud, S. "Group Psychology and the Analysis of the Ego." *Standard Edition of Complete Psychological Works of Sigmund Freud* Vol. 18. London: Hogarth Press, 1957.

_____. *Totem and Taboo.* New York: Winston, 1950.

Gendlin, E.T. "The Experiential Response." In *Use of Interpretation in Treatment*, E.J. Hammer, Ed. New York: Grune and Stratton, 1968.

Gibbard, G.S.; J.J. Hartman; and R.D. Mann, Eds. *Analysis of Groups.* San Francisco: Jossey-Bass, 1974.

Hall, C.S., and G. Lindzey. *Theories of Personality.* New York: Wiley, 1970.

Hammerschlag, C.A., and B.M. Astrachan. "The Kennedy Airport Snow-In: An Inquiry into Intergroup Phenomena," *Psychiatry* 34, August 1971, pages 301–308.

Lewin, K. *Field Theory in the Social Sciences.* New York: Harper, 1951.

Marram, G.W. *The Group Approach in Nursing Practice.* St. Louis: C.V. Mosby, 1978.

Maslow, A.H. *Toward a Psychology of Being.* New York: D. Van Nostrand, 1968.

Mills, T.M. *The Sociology of Small Groups.* Englewood Cliffs, N.J.: Prentice-Hall, 1967.

Mullan, H., and M. Rosenbaum. *Group Psychotherapy.* New York: Free Press, 1962.

O'Hearne, J.J. "How and Why Do Transactional Gestalt Therapists Work as They Do." *International Journal of Group Psychotherapy* Vol. 26, No. 2, 1976, pages 163–172.

Slater, P.E. *Microcosm.* New York: Wiley, 1966.

Perls, F. *The Gestalt Approach and Eye Witness to Therapy.* New York: Bantam Books, 1976.

Polster, E. and M. *Gestalt Therapy Integrated.* New York: Random House, 1974.

Slavson, S.R. *Child Centered Guidance of Parents.* New York: International Universities Press, 1974.

Weiss, R.S. "Transition States and Other Stressful Situations: Their Nature and Programs for Their Management." *Support Systems and Mutual Help: Multidisciplinary Explorations,* G. Caplan and M. Killilia, Eds. New York: Grune and Stratton, 1976, pages 215–231.

Wertheimer, M., and W. Kohler. "Gestalt Psychology." *Contemporary Schools of Psychology.* New York: Ronald Press, 1968.

Yalom, I. *The Theory and Practice of Group Psychotherapy.* New York: Basic Books, 1975.

4

Theoretical Frameworks: Interpersonal Groups

Ellen Hastings Janosik

In psychoanalytic and gestalt-existential groups attention is given to intrapsychic processes, since it is assumed that improvements in daily living are a consequence of intrapsychic change. Interpersonal groups are organized on the premise that corrective interpersonal transactions can alter the inner psychological experience of members. Such groups encourage relationships which teach and reinforce the accurate transmission and perception of meaning. Goals of interpersonal groups are often nonspecific and may consist of learning to be more comfortable with others or more skillful in expressing thoughts and feelings. In some respects every group, regardless of the framework used, represents an interpersonal field. There-fore concepts appropriate for communication-interactional groups may be ap-plied to various didactic, community, or family groups.

COMMUNICATION-INTERACTIONAL FRAMEWORK

Interpersonal communication may be described as an intricate process of human interaction and relatedness which transcends speech and language. Every communication act involves multiple messages and exists on multiple levels which are influenced by the sender, the recipient, and the context in which communication takes place. A concept essential to communication is *feedback,* which implies that change in an organism occurs because of the response of others to a previous message or performance. Feedback in human communication is important because it permits messages to be redirected to the source or sender. Thus feedback has the power to sustain or modify subsequent communication and interaction (Weiner, 1949).

Satir (1967), who used communication principles in the treatment of dysfunctional families, described communication as an exchange process permitting individuals to relate in the interpersonal field. Relatedness refers to the emotional, perceptual, and cognitive capacity of one individual to become involved with others (Rouslin, 1973). Transactions and interactions are part of communication, as are words, kinesics, and symbols. Proponents of communication-interactional group frameworks believe that learning and achievement do not precede but follow functional communication and interaction. Functional communication means the ability to transmit messages clearly and directly, to clarify and rephrase when necessary, and to receive and respond to feedback. Dysfunctional communication is characterized by indirect, unclear, or incongruent messages and unresponsiveness to feedback.

Communication includes messages which are denotive and explicit as well as connotive and implicit. Connotive communication is individualistic and is influenced by previous experiences of sender and receiver. Consequently, the possibility of misinterpretation is great, and the message received may not be the message sent. Human communication depends upon *metacommunication* for comprehensible interpretation. Metacommunication transmits additional information about the message being sent. The individual who says "thank you" but is grim-faced and angry while speaking is employing a form of metacommunication which is not congruent with the words but which accurately reflects the affective state of the sender. The recipient must then decide whether to respond to the message or the metamessage. All the participants in the communication process share responsibility for the consequences.

In working with family groups Satir uses a *model analysis,* which identifies the role models who drew up the blueprints used by other family members to interpret and respond to communication. Even though the blueprint is obsolete, it is followed reflexively by many individuals. Because of opportunities for feedback the interpersonal group provides a responsive milieu in which group members may help point out the uselessness of the blueprint and the need to develop new methods of relating.

Anxiety and Self-Esteem

Although interpersonal groups deal with behaviors in the here and now, it is difficult to understand human behavior without including the role of anxiety in interpersonal relationships. The work of Sullivan (1953) on anxiety and self-esteem as outcomes of past interpersonal experiences has broadened the usage of communication-interactional concepts in group work. Belief that anxiety arises in interpersonal relationships to threaten feelings of personal security is compatible with the communication-interactional framework. Although schooled in psychoanalytic theory, Sullivan departed from the idea of prede-termined biological needs in favor of interactional patterns which individuals establish early in life through experiences with significant persons. The mother-child relationship is described as both a source of anxiety and a means of relieving anxiety for the participants.

Psychoanalytic theorists regard interpersonal behaviors as the re-sult of transferences which are the legacy of childhood relationships. When group interactions are viewed in this way, personality reconstruc-tion and early experiences are highlighted. For a group organized ac-cording to a communication-interactional framework, the major ob-jective is the observation and modification of interpersonal behaviors without undue concern for their origin. Whether a group is composed of hypertensive patients, expectant mothers, or single parents, com-munication-interactional principles help assess the behaviors used by members to alleviate anxiety generated during interpersonal encounters.

Sullivan attributed much human dysfunction to inadequate com-munication, and he equated anxiety with threats to interpersonal security which lower self-esteem. Interpersonal relationships form the sense of self. In later life negative concepts of self may be revised by positive relationships with peers who provide supportive feedback. Thus early influences which were derogatory may be eradicated by later relationships which are gratifying. The interpersonal theory of Sullivan is indebted to social psychologists who contend that indi-viduals cannot be understood apart from their social environment. In a communication-interactional group, remedial action takes place in a setting in which members can safely observe, react, and comment. The comments and reactions of group members may be considered analogous to peer influences on adolescents, who need to be reassured and taught by friends, because friends are more accepting than parents

(Guttmacher, 1973). Being included in a cohesive interpersonal group allows members to test limits, observe styles of relating, and give as well as receive feedback.

Although the findings are ambiguous, the disruptive effects of anxiety have been confirmed by researchers (Sarnoff and Zimbardo, 1961) who found that the desire to affiliate with others increased as fear increased, but decreased as anxiety increased. Subjects who experienced anxiety, rather than fear, preferred isolation to affiliation. The findings support the empirical data of Sullivan that human behavior moves toward collaboration and mutuality unless blocked by anxiety. In a well-known study of five thousand junior and senior high school students, high anxiety levels correlated with low self-esteem (Rosenberg, 1962). High levels of anxiety have also been correlated with day dreaming and fantasizing, activities which contribute to social isolation (Singer, 1966).

The communication-interactional group leader considers anxiety an intervening variable which is affected by the impact of others in the interpersonal field, and in turn affects personal feelings of worth and confidence. The group leader is responsible for regulating group and individual levels of anxiety so that motivation to change is present but discomfort is not excessive. Tolerable levels of anxiety can mobilize and energize; anxiety which is intolerable overwhelms and disrupts (Leavitt, 1967).

Security Operations

Three communication modes have been described by Sullivan: *prototaxic communication,* which antedates language and symbolization; *parataxic communication,* in which language and symbolization are unique and idiosyncratic; and *syntaxic communication,* which is understood and consensually validated by others. Transferences, which are idiosyncratic distortions, belong in the category of parataxic experience and may be corrected through consensual validation by the group.

During interpersonal encounters which produce great anxiety, many individuals resort to *security operations* which reduce anxiety but distort reality. Two security operations presented by Sullivan are *selective inattention* and *focal awareness.* In selective inattention, information is deleted by the recipient of the message. This allows the individual to refuse those parts of the communication which contradict prior expectations, convictions, or beliefs. In focal awareness the individual attaches enormous significance to any aspect of communication which confirms prior expectations, convictions, or beliefs.

An individual who expects to be rejected by a group may be inattentive to evidence of interpersonal acceptance and interpret the most cordial message as confirmation of the expectation. Another individual, less sensitive to rebuff, may misinterpret or be unaware of dissenting or distancing behaviors in interpersonal transactions. Selective inattention causes convenient amnesia about certain details. Focal awareness results in interpretations which amplify some details and ignore others. Often these two security operations are used in conjunction with one another to maintain feelings of interpersonal comfort by reshaping reality.

There are two interventions which effectively counteract selective inattention and focal awareness: consensual validation from group members, and feedback from group members and the leader. Unless the leader can elicit corrective responses from the group or provide them in the form of leadership interventions, the group experience will be perceived in an unrealistic manner. This will reduce the anxiety of the members, but preserve the maladaptive communication and interactional patterns. A group leader who recognizes that security operations are in effect must examine the causes of anxiety and be prepared to reinforce functional communication to the point of being redundant, if necessary.

The effect of anxiety and lowered self-esteem on communication is substantiated by Virginia Satir (1972), who observed that persons under stress adopt any of four types of response when their self-worth is questioned: 1) blaming, 2) placating, 3) computing, and 4) distracting. All of these responses represent security operations by persons who fear criticism, exclusion, or failure. The "blamer" fears being held responsible for whatever happens and projects responsibility onto others. By accusing others the blamer manages to avoid admitting errors which may have been committed. The "placator" is afraid of the anger of others and avoids this through self-deprecating behavior. By belittling personal worth and importance the placator hopes to avoid confrontation and to be left alone. The "computer" adopts an attitude of calmness and detachment, which permits cognitive but not emotional involvement. This behavior is unlike that of the "distracter," who avoids dealing with essentials by moving rapidly from one tangential point to another. Satir agrees with Sullivan that communication patterns are learned in childhood, and that dysfunctional communication can be rectified by later interpersonal experiences which demonstrate the value of congruent communication appropriate to the situation. Functional communication is specific to the events being considered; dysfunctional communication is nonspecific, diffuse, and generalized.

Leadership Functions

There are several aspects of functional communication which interpersonal group leaders must consider. Anxiety is an interpersonal variable that must be assessed continuously. One effect of a high anxiety level is an increase in the variability range of responses among group members, even though average group scores are unaffected (Sarason, 1957; Schwab and Iverson, 1964). This variability may be explained in part by the idiosyncratic defensive behaviors which anxiety provokes. The group member whose customary defense is obsessive-compulsive behavior may become more rigid and constricted when anxious, while another member may become clinging and demanding. The wide variability of individual responses to anxiety complicates the assessment functions of the leader and is an argument for comprehensive preliminary interviews with prospective members in order to establish their behavioral baselines.

When assessing individuals in a clinical setting, the following observations may be used to ascertain when and how anxiety intrudes on the flow of communication (Sullivan, 1953).

- At what point during communication is an important subject or topic changed?
- When do security operations, in the form of defensive behaviors, appear?
- How and when do somatic manifestations of anxiety intrude?

Characteristics of functional communication have been outlined by a number of theorists whose precepts are excellent guidelines for assessment of group communication and interaction. The first precept is that it is impossible not to communicate. When nothing seems to be happening, something is actually happening (Birdwhistell, 1970; Watzlawick, 1964; Ruesch, 1961). There is no such thing as an absence of communication. Unresponsiveness in the form of silence constitutes a loud response. The individual who does not answer a question or a letter is communicating with the sender nonetheless. To understand what is being communicated it is also necessary to understand what is not communicated. The unanswered letter and the unanswered question may indicate indifference, incapacity, or a form of security operation. Frequently the details *not* contained in a message are more significant than those which are (Pittenger, Hockett, and Danehy, 1960).

Persons engaged in the communication process have an obligation to clarify meanings, to maintain congruence, and to avoid the blaming, placating, computing, and distracting which are used to conceal personal vulnerability rather than reveal meaning (Satir, 1967). If group members are unable to establish clear communication, the leader must intervene. Table 4-1 outlines functional and dysfunctional transactions in a communication-interactional group.

CLINICAL EXAMPLE: SECURITY OPERATIONS IN A GROUP FOR DIABETIC PATIENTS

In a long-term group sponsored by an out-patient medical clinic, six female diabetics met twice a month after their clinic appointments. The group leader was Ruth Allen, a clinical nurse specialist. All the group members were married homemakers between the ages of thirty and fifty who had been invited to join the group because their disease was either labile or only recently diagnosed. The group was open-ended, with members joining and terminating as indicated by the stability of their physical condition. The purpose of the group was to help provide continuity of care in a supportive interpersonal setting in which didactic material could easily be presented.

The senior group member was Mrs. Drew. A grossly overweight woman, Mrs. Drew had been attending the medical clinic for ten years,

Table 4-1   EFFECTS OF FUNCTIONAL AND DYSFUNCTIONAL COMMUNICATION

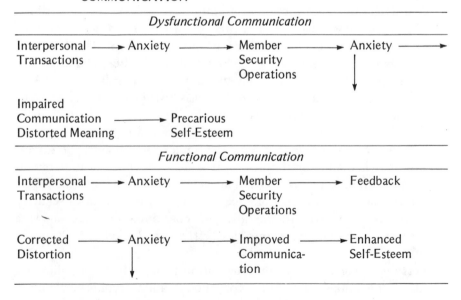

but had recently been invited to join the group because of the lability of her diabetes. The relationship of Mrs. Drew with the group leader had always been friendly during dyadic interactions. Ruth Allen, therefore, was surprised and dismayed to find that Mrs. Drew became a problem in the group situation. Even though Mrs. Drew was grossly overweight and her condition unstable, she seemed to vie with Ruth for leadership of the group. This was done by constantly challenging Ruth's professional judgment and expertise. In the meetings Mrs. Drew presented herself as the real expert on diabetes, indicating that only she could tell it like it was. Through her words and manner Mrs. Drew conveyed the idea that her experience as a diabetic made her a more reliable authority than Ruth, whose knowledge came from books. Although Ruth tried to avoid open confrontation with Mrs. Drew, she found that her sound teaching was being undermined and that some of the members were being misled by Mrs. Drew's statements.

Because she feared that the group was jeopardized by the contest for leadership, Ruth asked help from a staff consultant on group dynamics. The consultant agreed to observe the meetings through a one-way mirror. Since this observation had not been part of the group agreement, Ruth presented it to the members for approval. She explained that this was her first experience in leading a group and that she wanted consultation to improve her leadership skills. The members agreed to the observation, although Mrs. Drew said that the group itself could probably identify Ruth's weaknesses for her.

In observing the group sessions the consultant confirmed her own initial suspicion — Ruth's interactions with Mrs. Drew were inconsistent. By the time the consultation was requested, Ruth's reaction to Mrs. Drew was one of sheer rage. Ruth felt her status and credibility were being threatened by Mrs. Drew. This caused Ruth to dwell on Mrs. Drew's deficiencies and to see the woman as a malicious agent rather than a group member (*blaming*). The first objective of the consultant was to place Mrs. Drew's behavior into an interpersonal framework, which made it part of the total group interaction. Based on her observations the consultant made the following assessment.

1. Mrs. Drew was embarrassed by being the senior member: she had been attending the clinic the longest and had been diagnosed as a diabetic during her high school days. The lability of her diabetes and her obesity frightened and humiliated her. Despite her extensive knowledge of diabetes she was afraid that the other members of the group did not respect her. This made her acutely anxious. Her anxiety and low self-esteem caused her to attempt an alliance with the leader rather than with group members, from whom she feared rejection. Her annoying behavior was motivated by her wish to be allied with Ruth and to win Ruth's respect (*isolation from fellow members; affiliation with the leader*).

2. Although angry at Mrs. Drew, Ruth seemed to be relieved by sharing the leadership responsibility with her. When the group members fell silent, Ruth sent nonverbal messages to Mrs. Drew requesting her to take over. The nonverbal messages included nodding, smiling, and glancing at Mrs. Drew whenever Ruth was unsure of what to say next (*metacommunication*). This allowed Mrs. Drew to think that Ruth welcomed her contributions.

3. Mrs. Drew was exploited by the other group members who rewarded her verbosity and used it to avoid becoming more involved with each other. The members frequently referred to Mrs. Drew's extensive knowledge and experience with diabetes (*placating*).

4. Although Ruth was glad to relinquish leadership to Mrs. Drew at times, she resented doing this. When Mrs. Drew assumed leadership, Ruth doubted her own ability to sustain the group. Ruth gave many double messages to Mrs. Drew. On one level she signaled to Mrs. Drew for assistance. On another level she considered Mrs. Drew an intruder. After trying unsuccessfully to be consistent, Ruth became angry with Mrs. Drew (*ambiguous communication*).

Since the purpose of meeting was to help members handle their diabetes, the consultant suggested that Ruth distribute leadership functions among all the members, rather than continue turning to Mrs. Drew. Competition between two persons is a form of pairing which often interferes with the group task. To weaken the pairing with Mrs. Drew, Ruth asked all the members to identify for the group their most urgent concerns. At the suggestion of the consultant, Ruth told the group that she had depended too much on Mrs. Drew and needed to hear more from other members (*feedback*). Ruth also explained that having diabetes did not, automatically, make one an expert, and asked members to confirm this through their own experiences (*consensual validation*). She stressed that bringing their concerns to the group was the best way to learn and to work together.

Because Mrs. Drew found the group experience anxiety-provoking, she tried to protect her self-image. This caused her to avoid involvement with fellow members and to align herself with Ruth, whom she trusted. With the aid of the group consultant, Ruth became aware of the mutual anxiety which motivated the struggle between herself and Mrs. Drew. Interventions were planned to restore Mrs. Drew's self-confidence and to make Ruth's leadership consistent. Ruth explained to group members that diabetes mellitus was a disease with many ramifications, and that no one was a failure because the disease was not stabilized. Once Ruth accepted Mrs. Drew's interpersonal needs as sincere, she was able to modify the leadership inconsistencies which came from her own insecurity. By looking at the reciprocal nature of communication and interaction between Ruth and Mrs. Drew, the consultant helped Ruth to plan interventions which persuaded Mrs. Drew that interpersonal security lay in group membership rather than in a contest for leadership.

CRISIS FRAMEWORKS

Theory

Crisis intervention, whether offered to individuals or groups, deals with human reactions to contemporary, reality-based problems. Crisis theory is founded on the observation that human reactions to stressful events are remarkably similar, even though the nature of the stress and of the persons involved may vary. Hazardous events, developmental or situational, cause problems which individuals try to solve through their usual coping skills. When customary coping behaviors fail to bring relief, the result is tension, confusion, and feelings of inadequacy, all of which reduce the problem-solving ability even more. Crisis-ridden persons are so disorganized that feelings of helplessness overpower rational processes (Dixon, 1979). It is possible for individuals to be in crisis without experiencing subjective distress. Whether subjective distress is present or not, the goal of crisis intervention is to find a solution rather than eliminate the distress.

For every person, crises are recurrent and inevitable during the life cycle. Erikson's contribution to crisis theory was to enumerate the developmental or critical tasks which must be accomplished for growth to continue. The identity crisis of adolescence is a developmental task which has received wide attention (Blos, 1979). Midlife stresses, such as the *empty-nest syndrome,* are treated as hazardous events which have the potential for crisis (Kuhn and Janosik, 1980). At times crisis may be attributed to the developmental stage of the individual; at other times it may stem from situational causes, or a combination of developmental and situational factors. Stressful situations include bereavement, change in marital status, and social or geographic mobility (Weiss, 1976). Whether or not these events become actual crises depends on the coping skills of the persons involved and the supplies available in the social field.

Lindemann   Crisis theory is founded on the seminal work of Lindemann (1944). He observed that persons who responded to the loss of a loved one with painful grieving were better able to avoid more serious psychological disturbances later. The phrase *grief work* was applied to the mourning process, which was seen as painful but necessary. Caplan (1964) elaborated on the work of Lindemann, and outlined a sequence which often leads to crisis. First, individuals encounter a hazardous event which is impervious to their usual methods of coping. Failure of usual coping measures leads to a state of disequilibrium, the outcome of which is uncertain. Crisis entails both a danger and an opportunity. There is danger that dysfunctional resolution of the crisis will weaken previous coping skills, but there is also opportunity for functional resolution of the crisis to strengthen previous coping skills. Crisis is self-limiting in the sense that resolution — adaptive or maladaptive — is reached within a period of four to six weeks. When crisis theory is employed, therapeutic intervention is limited to the crisis situation. Crisis work differs from other types of therapies because its preoccupation is with the precipitating event, with the coping skills of the persons involved, and with the resources available in the social field. This is equally true of individual and of group crisis intervention. Selection of individuals for crisis groups is based on the availability of suitable groups and on the preliminary assessment of the individual as capable of benefiting from a group approach. There are individuals so demoralized by crisis that group treatment is not offered. For others, initial individual counseling is made available for several sessions, at which point group treatment may be recommended.

The recurrence and inevitability of crises are best explained in the language of systems theory. Any functioning organism is a permeable or semipermeable system which is subject to stresses leading to disequilibrium. Normally a functioning system maintains a steady state of exchange between environmental input which is acceptable to the system and output from the system which is acceptable to the environment. When internal or external pressures mount, the resultant stress overwhelms the adaptive capacity of the system. Adjustment between the system and the environment is interrupted: the system becomes disorganized and a period of disequilibrium follows. Disequilibrium brings about dysfunction or malfunction of the system. Crisis is not a form of mental disorder, and may ultimately be a source of additional strength. It is undeniable, however, that many behaviors of persons in crisis resemble forms of psychiatric disorder, and that some individuals and families are better equipped than others to handle change and crisis.

Caplan   Caplan (1963) considered crisis work a form of primary prevention and advised the use of crisis intervention to improve mental health and prevent psychiatric illness. Anticipatory guidance for persons known to be facing impending change is an admirable utilization of the principles of crisis work. Persons facing retirement, attending prenatal clinics, beginning school, or leaving college all face role changes which may precipitate crisis. Three major types of crisis were identified by Caplan: loss of satisfaction of basic needs through death of a loved one or loss of body integrity through illness; threatened or perceived loss of any of the foregoing; and challenges or changes for which individuals feel unprepared, such as job promotion, parenthood, or marriage.

Group Work

Persons in crisis are in need of social supplies which supplement their usual supports. Unfortunately, the disorganization which accompanies crisis prevents individuals from obtaining supplemental support without guidance. Crisis groups, by affording participants a temporary sense of community where they can find and offer help, persuade members that their needs are not abnormal. Restoration of feelings of belonging is important to crisis-ridden persons, who feel lost and alienated. Since the period of crisis lasts four to six weeks, participation in a crisis group is invariably short term. Often the crisis group is ongoing, but members contract to attend no more than eight meetings. If termination seems premature after eight meetings, other arrangements are made. While attending a crisis group individuals are usually responsive and motivated — a result of the disequilibrium they experience. The minimum goal of intervention is the resolution of the immediate crisis and restoration of the ability to function near precrisis levels (Aguilera and Messick, 1974).

The short time in which members attend crisis meetings engenders a sense of urgency. There are some leaders who believe that crisis groups are not cohesive because of their brevity, but others assert that the ongoing, open-ended nature of such groups insures that a nucleus of cohesive members is always present. One method of increasing group cohesion is to select members whose crises are similar or to select members with previous bonds and ties. College students attending the same institution have a common bond, regardless of the exact crisis they face. Newly divorced persons may come from diverse backgrounds but they share the common problem of building a new life. Pregnant teenagers must confront a situational crisis (unwed pregnancy) superimposed on a developmental task (adolescence). Such commonalities build cohesion even in a very brief group experience.

Definition The definition of a crisis group is clear and its goals are circumscribed in scope and purpose. A crisis group is a gathering of individuals who meet for a limited number of sessions with a designated leader in order to work on critical issues currently facing the members. The problems may be similar or dissimilar. Crisis intervention is applied impartially to members selected for the group. Even when every crisis in the group is similar, there are differences because members bring different coping skills and social resources to the group. This does not influence adherence to the crisis framework.

Goals When individuals are invited to join a crisis group the avowed purpose is to work on the stressful event identified as a crisis. During preparatory assessment meeting(s) the precipitator is identified and the crisis event delineated. Sometimes an individual's perception of the problem differs from that of the nurse making the preliminary assessment. Discrepancies between the nurse's assessment and that of the prospective member should be negotiated. Failing this, discrepancies should be brought to the attention of the group member. This is extremely important in these groups because attention is restricted to the critical event.

The Participant In preliminary meetings between counselor and prospective group member an agreement is reached that hazardous circumstances have precipitated a crisis which is amenable to group intervention. When all the members of a crisis group share a common problem, the general nature of the problem is divulged to prospective members during the preparatory interviews, without breach of confidentiality. If the problems of the group members are diverse, the prospective member may be informed only that group members have "problems in daily living" which will be dealt with in the group. Either explanation persuades prospective members that they need not feel isolated, because the group is made up of people much like themselves.

The Leader The leader of a crisis group is vigorous and directive, and group members are considered active contributors whose suggestions have merit. Sometimes members may digress to issues not relevant to their immediate problems, at which point the leader may intervene. Since the average number of meetings attended is six, the leader can cite time pressures as justification for keeping group members involved with the task. Many crisis group leaders resemble stage managers or directors, who carefully assess the ability and performance of members. Quiet members are encouraged to participate and dominant members are controlled. All members of the group are expected to follow the precepts which guide crisis work.

Problems Aguilera and Messick (1974) agree that crisis groups present problems even for experienced leaders. When members are undergoing diverse crises, the leader may find it difficult to prevent the content of the meetings from digressing into areas unrelated to crisis. A way of avoiding this is to organize the group around a common problem. When the critical problem is shared by the members, group pressure may be sufficient to hold members to relevant subjects.

Comparatively little systematic research has been done on crisis groups, but Morley and Brown (1968) list advantages and disadvantages of crisis groups, a few of which follow:

Advantages of Crisis Groups	*Disadvantages of Crisis Groups*
• Crisis groups are acceptable to persons who might otherwise refuse help.	• Crisis groups emphasize group content rather than group process.
• Crisis groups use nonthreatening terminology and avoid psychiatric labels.	• Crisis group intervention may remain at superficial levels.
• Crisis group goals are limited and specific; self-help is emphasized and regression averted.	• Activity and directiveness of crisis group leaders may inhibit spontaneity among members.
• Crisis groups are open-ended but time-limited.	• Crisis group cohesion may be questionable, due to the brevity of the group experience.
• Crisis groups provide prevention in the form of anticipatory guidance.	• Crisis group members who are unready to terminate must establish new group or individual relationships.

Crisis group work is particularly adaptable to the nursing process. Some knowledge of psychological dynamics underlying human reactions to crisis is essential, but intervention is limited to alleviation of symptoms. Chronic problems and concerns cannot be addressed within the time and contractual constraints of the crisis intervention framework. Persons joining a crisis group feel incompetent because of overwhelming circumstances, but the group helps put individuals in touch with resources which have been ignored or forgotten. The disorganization produced by crisis makes individuals lose their ability to deal rationally with their situation. Therefore the crisis group must first assist its members to gain an intellectual understanding of the crisis. Following this, members are encouraged to express feelings, to develop additional coping skills, and to restore social supports (Aguilera and Messick, 1974). Crisis groups are limited in time and restricted in scope, but operate in four dimensions: cognitive, affective, instrumental, and social.

CLINICAL EXAMPLE: LEADERSHIP AND TASK COMMITMENT IN A CRISIS GROUP

The basic course in psychiatric/mental-health nursing was required of all seniors in a baccalaureate nursing program. As part of the clinical component of the course, ten of the senior nursing students were assigned to an acute-care psychiatric in-patient facility for three months. In previous years students complained that this particular clinical placement was stressful. Some students assigned to the facility proved unable to fulfill the clinical requirements and had to repeat the course the following year. A few students with otherwise satisfactory records dropped out of the nursing program during this clinical placement.

The nursing faculty considered the problem a serious one. On the one hand, the acute-care facility offered a rich learning experience and the majority of students were able to take advantage of it. On the other hand, the placement evidently made demands which some students were unable to meet. Despite careful selection of students and good clinical teaching, there were always students who performed poorly and became discouraged. The problem was discussed at length by the nursing faculty. They concluded that the students were psychologically unprepared for this clinical experience and that no organized support was available to them. The nursing faculty decided to ask Mrs. Beck, a team leader at the acute-care facility, to meet weekly with the students assigned there. Mrs. Beck was a nurse accustomed to leading short-term, task-oriented groups which helped prepare patients for discharge.

Participation in the meetings was voluntary. The leader was selected for her leadership skills and because she was not an authority figure for the students. Group confidentiality was pledged, especially with regard to nursing faculty and hospital administration. The stated group purpose was to give anticipatory guidance to help students deal with their feelings about psychiatric illness and psychiatric nursing. As planned by the nursing faculty and implemented by Mrs. Beck, the group was a form of primary prevention.

Hour-long weekly meetings were scheduled for eight weeks and were held in a conference room at the psychiatric facility. At the first meeting Mrs. Beck expanded on the rationale for the group and disavowed any connection between herself as group leader and the nursing faculty or personnel. The crisis intervention format was described, and the group leader then began to disclose her own feelings about working in the psychiatric facility, describing how her feelings had changed over time. She suggested that members might like to discuss methods of adjustment which had worked for them in other clinical placements, and to look for ways to adapt these to the present clinical setting.

Group cohesion was evident even in the first meeting because of relationships already present among the students and because of shared feelings about the clinical placement. The first four meetings were effective in uncovering some of the students' concerns. Under Mrs. Beck's leadership the group began to problem-solve together. In the second meeting Kitty Sawyer confided that she had grown up with a manic-depressive brother and described the reactivation of old feelings when she had to interact with a manic patient. Kitty's uncertainty about her ability to get through the clinical placement elicited advice from the group. Among the suggestions made by her classmates was the possibility that expanding her knowledge of manic-depressive illness might make this problem less upsetting to her. During the fourth meeting Jennie Brice, a student with an alcoholic mother, talked of feelings which made her unable to be therapeutic in her interactions with alcoholic patients in the unit, particularly females. Again the group was supportive and concerned. At this point Mrs. Beck noted a lowering of anxiety among most of the students (*content consistent with group goals*). During the fourth meeting Mrs. Beck told the group that the nursing faculty realized that not every student could work with every psychiatric patient, and she suggested that Kitty and Jennie could request assignments to patients with whom they felt comfortable.

Clara was an interested, participating member in the first meetings but was silent in the session when Jennie talked about her mother's alcoholism. Early in the next meeting Clara told the group she had a personal matter to discuss. Although Clara was usually composed, her manner of speaking became hesitant and agitated. Because the group had responded so warmly to Kitty and Jennie, Clara said she felt brave enough to talk about her problem. After a few false starts Clara blurted out the information that she was uncomfortable with her sexual identity and was contemplating transsexual surgery so she could live as a male. She said she had tried lesbian relationships, but they were not satisfying. She considered them inadequate and unnatural, although there were several women whom she had loved. Furthermore, the revelations of Kitty and Jennie had made her feel very protective toward them, and this in turn had aroused a sexual response in her. "This is a real problem for me," Clara went on. "I know it's a heavy thing to lay on the group, but I love all of you so much. You people are so beautiful that I want to tell the truth to you. It feels good to be able to take off the mask" (*content inconsistent with goals*).

There was stunned silence for a few minutes after Clara's remarks, but the group rallied. Questions were asked about Clara's family history and personal life, which she answered with growing ease. It seemed to Mrs. Beck that in spite of Clara's turmoil there was a covert satisfaction at being the center of attention. After watching the proceedings for a short time the group leader intervened, choosing her words carefully.

"I feel very sympathetic about Clara's dilemma and think she has been courageous in talking about it. However, I am not sure this group is able to respond to such a complicated problem. We are limited to three more meetings and our agreement is to discuss feelings related to this clinical placement. If we try to help Clara, it means we can't meet our commitment to the group. It also means we are being unfair to Clara, who needs more help than this group can provide. I'd like to ask Clara and the rest of the group to trust me to find help for Clara while she considers this important decision. We can talk about this later, Clara, and I promise to be available to you. Now perhaps we can use the remainder of the meeting to finish the work we have started — how to get the most out of this clinical placement" (*redirection to group goals*).

The leader's purposeful intervention was received with signs of relief from the group. One student said she felt bad for Clara, but knew that she was out of her depth in trying to give advice. Another member confessed to mingled sympathy and resentment toward Clara, saying, "This is too large a burden to put on us. At first I was just angry with you. I didn't know what to say and I was relieved when Mrs. Beck got us off the hook. Right now I don't feel angry with you, Clara. I just feel very sorry and hope you can get the help you need."

Mrs. Beck followed this by remarking on the honest emotions the group was able to express. "This is a sign we trust each other and that we have grown. Let's use this trust to return to our original purpose, since there are people better qualified than we to respond to Clara. Clara has trusted us and we can help her most by remembering our agreement about confidentiality. She and I will meet later to consider obtaining help from other sources" (*structure for the group; reassurance for Clara*).

SUMMARY

Interpersonal groups are predicated on the assumption that learning and achievement follow adaptive communication and interactional patterns. Interpersonal groups provide a mechanism through which group members may give and receive feedback and consensually validate their perceptions of what is occurring in the interpersonal field. Four common patterns of maladaptive communication were enumerated and examples given. These included blaming, placating, computing, and distracting. The role of anxiety in facilitating or disrupting group interaction was described at length, as were leadership functions in this area.

An explanation of crisis theory preceded the section on crisis group work. In applying crisis theory to group work the advantages and limitations of this group approach were described. The necessity of adhering to specific goals and to a time-limited framework was strongly advised for the leader of crisis groups.

REFERENCES

Aguilera, D.C., and J.M. Messick. *Crisis Intervention Theory and Methodology.* St. Louis: C.V. Mosby, 1974.

Birdwhistell, R.L. *Kinesics and Content: Essays on Body Motion Communication.* Philadelphia: University of Pennsylvania Press, 1970.

Blos, Peter. *Developmental Issues.* New York: International Universities Press, 1979.

Caplan, G. *Principles of Preventive Psychiatry.* New York: Basic Books, 1964.

_____. "Emotional Crises." In *Encyclopedia of Mental Health*, A. Deutsch and H. Fishbein, Eds. Vol. 2. New York: Franklin Watts, 1963, pages 521–532.

Dixon, S.L. *Working with People in Crisis.* St. Louis: C.V. Mosby, 1979.

Guttmacher, J.A. "The Concept of Character, Character Problems, and Group Therapy." *Comprehensive Psychiatry* Vol. 14, No. 6, November/December 1973, pages 513–522.

Kuhn, K., and E.H. Janosik. "The Post Parental Family." In *Family-Focused Care*, J.R. Miller and E.H. Janosik, Eds. New York: McGraw-Hill, 1980.

Leavitt, E.E. *The Psychology of Anxiety.* New York: Bobbs-Merrill, 1967.

Lindemann, E. "Symptomatology and Management of Acute Grief." *American Journal of Psychiatry* 101, 1944, pages 141–148.

Morley, W.E., and V.B. Brown. "The Crisis Intervention Group: A Natural Mating or a Marriage of Convenience." *Psychotherapy, Theory, Practice, Research* 6, Winter 1968, pages 30–36.

Pittenger, R.E.; C.F. Hockett; and J.J. Danehy. *The First Five Minutes: A Sample of Microscopic Interview Analysis.* Ithaca, N.Y.: Martineau, 1960.

Rosenberg, M. "The Association Between Self-Esteem and Anxiety." *Journal of Psychiatric Research* 1, 1962, pages 135–151.

Rouslin, S. "Relatedness in Group Psychotherapy." *Perspectives in Psychiatric Care* Vol. XI, No. 4, 1973, pages 165–171.

Ruesch, J. *Disturbed Communication*. New York: W.W. Norton, 1961.

Sarason, I.G. "Effects of Anxiety and Two Kinds of Motivating Instructions on Verbal Learning." *Journal of Abnormal and Social Psychology* 54, 1957, pages 166–171.

Sarnoff, I., and P.G. Zimbardo. "Anxiety, Fear, and Social Affiliation." *Journal of Abnormal and Social Psychology* 62, 1961, pages 356–363. Reprinted in *Interpersonal Behavior in Small Groups*, R.J. Offshe, Ed. Englewood Cliffs, N.J.: Prentice-Hall, 1973.

Satir, V. *Peoplemaking*. Palo Alto, CA.: Science and Behavior Books, 1972.

————. *Conjoint Family Therapy*. Palo Alto, CA.: Science and Behavior Books, 1967.

Schwab, J.R., and M.A. Iverson. "Resistance of High Anxiety under Ego Threat to Perception of Figural Distortion." *Journal of Consulting Psychology* 28, 1964, pages 191–198.

Singer, J.L. *Day Dreaming: An Introduction to the Experimental Study of Inner Experience*. New York: Random House, 1966.

Sullivan, H.S. *The Interpersonal Theory of Psychiatry*. New York: W.W. Norton, 1953.

Watzlawick, P. *An Anthology of Human Communication*. Palo Alto, CA.: Science and Behavior Books, 1964.

Weiner, N. *Cybernetics*. New York: Wiley, 1949.

Weiss, R.S. "Transition States and Other Stressful Situations: Their Nature and Programs for Their Management." In *Support Systems and Mutual Help: Multidisciplinary Explorations*, G. Caplan and M. Killilia, Eds. New York: Grune and Stratton, 1976.

5

Aspects of Group Development: Stages and Levels

Ellen Hastings Janosik

Group development refers to the entire life cycle of the group as it is generated, mobilized, and ultimately depleted by its participants. Some groups enjoy a long, productive life span, some do not survive infancy, and still others reach maturity, but function at less than optimum capacity. Each group session is unique and cannot be duplicated by that group or any other. It is, however, possible to assess aspects of group development by observing patterns of prevailing behavior, contrasts in group problem solving, and levels of group interaction.

FACTORS IN GROUP DEVELOPMENT

One aspect which deserves attention is the stage at which the group is functioning. Clusters of prevailing behaviors evident at a particular time help indicate the current stage of development. During their first meetings groups are concerned with survival, and the *curative factor* of *universality* is crucial as members search for commonalities. Universality is described by Yalom (1974) as the recognition that other group members have similar problems and experiences, and that the concerns of any one member are not unique but are shared by others. *Instillation of hope* and *interpersonal guidance* are other factors important to the survival of the immature group. *Cohesion* is an essential factor throughout the life of the group, but it changes in nature as the group matures. At first cohesion is actively pursued by members, and the pursuit often takes the form of well-meant suggestions exchanged among members. Gradually the cohesion among members becomes deeper and more pervasive. There is less concern with offering glib advice and more evidence of *altruistic* caring. (The above factors are discussed at greater length in Chapter 6.)

Accepting the premise that groups go through stages of development helps leaders and observers interpret various events as constructive rather than destructive. All groups must deal with issues of dependency, authority, and intimacy. Understanding the inevitability of certain conflicts means that hostility toward the leader, for example, is not deemed personal but is seen as directed toward the leader's role. When groups are assessed as functioning at a particular stage of development, otherwise questionable actions are considered maturational.

There is a danger that rigid adherence to a scheme of developmental stages may cause observers to identify only notable demarcations in group behavior and to ignore subtler changes. Undue regard for sequential development may cause observers to discount the overlapping, recurring conflicts in groups which the pendular life cycle model explains so well. There is merit in recognizing stages of group development, but there are hazards in taking them too literally (Yalom, 1974). Awareness of regressive and progressive forces in groups eliminates surprise when "settled" issues are resurrected, and mitigates belief that groups always develop in predictable stages. As a rule, clear demarcation of developmental stages is more conspicuous during the first and last periods of group life. In the middle stage, recurrent conflicts frequently arise and intervals of rapid growth or developmental lag appear.

In depicting successive stages of development, only general features can be included. Behaviors which are said to typify stages of development imply that the group moves as one through the stages. Actually, this is seldom true. Despite clusters of prevailing behaviors, not every member is functioning in the same way at a precise moment. For instance, most leaders are challenged at some point by the members, but the challenge is rarely issued simultaneously by every member. Instead there are factions which challenge and factions which defend the leader. A minority of members may be reluctant to commit themselves to any faction and therefore avoid controversy altogether. Because of this variability the leader must be alert to individual dynamics as well as to group dynamics and attend not only to the members who have taken sides in the prevailing struggle but also to those who have not. Often, passive members avoid joining a group confrontation by remaining in a condition of dependency from which the majority has advanced (Fried, 1972). Thus a scheme which distinguishes stages of group development can also be used to assess the movement of individual members against the movement of the group.

INITIAL STAGE

A range of schemata is available for delineating the stages of development, and several variants are described in Chapter 2. Dividing group development into three stages — initial, middle, and final — has the advantage of wide applicability. Within these three major stages, certain phases have been identified. The first phase of the initial stage of development is a time of *inclusion* in which group members are concerned with being accepted and belonging. The inclusion phase is marked by hesitant and tentative behavior, as members turn to the leader for guidance and gratification of needs. As noted previously, many groups symbolically restore the original family configuration. Feelings of rivalry develop among members, as each one wishes to be the special child but fears the results if the fantasy becomes real. All members hope for a secure place in the group and for the favor of the leader, but are apprehensive that one or another hope will be unfulfilled.

Inclusion Phase

The underlying feelings of the members are similar, but behaviors may differ. Many members use behavioral and verbal language which directly expresses what they want from the leader and the group, but others use language which conceals their desires. Some members are afraid of being excluded should they incur the displeasure of others and seek inclusion by being compliant or obsequious. Other members, just as eager to be accepted, may engage in actions which test the group and its purpose even in this early phase. During the inclusion phase most members believe that the leader is wise and powerful, and compliant behaviors which result are fairly easy to assess. Individual conflicts around dependency may be expressed in paradoxical ways which are more difficult to understand. It is always useful to observe the prevailing behaviors of the group and of the individual members.

This is enlightening for the leader using dynamic and behavioral assessment to plan future interventions. In dealing with their conflicts around dependency, overtly dependent members are likely to be clinging and ingratiating. In contrast, counterdependent members may exhibit testing or distrustful behaviors to conceal their wish to be dependent, and maneuvers which seem negative may well hide a desire to be accepted and included. Assessing behavioral manifestations of dependency and counterdependency as two sides of the same coin eases the work of the leader in planning legitimate interventions.

During the inclusion phase of a group, politeness and triviality are employed to control anxiety and preserve interpersonal comfort. Silence can be anxiety-provoking, so there is an inclination on the part of members and even the leader to replace silence with idle chatter. Since disagreement creates anxiety, there is a tacit conspiracy to avoid controversy if possible. Members look for similarities among themselves in order to find a substitute for the cohesion the group needs. There is much advice-giving, which is not helpful in itself but testifies to the goodwill of members. Like the search for common interests, advice-giving is unimportant except as a substitute for cohesion, which has not yet developed. During the inclusion phase the major issue for group members is whether to be in the group or not (Schutz, 1966).

Power Phase

After the inclusion issue has been surmounted, the struggle for individuation and status begins. This is the power phase of the group during which the chief concern of members is who shall be on the top and who shall be on the bottom (Schutz, 1966). The members enter the group and then become conscious of what joining the group means. Now a majority of the members begin to assert themselves, challenging each other, but especially the leader. The contest is between virtually all members, as well as between the leader and factions in the group. Advice-giving and solicitude may continue, but are qualitatively different. Protocol and social constraints are weaker. Advising is no longer a testimony of altruism or mutuality, but is offered as evidence of one's own superiority (Yalom, 1974).

During the inclusion period, members think the power of the leader is unlimited. When the group learns that its expectations of the leader are unrealistic and that all needs will not be met, members often rebel against the leader, compete with other members, and insist on individuation. In contending for position and power in the group, some members are more active than others, and this is an excellent state of affairs. When all group members enter the power struggle at the same time and challenge the leader, group anxiety can become extreme. This is an argument for selecting group members whose strengths and coping behaviors are heterogeneous. The effect of a concerted attack against the leader produces great anxiety in the members and may be devastating for a neophyte leader, no matter how well prepared.

Concern has been voiced by group theorists when the leader is attacked too vigorously (Fried, 1972). A suggested alternative is to encourage members to attack an internal or external scapegoat, but this is a questionable tactic. Surely the leader is in a better position to withstand attack than a group member, whose psychological strength and knowledge of group dynamics may be limited. The progression of group members from passive dependency to active striving is desirable. Rather than resent the emerging strength of the group, the leader should weigh and reinforce certain challenges to authority. When the group questions, criticizes, or evaluates the leader, it is likely that a necessary challenge is being issued. Prevailing rebellious behaviors usually mean that the group is trying to recover the autonomy which was relinquished during the inclusion phase of development.

The initial stage of group development can be divided into an inclusion phase and a power phase. The first is a symbiotic phase representing the urge to merge with the group (preoedipal), while the second is a competitive phase representing the struggle for individuation (oedipal). In Tuckman's well-known scheme (1965) the initial group phase includes the periods of *forming* and *storming*. This initial stage of group development also encompasses the first three stages of psychosocial development described by Erikson (1963). In collective terminology, the first group issue relates to dependency and inclusion, and the second group issue relates to power and authority. Both issues must be confronted during the initial stage of group development.

MIDDLE STAGE

The middle stage of group development can be divided into the *near or far* phase of group life, in which the unresolved conflict is one of intimacy, and the *work* phase, which is characterized by cohesion and cooperation (Schutz, 1966). At this point boundaries have been established and there is awareness of unity and wholeness. Moving into a productive working phase does not mean an absence of tension; some tension persists among members and surrounds the task as members continue to reconcile need-gratification with task productivity.

Primary and Secondary Tasks

Groups are faced with primary and secondary tasks. The primary task is the purpose or purposes for which the group was organized. The secondary task is group maintenance, which insures the security and gratification members need for the group to survive long enough to complete the primary task, whatever that may be (Rioch, 1975). To accomplish their primary task, groups must perform adaptive functions which represent accommodation to external demands and to the group task. For example, the group must adapt to the system it exists in and to the external roles and limitations of group members. Nursing students performing an assigned task together must work within the constraints of the student role and the educational standards of the school. To accomplish secondary tasks related to group maintenance, integrative functions are required. The integrative functions represent responses to internal circumstances. In the group, personal animosities and attachments must be replaced by new alliances which will allow the group to survive. The first stage of group development is largely integrative; during the middle stage, integrative and adaptive functions are performed concurrently. New relationships established on behalf of group survival are usually temporary in nature, rarely lasting beyond the point of usefulness.

In some groups the secondary goal of personal satisfaction automatically follows attainment of the primary goal or task for which the group was organized. This might be true of a football team whose members find primary and secondary goals confluent, so that distinctions are unwarranted and unnecessary. But, for a group composed of recovering drug addicts whose primary task is to avoid readdiction, the members must make a concentrated effort to achieve the secondary goal of security and gratification. Alcoholics Anonymous (AA) programs recognize the contribution of the secondary task to the mastery of the primary task, and, therefore, AA programs stress group-maintenance functions. Few groups accomplish the primary task easily or expeditiously if the secondary task is neglected or left to chance.

Problem-Solving Methods

A satisfactory way of assessing group development during the working stage is to examine its problem-solving methods. The duality of group life necessitates accommodation between progressive and regressive urges to complete or avoid the task. This helps explain the way groups return to the same problem, approaching it each time from a different perspective and exploring it in greater detail. Distinctions have been drawn between *enabling* solutions and *restrictive* solutions to group problems (Whitaker, 1976). Restrictive solutions relieve group anxiety and maintain interpersonal comfort, but avoid the real issues. Enabling solutions require exploration of the issues, open communication, and avoidance of superficial advice.

Restrictive problem-solving can occasionally be functional in groups by maintaining a semblance of cohesion which can later be directed to the primary task. A group which is still in the initial stage or whose capabilities are untried may be unready to engage in enabling solutions. The movement of a group into a working phase may be sudden or gradual, with some members more prepared than others to undertake the primary task. While beginning the task, a work group may employ restrictive solutions. Most of the solutions in the repertoire of a group are a combination of restrictive and enabling activities, although groups demonstrate prevailing patterns of behavior which change over time.

Restrictive Solutions

Issues arise which induce leaders to support restrictive solutions, but this should not occur inadvertently. If the leader believes that group anxiety is excessive, interventions should be planned which will not engender more anxiety. *Clarifying, restating, or summarizing* are interventions which can be used to support restrictive solutions if that is what the group seems to need. Leadership support of restrictive solutions is less defensible when it is inadvertent. Personal wishes of a leader to be liked or admired may reinforce restrictive solutions which are dysfunctional. Group solutions, enabling or restrictive, often require the participation of the leader, and should be within the leader's conscious awareness.

Restrictive solutions are more evident in the initial stage. Dependency behaviors of the inclusion phase represent restrictive solutions, whereas the challenging behaviors of the power phase represent enabling solutions. As the group becomes mature and willing to address the task, reliance on restrictive solutions lessens. What members want during the inclusion phase is to be accepted, to feel safe in the group, and to avoid the primary task for awhile.

Collusive Defenses Group members at times resort to collusive defenses which are almost always restrictive. Collusive defenses take the form of collective agreement to avoid certain topics, or to use humor and small talk to camouflage more important matters. Talking about unrelated subjects, intellectualizing, or permitting one or two members to monopolize a session are all forms of collusive defensiveness. Looking to the leader for guidance is another collusive tactic which does little except help the group avoid risk.

Enabling Solutions

Distinctions between restrictive and enabling solutions are unlikely to fit into a developmental scheme. Enabling solutions may be adopted in the initial stage of group development and restrictive solutions may be used by productive groups in a working phase. In open-ended cohesive groups like *Make Today Count,** enabling solutions continue as new members enter the group. Group boundaries expand to enclose the new member, who is offered whatever resources are available. In less cohesive groups, admission of new members may cause reversal to restrictive solutions as the group tries to preserve interpersonal security while dealing with expansion of its boundaries.

It is not always easy to differentiate restrictive and enabling solutions. One way to assess group solutions is to weigh them against the primary task functions of the group. If the solution allows the group to evade a primary task, it is probably restrictive. When group anxiety is high, a restrictive solution may be advisable even if task accomplishment is temporarily halted. The group which engages only in restrictive solutions imperils its survival, for the primary task is the reason for its existence.

A group in a working phase has a shared history which helps establish and maintain cohesion, even though members came together as strangers. The working group has survived the inclusion and power strivings of the initial stage and has demonstrated to the members that the group can withstand stress. For participants the working phase is a rewarding period in which the creative energy of the group is applied to the task. Problematic issues may require specific interventions, but conflict is not likely to be diffuse. Alliances and coalitions may form which seem to impede progress. Tensions between members may mount, or resistance to the task may appear, but these conditions are usually responsive to strategy based on the group contract and the theoretical framework on which the group is founded. The leader may be less active than before, because leadership can now

---

*Make Today Count is a national self-help group organized for cancer patients and their families.

be shared with the group, although the leader should continue to monitor and regulate. The middle stage of group development parallels the *norming* and *performing* stages described by Tuckman (1965) and the four Eriksonian stages whose critical tasks are Industry versus Inferiority; Identity versus Role Confusion; Intimacy versus Isolation; and Generativity versus Stagnation (Erikson, 1963).

FINAL STAGE

As in every therapeutic interaction, termination begins with the first planning and is an important part of the group contract. In open-ended groups termination may be an individual matter; in closed groups the group terminates as a unit. Premature termination occurs when a member drops out or when a group disbands without completing its primary task. Even though termination has been explained to members during preparatory sessions and alluded to during meetings, it remains a painful event for which the participants are unprepared. This element of unexpectedness which members attach to termination is a form of denial.

Disengagement and Dissolution

A constructive way of dealing with the final stage of a group's existence is to conceptualize two phases: disengagement and dissolution. The period of disengagement usually precedes the actual dissolution of the group and is a time during which, if the final stage is marked by a phase of disengagement, issues relevant to the dissolution are discussed and members are less able to deny the approaching end and more inclined to permit beneficial grief work. By treating termination as biphasic, the group is more likely to devote sufficient time to the termination process.

With termination at hand, bonds of affection between members may weaken. Regressive forces may again dominate the group for a time. Problems around authority reappear, and it is common for members to show anger toward the leader (Sampson and Marthas, 1977). This hostility should be interpreted as a way of assuaging grief. Avoiding the issue of termination is a restrictive solution of dubious value. Members should be encouraged to talk about what the group experience has meant. Appropriate leadership interventions encourage reminiscing, review progress, and evaluate success or failure. Members and leader benefit by acknowledging and sharing the pangs that accompany termination.

Intensity of the grieving process depends on many factors, including the nature of the task and the gratification obtained by group members. The longevity of a group and its importance to the members affect the impact of termination. Members often attempt to deal with termination by arranging additional meetings or by celebrating the last session by eating together. Such manipulation of the group contract calls for careful assessment of underlying motivation. Reminding members of the group contract is helpful in dealing with evasive or manipulative ploys. Eating together is permissible, but not if the ritualistic dining is a way to avoid terminating. Termination is a time-consuming process which should neither be hastened nor prolonged if group members are to feel a sense of closure. The separation of members and the dissolution of the group resemble the last stage of psychosocial development in which the critical task is Ego Integrity versus Despair (Erikson, 1963).

LEVELS OF INTERPERSONAL PROCESSES

Stages of group development show successive change in the prevailing behavior of groups, but there is another method of assessment. Interpersonal processes of groups have been organized into five categories, each of which is governed by its own principles (Mills, 1967). The designated levels of group processes are *behavior, emotion, norms, goals,* and *values.* Behavior refers to overt actions performed in the presence of others in the group. Emotions are drives and feelings members have about the leader and one another, and about events in the group. Norms consist of standards applied to acceptable and unacceptable conduct in the group. Goals are opinions about what the group should do and how it should be done. Values are ideas about what the group is and what it should become.

According to Mills, newcomers enter a group and learn progressively to interact on all levels. As members move from unsophisticated interpersonal levels to sophisticated ones, their subjective experience of the group changes. When interpersonal processes are categorized according to levels instead of stages, it is possible to assess whether the group is functioning only on behavioral and emotional levels or on more advanced levels, where norms, goals, and values have been constructed. In this formulation the interpersonal processes of individual members and of the group as a unit may be compared. A mature group may be functioning on four or five levels, but this may not be true of every group member.

Behavior

Group newcomers may seem to be operating on all levels of group interaction, but their behavior is merely imitative. The group has an emotional impact on newcomers and newcomers have an emotional impact on the group. But until new members understand and accept group norms, goals, and values, there are deficits in their knowledge of the group. The new member is an avid observer of the behavior of the others, since the newcomer must adjust to patterns of social activity which are not yet understood. Although the newcomer observes social patterns, classifies other members, and copies behavior, there is no genuine comprehension of the meaning which the group attaches to behavior and events.

Emotion

Members do not discard idiosyncratic needs and feelings upon entering a group. Most intragroup transactions take place with the hope that personal feelings and needs will be gratified. Within group boundaries, individual needs and feelings cannot exist in isolation but influence and are influenced by what happens in the group. This complex interplay between members and leader, and among members results in the configuration called group emotion. The components of the configuration include: individual needs and drives; feelings of frustration or satisfaction with the group; personal attachments and animosities; and attachment to or alienation from the whole group (Mills, 1967).

Focal Conflict Many leaders work effectively with groups without really understanding the dynamics of group emotion. The basic-assumption groups of Bion (1959) are groups whose behavior is motivated by yearnings for dependency, fight-flight, or pairing. The investigation team of Whitaker and Lieberman (1964) use the term *focal conflict* to describe the shared feelings of group members. One illustration of a focal conflict is the wish of group members to be favored by the leader combined with a fear of the consequences of being favored. Members often try to resolve the focal conflict by trying to be more alike and less distinguishable so that neither the wish nor the fear is realized. Teachers are sometimes able to recognize a focal conflict among groups of students, some of whom wish to excel but fear that attracting favor through excellence means expulsion from group ranks. The price exacted for being the "teacher's pet" is more than many students are willing to pay.

Research into group emotion is difficult from a technical point of view, but early studies suggest that individual and collective emotions may be inferred from systematic analysis of what is said and done in the group. The investigations of communication experts Birdwhistell (1952), who coded body-language movements, and Torrance (1955), who used projective story-telling techniques to study group emotions, provided some techniques used in this area. Although difficult to investigate, group emotion may be considered an authentic presence which affects the ability of the group to accomplish the primary task and the secondary task of group maintenance. Members who do not progress beyond the behavioral and emotional levels of interpersonal processes lack cognitive and instrumental appreciation of what the group is all about.

Norms

Norms are pressures toward conformity established through collaborative actions and shared expectations of the group (Cartwright and Zander, 1960). Norms evolve over time, are shaped jointly by members and the leader, and represent spoken or unspoken standards held by the group about what is appropriate or inappropriate. Although norms are not rules, they are ideas or opinions held by the group about rules. This does not mean that norms are less binding than rules, for often the opposite is true. Unlike rules, which tend to be specific, norms are subject to many distinctions and qualifications which permit them to be applied unequally among members. Behavior considered acceptable from one member may not be condoned coming from another. Because norms are implicit standards or ideas with multiple ramifications, they are considered cognitive and cultural attitudes different from behavioral or emotional levels of interpersonal transaction.

Goals

A group goal consists of shared ideas about what the group should do and how to do it. Individual goals and group goals are not necessarily congruent, but it is important that they be compatible. Members of a relay track team may accept the team performance as a group goal, but some of the team members may want to compile outstanding individual records as well. In this situation the group goal and the individual goal are not incompatible, unless the individual goal has priority. If team practice sessions are missed in order to perfect individual skills, the goals are no longer compatible. Group goals often require the subordination of individual ones, so it is advisable for group goals to be as precise as possible.

As groups begin to enjoy success in achieving goals, the commitment of members grows stronger. Groups which experience feelings of accomplishment become confident, knowledgeable, and cohesive. Members of successful groups are thought to be: more committed to group goals, more able to communicate openly, more inclined to coordinate group activities closely, and more positive in their feelings for one another. The "spiral" effects of success raise the question of whether the positive feelings of functional groups are an effect or a cause of their success (Mills, 1967). In general, groups which successfully reach their goals not only develop positive attitudes toward the group but also raise their aspirations for future achievement, thus proving the adage: Success breeds success.

Values

Some successful groups may never reach the interpersonal level of values, nor should they. Short-term groups and those organized around a simple primary task do not need to advance to this level. A long-term group such as an interdisciplinary health team charged with providing patient care might devote a great deal of time to group values with the intention of changing the purpose, composition, and modus operandi of the group. Groups function on the level of values only if an *executive* appears who is able to bring about group consciousness and influence what the group is to become.

The Executive Role An example of an individual moving into an executive role in the group is that of the member who works with a hospital auxiliary committee to plan a fund-raising event for the children's wing and eventually begins to evaluate group activities. In previous years the fund-raising event had been a lavish dinner dance enjoyed by those who attended but producing little revenue for the hospital department which was the alleged beneficiary. Although the committee had been functioning for years, no one had ever remarked on the incongruity between the primary task and the way it was accomplished. The person who performed the executive role was the member who stepped back from the proceedings to ask, "What is the purpose of this group?" "How well are we meeting our purpose?" "What should the group become in order to serve more effectively?"

Since any member who moves into an executive role questions the status quo, feelings of annoyance toward the executive are aroused in other members. Because the security and comfort found in the group is endangered, the executive member may be treated as a malcontent. A group leader may sometimes function as executive. Since the leader is committed to the primary task, it is often a rank-and-file member who incites the group to examine its values. Any individual assuming an executive role comprehends the behavior, emotion, norms, and goals of the group but functions independently of these levels, if necessary, in order to clarify or modify group values (Mills, 1967).

CLINICAL EXAMPLE: LEADER COLLUSION IN RESTRICTIVE PROBLEM-SOLVING

A group of pregnant teenagers met regularly with a nurse assigned to the obstetrical service of an urban medical center. One primary task of the group was to prepare its young members for labor and delivery, and to assist them with early parenting. Another primary task was to help them interact with one another both as adolescents and as expectant mothers. The group, composed of ten members, was time-limited and closed to new members after the first three meetings. When prospective members came for their first antepartal appointment, the group was described to them and they were invited to join. Most of the girls entered the group during their fourth month of pregnancy. After the members had given birth, they continued to attend the meetings, bringing their infants with them. The group was scheduled to meet until every one of the ten members delivered. This meant that the life expectancy of the group was about six months. Selection criteria for the group consisted of the following: 1) all members were primipara between the ages of thirteen and seventeen, 2) all members attended the antepartal clinic and expected to be delivered at the medical center, and 3) all members were unmarried schoolgirls who planned to keep their babies.

The group leader was an excellent maternity nurse and a good teacher. By means of films, diagrams, and discussion the leader taught the members the mechanics of labor and delivery. Childbirth exercises were practiced, questions about delivery were answered, and the group members were well prepared for labor and delivery.

Although extremely familiar with the care of expectant mothers, and relatively familiar with group dynamics, the leader lacked experience in facilitating peer interaction. Therefore she avoided discussions of feelings about adolescence and motherhood and limited group interaction to cognitive material.

The common bond of pregnancy brought the adolescent members together and helped build cohesion. Friendships flourished and the group showed concern for members as their delivery dates neared. Those who had already delivered and returned to the group intuitively avoided remarks that would frighten the girls who were still pregnant. Although the members were unsentimental and affected a veneer of toughness, they were tender with one another. Attachments to the group were very strong. This was shown by regular attendance and by active participation of the members before and after the birth of their infants.

When all the members were pregnant the leader had been held in awe and respected as an authority figure. The leader's unwillingness to deal with feelings reinforced the group norm of dealing only with facts. As more members delivered and brought their babies to the meetings, however, the inhibiting power of the leader diminished. Members began to talk about what it was like to be a teenage mother, and seemed bored when the leader insisted on factual content. The slides and films shown by the leader, which had formerly been viewed with rapt attention, were now belittled. Initially the group had seemed cohesive and united, now there were two factions. Group members who had already delivered became hostile toward the leader but remained sympathetic toward other members. Pregnant members continued to be attentive to the leader but obviously enjoyed the defiant behaviors of the rebellious faction.

One of the members, Sharon, attended meetings faithfully before and after the birth of her baby. She was accepted in the group, but, unlike the others, she did not seem happy after her baby was born. Nurses working in the maternity unit were worried about Sharon's behavior toward the child, and informed the group leader of their concerns. It was not long until Sharon's rough way of treating her baby was noticed by the other group members, one of whom said, "I'm sure glad I'm not your baby, Sharon." At this Sharon shrugged her shoulders and replied, "My baby is nothing but a bad old boy. He ain't pretty like your girl. He is just a mean, ugly baby."

In an effort to be honest but still comfort Sharon, the nurse leader intervened rather firmly, "How can you say such a thing, Sharon? All healthy babies are pretty no matter what they look like, and your little boy has so much personality." Unwittingly the leader had confirmed Sharon's statement that her baby was not pretty, thereby leading the group into a restrictive solution. The clumsy but well-meant intervention was taken up by members who pointed out some of the baby's good points, such as his strength and size. Sharon's response was to shake her head in sullen disagreement and say nothing.

Sharon had already been suffering from a poor self-image when she became pregnant. Other girls in the group continued to see the putative father of their child during pregnancy, and to receive emotional if not financial support. This was not available to Sharon, who had been deserted by her baby's father. Throughout her pregnancy Sharon was bitter and disillusioned. She believed herself completely unattractive and thought no man would ever want her on a permanent basis. When she gave birth to a baby boy instead of the girl she wanted, Sharon was disappointed, and she devalued the child as she devalued herself. She projected her feelings of worthlessness and inferiority onto the baby, and this interfered with her mothering activities. Sharon needed help with her low self-esteem, and this could well have been provided by a peer group.

When the group revealed itself as willing and ready to deal openly with Sharon's problematic mothering behavior, the leader felt uncomfortable and retreated into benign authoritarianism. As a result the group did not explore Sharon's feelings of inferiority but engaged in a restrictive solution which disregarded the negative self-image which was Sharon's real problem. An enabling solution might have been found by the group had the leader intervened with some thoughtful, exploratory questions. "Do you think your baby is ugly because he is a boy, Sharon, or because he is yours? You really seem to feel bad. Can you tell us more about it?"

The teenage mothers' group had two purposes, one of which the assigned leader handled competently. For the most part, groups such as this, with two diverse tasks, are better served by a coleader arrangement, unless one person possesses sufficient skills to facilitate both purposes. In a coleader arrangement one nurse might take responsibility for presenting cognitive material, while a nurse with a different background might take responsibility for affective material. The task or instrumental leader would function as teacher or coach for labor and delivery. The socioemotional leader would be responsible for psychological issues such as Sharon's devaluation of herself and her child. Thus both tasks would be addressed and each leader provide feedback to the other. Excellent coleadership can be provided by dividing responsibilities so that an instrumental leader is working in tandem with a socioemotional leader. Such an arrangement would reduce the incidence of restrictive solutions in both cognitive and affective domains.

SUMMARY

Group development may be examined from the vantage point of group stages and group levels (Table 5-1). Group stages of development are classified as initial, middle, and final. Each of the three stages is biphasic in nature. The initial stage of group development is divided into an inclusion phase and a power phase. During the middle stage of group development, issues of intimacy are resolved first, issues of cohesion and cooperation are resolved later. The final or termination stage should attend to issues of disengagement before the dissolution of the group takes place. In general, groups have access to two types of problem-solving methods — restrictive solutions and enabling solutions. Appropriate leader interventions in response to both types of problem-solving are suggested.

The second vantage point for assessing group development consists of examining five sequential levels of group process which are designated as behavior, emotion, norms, goals, and values of the group. When group processes are assessed as levels instead of stages, it is pos-

Table 5–1   STAGES, LEVELS, AND CRITICAL TASKS OF GROUP
DEVELOPMENT

Stages	Phases	Prevailing Behaviors	Interpersonal Process Levels	Critical Psychosocial Tasks
Initial Stage	Inclusion	Dependent Testing Tentative	Behavior Emotion	Basic Trust versus Mistrust
	Power	Challenging Competitive	Behavior Emotion	Autonomy versus Shame and Doubt
				Initiative versus Guilt
Middle Stage	Intimacy	Cohesive Sharing	Behavior Emotion Norms	Industry versus Inferiority
	Work	Coherent Cooperative Productive	Behavior Emotion Norms Goals	Identity versus Role Confusion
				Intimacy versus Isolation
				Generativity versus Stagnation
Final Stage	Separation	Evaluative Disengaging	Behavior Emotion Norms	Ego Integrity versus Despair
	Dissolution	Life Review Grief Work	Goals Values	

sible to decide whether the group is functioning only on behavioral
and emotional levels, or on more advanced levels at which norms,
goals, and values have been established. In this formulation the interpersonal processes of individual members and of the group as a whole
may be compared. A mature group is perceived as having progressed
to all levels of group development, but this progression may not characterize every group member, some of whom may exhibit developmental lags.

REFERENCES

Bion, W.R. *Experiences in Groups.* Basic Books: New York, 1959.

Birdwhistell, R.I. *Introduction to Kinesics.* Louisville, KY.: University of Ken-
tucky Press, 1952.

Cartwright, D., and A. Zander, Eds. *Group Dynamics.* Evanston, IL.: Row, Peterson, 1960.

Erikson, E. *Childhood and Society.* New York: W.W. Norton, 1963.

Fried, E. "Individuation Through Group Psychotherapy." In *Progress in Group and Family Therapy,* C.J. Sager and H.S. Kaplan, Eds. New York: Brunner/Mazel, 1972.

Mills, T.M. *The Sociology of Small Groups.* Englewood Cliffs, N.J.: Prentice-Hall, 1967.

Rioch, M.J. "Group Relations: Rationale and Technique." In *Group Relations Reader,* A.D. Colman, and W.H. Bexton, Eds. Sausalito, CA.:, 1975.

Sampson, E.E., and M.S. Marthas. *Group Process for the Health Professions.* New York: Wiley, 1977.

Schutz, W. *Interpersonal Underworld.* Palo Alto, CA.: Science and Behavior Books, 1966.

Torrance, E.P. "Perception of Group Functioning as a Predictor of Group Performance." *Journal of Social Psychology* 17, 1955, pages 271-282.

Tuckman, B.W. "Developmental Sequence in Small Groups." *Psychological Bulletin* 63, 1965, pages 384-399.

Whitaker, D.S. "A Group Centered Approach." *Group Process* 7, 1976, pages 37-57.

————, and M.A. Lieberman. *Psychotherapy Through the Group Process.* New York: Atherton Press, 1964.

Yalom, I.D. *Theory and Practice of Group Psychotherapy.* New York: Basic Books, 1974.

6

Process and Content: Distinctions and Implications

Veda Bowler Boyer

In order to lead a group effectively a leader must have a working knowledge of the concepts of *process* and *content* in order to gather and interpret data.

Content and Process are the basis of group assessment and strategy, regardless of the theoretical framework being used. This is not to say that these are the only concepts relevant to leading and understanding groups. Bascue (1978) suggested that it was imperative for leaders to select a specific conceptual model in order to diagnose and treat a group. Analysis of content and process, combined with a theoretical model, helps the leader to orchestrate group interaction (Tauber, 1978).

CONTENT AND PROCESS DEFINED

Content refers to substantive or factual material brought up in the group. It is observable, explicit material apparent in group interactions. In simple terms, content may be identified as *what* is transacted in the group. The content of an interaction may be determined by noting what was said or not said, by whom and to whom, and whether responses were verbal or nonverbal. Systematic analysis of content information allows one to establish hypotheses about what has occurred. These hypotheses are assumptions or inferences which can be refuted or validated by gathering more content information or by directly confronting the group with the hypotheses (Sampson and Marthas, 1977).   There is an interdependent relationship between group content and process.   Frequently, content information leads to the formulation of process-oriented questions such as *why* and *how* interactions occurred. Content may be used to understand process while process provides a matrix for interpreting content (Luft, 1963).

Group process includes covert acts, feelings, and unexpressed thoughts. It may also be described as the emotional nuances, unconscious goals, and intrapersonal and interpersonal forces that influence the group's movement toward or away from its goals (Luft, 1963; Mills, 1967; Werner, 1970).   Group process directs attention to intragroup structures and relationships, conflict resolution, problem-solving, behavioral patterns, and to how these observable data fit together to establish the group as a viable, dynamic system (Sampson and Marthas, 1977). Process information answers such questions as: How do member interactions relate to each other? How does the group as a whole react to an occurrence? Why does the group respond in this manner?

Whitaker and Lieberman (1964) noted that by analyzing group process the leader is better able to help the group meet the needs of its members. Assumptions made by the leader concerning process must be validated against previous and subsequent events in order to correct erroneous or inadequate analysis of process.

Identifying facilitative and inhibiting forces present in group interaction enables the leader to devise strategies based on group dynamics. The analysis of content information uncovers themes, sequences, and patterns which reveal central issues affecting the work of the group.

Analyzing group content permits assumptions to be made about group process. When the assumptions are correct the interventions of the leader are more effective. Verification of process assumptions is essential and may be accomplished through ongoing observation and analysis of content. Examples of assumptions made about group process, based on thematic observations of content, are shown in Table 6-1.

A knowledge of process requires the ability to observe verbal and nonverbal behaviors, to formulate assumptions about the needs of members, to apply interventions, and to anticipate the results.

Table 6-1   THEMATIC CONTENT ANALYSIS AND PROCESS ASSUMPTIONS

Group Composition	Group Content	Process Assumptions
Hypertensive patients in an out-patient group	Prolonged indecisions about agenda and choosing a new location	Covert ambivalence about the group and a wish to be in control
Diabetic patients in a health-teaching group	Complaints about physicians and relatives who don't understand diabetes	Covert dissatisfaction with the leader and with group progress
Recent nurse graduates in a staff orientation program	Discussion of commuting, drivers' licenses, and car accidents	Covert fear of losing student status, of assuming a professional role, and of making errors
Pregnant adolescents in a childbirth-education group	Refusal to give up favorite junk food for a balanced diet	Covert expression of unmet needs for nurture or affection

Tauber (1978) identified several examples of process which call for analysis, including a member confronting a leader; one member confronting another; some members digressing or avoiding topics other members wish to discuss; a member of the group first reacting affectively; a response representing a typical group or individual reaction which others question; an action by a member which specifically states a need; a response which points out incongruities; a response which directly affects others in the group; a member or leader who seems to be structuring the group topic; and a member or leader who tries to impose ground rules on the contract.   By developing alertness to such interactions the leader is able to question why they occur and to determine the results they produce.

COMMUNICATION

The vehicle that impels or impedes group progress and intensifies or alleviates group conflict is communication. But what do we mean by communication? Communication is a dynamic process reciprocally sensitive to any social situation and is essential to understanding and being understood. The viewpoints, moods, decisions, and behaviors of individuals are affected by messages communicated in the social environment (Watzlawick, 1964). Communication is concerned with the transmission of emotions, attitudes, thoughts, and actions via verbal or nonverbal messages from sender to receiver. The receiver then interprets the meaning and reacts, thus becoming a sender in the communication process. Sender or receiver may be individual group members or the group as a whole (Hinsie and Campbell, 1977).

Communication includes verbal and nonverbal messages. There are two types of verbal communication: content, or what is said, and *paralinguistics,* or how content is vocalized (Egan, 1982). Paralinguistic cues include pitch, hesitation, intonation, and pacing of words, as well as sighs, grunts, groans, or other sounds distinct from actual words (Sampson and Marthas, 1977).

Nonverbal communication, such as facial expression, posture, movement, eye contact, and gestures, deals more with process than content; unless the nonverbal message is clearly denotative, such as sign language for the deaf or the precise hand movements of an umpire or referee. Most nonverbal communication gives information beyond the verbal dimensions of the message. Ekman and Friesen (1975) wrote that true feelings can be observed more through nonverbal behavior than through verbal messages. They identified emotions that may be determined solely by watching facial expressions. Kinesics, eye contact, behavioral attentiveness all give information about mood, degree of interest, positive or negative feelings, anxiety, and leadership status (Egan, 1982; Sampson and Marthas, 1977). There are five components present in verbal and nonverbal communication: 1) *denotative messages,* 2) *connotative messages,* 3) *metacommunication,* 4) *manifest (overt) content,* and 5) *latent (covert) content* (Marram, 1978; Reusch, 1961; Watzlawick, 1964).

Denotative messages and manifest content are expressed more through verbal than nonverbal communication. Denotative messages refer to the meanings assigned to words by the majority of persons sharing a language. Some words may have more than one commonly accepted meaning, but the specific meaning can be discerned by noting how the word is used in a sentence.

An example of a nonverbal denotative message is shown by a group member who makes the hand sign of a "T." Anyone familiar with basketball recognizes that the sign means "time out." Examining the connotative aspect of the message might explain why a signal from the sports world was used instead of a verbal request.

Some denotative messages, like the hand sign for "time out," are culturally or experientially derived. A group composed of members with shared culture or experience is more apt to avoid misunderstandings than groups that lack these common denominators. The leader must identify and clarify denotative messages which have cultural or experiential meanings unfamiliar to all the group members.

Manifest content is sent and received on conscious levels, and is audible or visible. In dealing with manifest content, one would note the purposeful intent of verbal and nonverbal messages being transmitted. For instance, group members may be consciously aware of one member's need to speak more assertively. When the member exhibits assertive verbal behavior, the group reacts by applauding. Manifest content may be verbal or nonverbal, but always expresses messages that groups or individuals are consciously trying to convey (Langs, 1973).

If a group leader were to limit observation only to the manifest content of communication, group behavior would seem incongruent or paradoxical (Yearwood-Grazette, 1978). One member may consistently talk about how valuable and interesting women are, but only address or respond to the men in the group. This is a situation in which manifest content must be examined in terms of covert process in order to learn how or why the incongruency exists.

Process Components of Communication   The process components of verbal and nonverbal communication represent forms of metacommunication, and are connotative or latent. Process components are less obvious and require that inferences or interpretations be made about the meaning of the message for receiver and sender.

Connotative messages carry a secondary meaning which is often emotional (Marram, 1978). For example, the word "mother" has an explicit definition, but also carries an affective meaning. The implicit or secondary meaning is different for different people. For one person the word "mother" connotes a nurturing, warm person; for another the word connotes a rigid, harsh disciplinarian. A hug may be defined as an embrace. Connotatively, a hug may mean consolation to one person and sexuality to another. The leader is responsible for aiding the group in understanding connotative and denotative aspects of communication.

Latent content is considered process because it sends messages through implicit cues such as voice intonation, facial expression, themes, sequences, evasions, and elisions. It is related to unconscious conflicts, fantasies, and feelings of the sender (Langs, 1973). The leader must collect verbal and nonverbal data over time in order to avoid premature interpretation of latent material. Premature interpretation to the group produces denial or intellectualization rather than insight. When interpretations are presented to the group, it should be done tentatively and in the form of suggestions or questions.

Metacommunication

Process and content subsume latent and manifest content which is incongruent or contradictory. Bateson et al. (1963) termed latent and manifest contradictions *double messages,* because the receiver must respond to two opposing messages while the sender is consciously aware of having sent only one. Metacommunication may be defined as a message about what is being communicated. An example of metacommunication is shown in the contrast between the following requests: "Close that door at once!" and "I'm cold, would you please close that door right away." Although both messages make the same request, the manner in which each is expressed is indicative of the nature of the relationship between sender and receiver (Yalom, 1975).

By analyzing communication and metacommunication, the latent content of the message is made more accessible. Verbal communication may express commitment to group goals, but lack of progress toward the goals indicates that at a deeper level there is a block or impediment. Such a discrepancy is related to the group's internal order and to the socioemotional needs of members. In order to resolve conflict around socioemotional needs, unconscious agendas must be explored. By persuading group members to examine discrepancies in messages which are being transmitted, the leader may guide the group to conscious awareness of impediments to progress toward stated goals (Sampson and Marthas, 1977).

Communication Structure   Group communication is not limited to immediate transactions between individual members. Over time, ordered arrangements or patterns are established which provide constancy and stability for the group even after membership has changed. These durable patterns are called communication structures, which, once established, endure as long as the group lasts. Examples of groups with enduring communication structures are fraternities, faculties, health teams, and business firms. To identify communication structures, one must look beyond psychological assessment of groups to discernible communication channels, problem-solving and decision-making tactics, and the locus of power within the group (Sampson and Marthas, 1977).

In observing communication structures a number of questions are germane. One is whether the group is an open or closed system. If the communication pattern can be affected by events or objects in the environment, it is a relatively open system. If all communication within the group is fixed and predictable, regardless of external influences, the group is a relatively closed system. A second question is whether the communication structure is characterized by directness or indirectness. If the members use person-to-person verbalization to convey messages, communication structure is fairly direct. If messages are relayed through progress notes, memoranda, audio tapes, or are transmitted only on administrative levels, the communication structure is an indirect system.

Variations in communication structure include *circular* arrangements whereby messages are distributed in a roundabout fashion (Figure 6-1); *chain* patterns, whereby messages are passed in sequential order; and *wheel* patterns, in which all messages travel outward to each spoke from a central point at the hub.

The circle communication structure is thought to be the most effective for complex problem-solving and member satisfaction; the wheel is considered the most efficient for simple problem-solving and the most controlled; and the chain is considered to be the most hierarchical (Sampson and Marthas, 1977).

Attraction Structure   Attraction structure deals with the tendency of people who like each other to communicate more often with each other. Yalom (1975) referred to attraction structure as part of group cohesiveness.

Power Structure   Power structure is another aspect of communication structure which can be determined by identifying the

Figure 6-1   VARIATIONS IN COMMUNICATION STRUCTURE

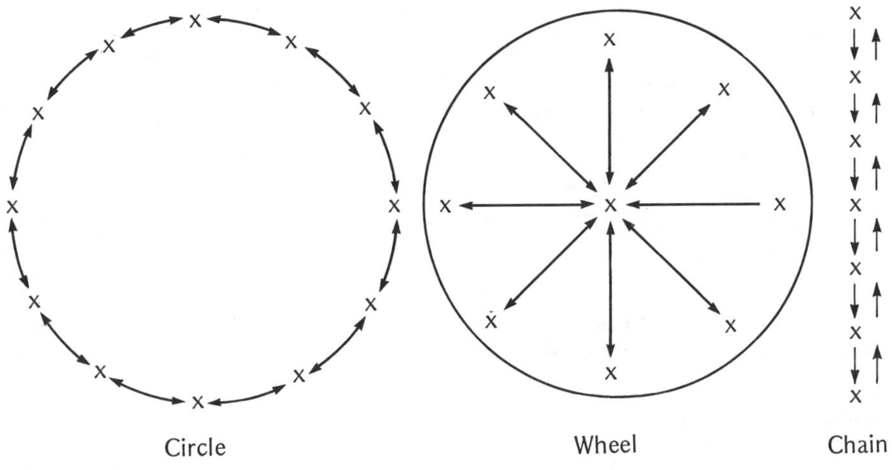

Circle   Wheel   Chain

member who is listened to most and the member who is listened to least. In differentiating attraction structure from power structure, one must consider the quality as well as the quantity of interactions between members. The person who is listened to with the greatest attention and deference is probably the person in the group with the most power and influence. This information is valuable in determining whether the ascribed authority figures (leaders) actually wield power or whether power has been achieved by one or more group members who have not been formally designated (Sampson and Marthas, 1977; Yearwood-Grazette, 1978).

Sometimes the identification of disruptive communication patterns does not lead to coping with dysfunctional communication structure but to the scapegoating or removal of a problematic member. By concentrating on communication structure in the group, individual personalities are not held responsible for communication failures. It is important to realize that characteristics of communication structure reside in the system rather than in any single individual. Communication structure provides a format for observing interactions of the group as a whole, and for devising strategies for altering maladaptive communication.

CONFLICT RESOLUTION

When people come together in groups there is always potential for conflict. In many groups there is a tendency to avoid conflict lest the group be unable to survive the stress (Glassner and Freedman, 1979). Group conflict is a phenomenon attributable to multiple opposing forces operating simultaneously (Werner, 1970). Whitaker and Lieberman (1964) defined group conflict as the result of unconscious wishes, desires, goals, or motives which are opposed by reactive fears of having these unconscious desires gratified.

The conflict between the wish and the fear of consequences if the wish is gratified leads to a search for solutions. When the eventual solution gratifies the disturbing wishes and alleviates the reactive fears, an *enabling solution* has been reached. When the reactive fears are alleviated by foregoing the gratification of the disturbing wish, a *restrictive solution* has been reached. Either solution may be appropriate, depending on the nature of the conflicting fears and wishes, and on the stage of group development. Enabling and restrictive solutions may be used by the group as a whole or by individual members. An extensive discussion of restrictive and enabling solutions related to the stage of group development may be found in Chapter 5.

Nuclear Conflict

Two types of conflicts have been identified by Whitaker and Lieberman (1964), in addition to two types of solutions. The first is nuclear conflict, which originates when the individual learns a maladaptive mode of coping with early conflicts, either developmental or situational. In later life, whenever similar situations or issues arise, the individual reverts to the same maladaptive behavior. An example is a member who leaves the group meeting whenever two members actively disagree. When the behavior is explored the member remembers leaving the house as a youngster whenever his parents became embroiled in a drunken brawl. The disturbing wish was to be powerful enough to make the parents stop fighting. The reactive fear was that mediating or becoming involved would unite the parents against him. The restrictive solution used in the group situation was motivated by disturbing wishes and reactive fears experienced when he was young and powerless. This prevented him from learning that disagreements are seldom resolved by running away, and that behavior appropriate in childhood was no longer necessary or adaptive. This member's sense of autonomy was threatened by fear of retribution. Consequently, whenever disagreement arose in his current interpersonal world, original anxiety was triggered. As long as this or similar manifestations of nuclear conflict are not dealt with in the group, the individual will continue to rely on habitual restrictive solutions.

Focal Conflict

The second type of conflict is the group or focal conflict described by Whitaker and Lieberman (1964). Unlike nuclear conflict, focal conflict originates in the current group interaction and is shared by all members. The focal conflict has no history outside the group, and a successful resolution can occur only if the reactive fears of all members are allayed and the solution is accepted by the whole group. Although some group members may be aware of the focal conflict, they may not be able to deal with it unless the leader intervenes. It is the leader's obligation to recognize focal conflict and assist the group in resolving it, since the group will return again and again to the issue until the conflict is resolved. An example of focal conflict might be the group's wish to regress and to turn to the leader for all decisions. Here the disturbing wish is to regress and the reactive fear is that separateness and individuality will be lost. In dealing with focal conflict, the following guidelines are advised: focus on here-and-now experiences within the group; recognize that unconscious, preconscious, and conscious levels of the same conflict may exist simultaneously and try to identify the level on which the group is operating; and guide the group away from the wish toward an enabling solution by formulating a hypothesis about what is happening in the group.

Commenting on here-and-now behavior precedes the exploration of motives, conscious or unconscious. An intervention which deals prematurely with focal conflict may be ignored, denied, or rejected by the group. Conflict resolution comes from helping the group to realize that opposing fears and wishes are legitimate, and that compromise between the two may be negotiated. The contrasting elements of nuclear and focal conflict are presented in Table 6-2 (Benne and Birnbaum, 1969).

Constructive Conflicts   Group conflicts may be either constructive or destructive in their end result. Constructive conflicts often arise out of competing loyalty of members toward outside groups, or among group members who are genuinely committed to group goals but disagree about priorities, procedures, or policies. Usually compromises can be arranged because commitment to the task is shared and the group as a whole benefits from the airing of different viewpoints.

Destructive Conflicts   Destructive conflicts often involve power and status struggles between group members rather than substantive issues. Occasionally, destructive conflicts reflect group frustration and tension over the group task; negative feelings about the task are displaced on fellow members.

Table 6–2   CONTRAST BETWEEN NUCLEAR AND FOCAL GROUP CONFLICT

Nuclear Conflict	*Focal Conflict*
Intrapsychic	Interpersonal
Held by one member	Shared by many members
Originate in past experience	Originate in here-and-now
Influenced by disturbing motives (wishes)	Influenced by disturbing motives (wishes)
Influenced by reactive motives (fears)	Influenced by reactive motives (fears)
Subject to enabling or restrictive solutions	Subject to enabling or restrictive solutions

Successful resolution of any group conflict is largely dependent on leader interventions. Productive group conflicts should be confronted and worked out. Nonproductive conflicts may sometimes be confronted directly, giving members a choice of ending the conflict or of exploring related motives and behaviors. In some instances nonproductive conflicts are best ignored or avoided. When conflicts have been resolved successfully, the following benefits ensue: lack of recurrence of the conflict; open expression of disagreements; exploration of the reasons for conflict; search for compromises; and discovery of creative solutions. When conflict is resolved successfully, cohesiveness is preserved and the group is able to tolerate differences (Longo and Williams, 1978).

Group content and process must be observed over time in order to understand the nature of group conflict. By concentrating on what is seen and heard, content information is collected. Group process data are used to analyze content in terms of how and why it occurs. Process data address the effects which group interaction has on goal attainment, and helps the leader intervene effectively. A group is more likely to devote energy to conflict resolution if it possesses cohesiveness and internal trust. The attributes may be considered in the context of group curative factors (Yalom, 1975).

CURATIVE FACTORS

Curative factors are interpersonal experiences which move the individual and the group toward a sense of well-being, productivity, and competence. Yalom (1975) identified curative factors as: 1) instillation of hope, 2) universality, 3) imparting and receiving information, 4) altruism, 5) corrective recapitulation of the primary group, 6) development of socializing techniques, 7) imitative behavior, 8) interpersonal learning, 9) group cohesiveness, 10) catharsis, and 11) existential factors.

Since curative factors have some abilities to decrease inhibiting forces and increase enabling forces in a group, they may be used to illuminate the concept of group process. By identifying these curative factors as variables of group process, observation, assessment, intervention, and evaluation may be based upon specific curative factors. In order to further differentiate content and process, each curative factor is explained as a content interaction, a process interaction, or a combination of the two.

Content Curative Factors

Imparting information is the only curative factor that can be classified as solely content. Direct advice, suggestions, or explanations about group interactions are expressed verbally and consciously. When information is given, emphasis is on what is being said. If the information is relevant, group members experience a decrease in the anxiety which accompanies lack of information. When the information gives the group assurance of predictability, members are better able to handle the group experience. Sharing information promotes common interests, which leads to group cohesiveness.

Process Curative Factors

Process-oriented curative factors include altruism, universality, corrective re-enactment of the primary group, imitative behavior, and group cohesiveness. When a group is functioning there may be no conscious awareness of the presence of these factors. Members may have a sense of belonging, security, well-being, and self-worth without understanding the reason.

The group leader often uses manifest verbal and behavioral content to encourage process-oriented curative factors. This is done by modeling or by commenting on interactions which depict, elicit, or reinforce certain curative factors. The leader may observe one member offering verbal support to a distressed member and intervene to acknowledge the action as having positive value to the group. The member receiving the verbal support might be asked to tell the group whether a feeling of being understood had been experienced.

When process curative factors are present in a group the leader may which to call attention to the interpersonal transactions producing the curative factors. By using the here-and-now group interactions to illustrate verbal and nonverbal manifest content, the leader may bring to conscious awareness the meaning such messages hold for sender and receiver. These interventions of the leader, which are sometimes referred to as process illumination, reinforce the positive impact of the curative factors and encourage their presence. Even when the meaning of group interactions is not consciously realized, the unconscious benefits continue. Nevertheless, conscious awareness aids in dynamic self-understanding of a corrective group experience (Egan, 1982).

Inhibiting Forces One of the most inhibiting forces present among new group members is the fear that their problems, thoughts, and impulses are unacceptable to others. These fears are expressed in thoughts such as, "If they really knew me, they would see how inept and how unlovable I am." Encouraging group members to share feelings of worthlessness puts to rest their fears of rejection. Fears of rejection are replaced by feelings of belonging and of universality. Leader intervention should assert that concerns which seem unique are merely part of being human. Comments which stress universality such as, "That sounds pretty human to me," reinforce the idea that the members have much in common.

During the course of the group experience, members may be reminded of how similar the group is to their primary or family group experience. The original family experience intrudes on the current group and reactivates old responses to unresolved family issues. When the group experience is contaminated by early memories, members use old coping mechanisms instead of finding new solutions. If stereotyped responses of members are challenged by the leader or the group, early conflicts can be re-enacted in ways which correct distortions and complete unfinished developmental tasks.

Imitative Behavior   Being freed of earlier conflicts is only one step in the process of learning new ways to interact. Realization that a preferred mode of interacting is dysfunctional may be accompanied by dread that one will not be able to change. Sometimes the familiar way of interacting is less threatening than searching for new ways. Imitative behavior offers a member a glimpse of what one might become without making a conscious decision to change. One or more group members may imitate the leader's style of dressing or behaving, or may imitate an admired member. Instead of deriding such imitation, the leader might comment on its positive aspects. The purpose is to encourage risk-taking and to open the group to change. The intervention of the leader is to reinforce observed functional behaviors resulting from the unconscious imitative process.

Cohesiveness   The curative factor of group cohesiveness is an important process-oriented concept. Cohesiveness can be an energizer, moving the group through norm setting, conflict resolution, interpersonal growth, self-awareness, and goal attainment. Cohesiveness is generated through a member's experience of being accepted and of being a valued member of the group. It encompasses the members' relatedness to one another and to the group leaders. This multilevel relationship must be characterized by warmth and unconditional acceptance if group cohesiveness is to be sustained (Egan, 1982; Truax and Carkhuff, 1967).

Group members who have a sense of relatedness to the group are more likely to respect the opinions of others, to be willing to explore interpersonal transactions, and to make changes compatible with group expectations and values. In order for a group to be successful, members must care enough for each other to endure the anxiety of dealing with change.

Interventions which increase group cohesiveness include statements which are "we"-centered, such as comments about how hard the group is working and how much is being accomplished. Interventions which extol honesty, nondefensiveness, and commitment to the task are effective and convince the group that it can handle all issues and remain intact. References to the shared history of the group and statements that the group contains resources which are available to any member also contribute to cohesiveness.

Content and Process Curative Factors

Curative factors which are both process-oriented and content-oriented include development of socializing techniques; interpersonal learning; instillation of hope; catharsis; and existential factors. In the presence of these factors, attention is directed to what is expressed consciously and how this is dynamically related to early life.

The strategy used in merging content with process is called *process illumination* (Yalom, 1975), *alternative frames of reference* (Egan, 1982), or *processing the here-and-now* (Sampson and Marthas, 1977). Regardless of its name, the strategy involves examination of interactions that have just taken place. The leader notes thematic behavioral patterns of the group, evaluates behaviors which promote or impede the group task, develops tactics for sharing these data with the group, and determines the effectiveness of interventions by assessing the awareness the group has of current issues and available alternatives.

Within the group and within individual members are forces which impede progress. One such force is a lack of ability to express oneself or to respond to the messages of others. These inabilities lock members into ineffective communication modes. Through process illumination from the leader and feedback from the group, members share information about behaviors and relationships in the group. The leader monitors feedback between members so that it is not detrimental to self-esteem and includes constructive suggestions.

The Group as a Microcosm of Society The curative factor of interpersonal learning is concerned with interpersonal relationships, corrective social experiences using the group as a microcosm of society. The need for interpersonal interactions with significant persons is fundamental. The way members see themselves reflected in the perceptions of others significantly affects self-esteem. The group is therefore a functional medium for molding behavior, through the approval or disapproval of fellow members. A number of forces influence the members' perception of group relationships. Interpersonal interactions are interpreted in ways that support an existing self-image or basic belief. Group members who think themselves unworthy will perceive interactions as rejecting or derogatory. An extreme form of interpersonal distortion is present when a group member withdraws from the reality of the interpersonal situation through delusions or hallucinations. When the interpersonal reality of a member differs from that of the group, the leader endeavors to decrease distortions through consensual validation which compares individual evaluations with the evaluations of the group. The leader may ask individual members to describe what is happening in the group and to compare these descriptions with those of other members. It often becomes. apparent that some members discount all perceptions which do not coincide with their own self-image. By reinforcing reality and challenging misperceptions, the leader helps members acquire a more accurate perception of self in relation to others.

Once members are convinced that the group will tolerate risk-taking, they feel free to disclose certain feelings and thoughts. This process of self-examination is an emotional and a cognitive experience. The affective component of self-disclosure should be accompanied by the acquisition of information and the development of insight.

Catharsis   The value of catharsis as a curative factor is dependent on its contribution to dynamic self-understanding and group cohesiveness. Catharsis alone does not produce lasting change. The content of catharsis indicates the nature of the problem, but does not automatically create self-understanding. Growth and change result from a processing of information accrued through here-and-now transactions in the group. Catharsis must be more than an affective experience if insight and interpersonal learning are to follow.

Interpersonal Relationships   The leader facilitates progress toward a corrective group experience whenever interpersonal distortions are challenged. As interpersonal exploration takes place, the leader begins to see how group members interact with persons outside the group setting. Since the group is a social microcosm, interpersonal relationships established in the family and carried into adult life are replicated in the group. Encouraging members to realize this and to use the safety of the group to try out new ways of relating may produce change which can be transferred to relationships outside the group.

During the process of interpersonal learning, the member first becomes aware of idiosyncratic distortions, learns to deal with them affectively and cognitively, and accepts responsibility for shaping the interpersonal world. Following this, the member begins to experiment with new behaviors and is rewarded with less anxiety and greater self-esteem. The need for concealing the real self is removed and the member is able to relate to others in a new dimension.

Instillation of Hope Success in one area promotes hope that other areas of life can be changed. Through instillation of this hope, members are freed to invest more energy in goal-oriented behavior. This is accomplished by calling attention to improvements other members have made and by citing verbal and behavior changes of the content of group interactions. Members who have coped successfully with any issue may be encouraged to share their experiences with other members who are beginning to confront similar issues.

Existential Factors When issues of self-determination, responsibility, freedom of choice, and the meaning of life are being addressed, the presence of existential forces is very valuable. These forces are activated when group members begin to search for answers to basic questions that do not have easy solutions. As the verbal and behavioral content of group interactions are experienced over time, the group faces the fact that its resources are not unlimited and that the group itself is not nirvana. There follows the realization that living always involves a certain amount of injustice, pain, and loneliness, and that death is inevitable. This knowledge encourages members to accept the disappointments and vicissitudes of life, and to be less concerned with trivialities.

The most important lesson learned from existential theory is that no matter how much guidance is provided by others, one is ultimately responsible for one's own life. In working with existential concepts, the leader imposes responsibilities on the group and discourages members from excessive preoccupation with unanswerable questions. At the same time group members are encouraged to accept the potential and limitations of the universal human condition.

In reviewing content and process as related to curative factors, it is useful to keep four distinctions in mind: 1) content is important as a source of data which can be collected and used over time to make assessments and plan strategies; 2) content in itself serves a function in giving the group a certain predictability, as is evident in imparting information; 3) process offers a mechanism for interpreting content data collected over time and helps the leader guide the group toward its stated goals; 4) process in itself serves a function by giving the group members a sense of belonging, undoing dysfunctional patterns of interaction, and freeing members to take risks and to support the risks taken by others.

CLINICAL EXAMPLE: CONTENT AND PROCESS IN A HEALTH COMMITTEE MEETING

An ad hoc committee composed of nurses and activity therapists convened to discuss intradisciplinary responsibilities for an expanded group program in the in-patient facility where all were employed. Until now all groups for patients had been organized and led by an activity therapist. The imminent expansion of the group program had motivated the nurses to use their regularly scheduled staff meetings to discuss the implications for nurses of the new group program and to define areas of work in which they wished to participate. The nurses were enthusiastic at the prospect of being involved in the program. Some of them had begun to read extensively in order to increase their knowledge of group theory.

A major area of interest to the nurses was interpersonal communication groups, even though they knew that a communication skills group, led by an activity therapist, had been meeting for some time. Designation of an ad hoc committee was made by the hospital administration.

An initial committee meeting was attended by eight persons, including three staff nurses and three activity therapists. The committee was chaired by the clinical nurse specialist and the supervisor of activity therapy. During the meeting, nurses sat to the left of the clinical nurse specialist; activity therapists sat to the right of their supervisor. The two coleaders of the committee sat side by side.

The stated task of the committee was to identify specific areas of expertise among the members in order to begin planning an expanded group program. The meeting was opened by the clinical nurse specialist, who explained the task. This explanation was followed by a long silence. Finally the silence was broken by an activity therapist who expressed strong opposition to having the group program of the unit "invaded" by nurses. A more tactful activity therapist said sympathetically that nurses already had so many important responsibilities that it was unfair to burden them further. At this point a staff nurse stated that activity therapists had no right to decide what was fair for nurses, and

that the job of the nursing staff would be much easier if activity therapists kept nurses informed of which patients were in what groups at a
given time, particularly when medications were due. A second nurse
asserted that the activity therapists wanted nurses to be restricted to
menial housekeeping tasks, although it was nurses who really met the
needs of patients. As anger mounted, accusations and counteraccusa-
tions were hurled between the subgroups.

The clinical nurse specialist and the activity therapy supervisor remained composed and did not join the argument. After a few moments
the activity therapy supervisor intervened to remark that some of the
concerns of both factions might be valid but they were distracting the
committee from its task. The clinical nurse specialist stated how much
activity therapists brought to current group programs, adding that it
was now important for everyone to be involved in the expanded group
program. The activity therapy supervisor nodded in assent and said,
"I have always been very proud of the way our two groups worked together in the unit. Our relationship is an example for the rest of the
hospital." The clinical nurse specialist then restated the committee's
task, and explained that outlining areas of expertise was not a prelude
to giving up effective work but a means of enhancing it, since "we can
meet the patients' needs by knowing what we do best."

The activity therapy supervisor suggested that each subgroup indicate
what aspects of group work were appropriate to one discipline or the
other, and what aspects of group work might be shared. The clinical
nurse specialist reminded committee members that groups could be
co-led by a nurse and an activity therapist willing to share their skills.
As group emotion gradually became less intense, an activity therapist
admitted being afraid of having to give up her favorite group. Upon
hearing this, a staff nurse reached out to touch the activity therapist,
saying, "We've always been able to work things out before, haven't
we?"

At the suggestion of the coleaders a nurse and an activity therapist
began writing on a blackboard a list of groups which might be led by
two nurses, a list of groups which might be led by two activity therapists, and a list of groups to which both disciplines might contribute
leaders. In a short time it became apparent that some groups, such as
health-teaching groups, should be led by nurses, whereas craft groups
should be led by activity therapists. The preponderance of groups,
however, including communication groups, could be led by coleaders
from either or both disciplines.

As the three lists lengthened, committee members realized that
there would be enough group work for everyone. With this realization, communication between the subgroups became entirely rational.
Restrictive problem-solving was replaced with enabling behaviors.
Tentative suggestions were made by nurses and activity therapists who

might conceivably lead groups together. As the session neared an end, the activity therapy supervisor reminded committee members to set up another meeting for the following week. A staff nurse and an activity therapist were given joint responsibility for devising the agenda. As the group began to disperse, the activity therapy supervisor commented that it was exciting to be planning such an innovative program. The clinical nurse specialist said that it was good to work with dedicated people. Hearing this, the committee members exchanged a few friendly glances as they left the room.

Table 6–3   CURATIVE FACTORS PRESENT IN THE COMMITTEE MEETING

Content Factors	
Imparting Information:	Leaders stated goals
	Leaders reassured subgroups
Interpersonal Learning:	Leaders modeled interdisciplinary cooperation through shared leadership
	Members stopped making accusations and began to problem-solve
Process Factors	
Instillation of Hope:	Leaders reminded members of cooperative endeavors in the past, indicating that the subgroups could work together
Universality:	Members knew that they all were paid employees with a responsibility for patient care and the reputation of the psychiatric facility to consider
Cohesiveness:	Leaders indicated to the subgroups that despite interdisciplinary differences, all were members of the same health team
Mixed Factors (Content and Process)	
Socializing Techniques:	Leaders were not drawn into the altercation, but expressed trust in each other
Imitative Behavior:	Members ultimately followed the example of the group leaders in working together
Existential Factors:	Leaders asked the group to make personal interests secondary to the welfare of the patients, whose needs were greater than their own

Source: Yalom, 1975

SUMMARY

This chapter provided the reader with a working knowledge of group process and content by differentiating between the two concepts. The case example indicated how intricately intertwined these concepts are with interpersonal communication, conflict resolution, and curative factors. The primary function of content is to transfer information and to point to process. Process deals with monitoring the group's movement toward its goal by facilitating or impeding this effort. The way content and process are analyzed depends on the interpersonal and intrapersonal theories of interaction one believes in. The curative factors identified by Yalom were described and classified as content-oriented, process-oriented, or a combination of the two.

REFERENCES

Bascue, L.O. "A Conceptual Model for Training Group Therapists." *International Journal of Group Psychotherapy* 28, No. 4, 1978, pages 445–452.

Bateson, G.; D.D. Jackson; J. Haley; and J.H. Weakland. "A Note on the Double Bind." *Family Process* 2, 1963, pages 154–161.

Benne, K., and M. Birnbaum. "Principles of Changing." In *The Planning of Change*, W. Bennis, K. Benne, and R. Chin, Eds. New York: Holt Rinehart & Winston, 1969.

Egan, G. *The Skilled Helper.* 2nd ed. Monterey, CA.: Brooks Cole, 1982.

Ekman, P., and W. Friesen. *Unmasking the Face.* Englewood Cliffs, N.J.: Prentice-Hall, 1975.

Glassner, B., and J. Freedman. *Clinical Sociology.* New York: Longman, 1979.

Hinsie, L.E., and R.J. Campbell. *Psychiatric Dictionary.* 4th ed. New York: Oxford University Press, 1977.

Langs, R. *The Techniques of Psychotherapy* Vol. 1. New York: Jason Aronson, 1973.

Longo, D.C., and R.A. Williams. *Clinical Practice in Psychosocial Nursing: Assessment and Intervention.* New York: Appleton-Century-Crofts, 1978.

Luft, J. *An Introduction to Group Dynamics.* Palo Alto, CA.: National Press, 1963.

Marram, G.D. *The Group Approach in Nursing Practice.* St. Louis: C.V. Mosby, 1978.

Mills, T.M. *The Sociology of Small Groups.* Englewood Cliffs, N.J.: Prentice-Hall, 1967.

Reusch, J. *Therapeutic Communication.* New York: W.W. Norton, 1961.

Sampson, E., and M. Marthas. *Group Process for the Health Professions.* New York: Wiley, 1977.

Satir, V. *Conjoint Family Therapy.* Palo Alto, CA.: Science and Behavior Books, 1964.

Tauber, L.E. "Choice Point Analysis — Formulation, Strategy, Intervention and Result in Group Process Therapy and Supervision." *International Journal of Group Psychotherapy* 28, No. 2, 1978, pages 163–184.

Truax, C.B., and R.R. Carkhuff. *Toward Effective Counseling and Therapy.* Chicago: Aldine, 1967.

Watzlawick, P. *An Anthology of Human Communication.* Palo Alto, CA.: Science and Behavior Books, 1964.

Werner, J.A. "Relating Group Theory to Nursing Practice." *Perspectives in Psychiatric Care* 8, 1970, pages 249–261.

Whitaker, D.S., and M.A. Lieberman. *Psychotherapy Through the Group Process.* New York: Atherton Press, 1964.

Yalom, I.D. *The Theory and Practice of Group Psychotherapy.* 2nd ed. New York: Basic Books, 1975.

Yearwood-Grazette, H.S. "An Anatomy of Communication." *Nursing Times* 74, 1978, pages 1672–1679.

PART TWO

Group Strategy and Techniques

7

Group Organization: Selection Criteria, Member Preparation, Contractual Issues

Lois Koch Marvin

The decision to offer health care on a group basis may originate among prospective group members who are aware of their own needs and can organize a group to meet their requirements. More often, however, prospective group members are ignorant of the possibilities inherent in a group approach to health care. Therefore it is usually the nurse or other health professional who must identify target needs or recognize target populations amenable to group intervention. Nurses who decide that the needs of certain clients are best served in the context of group interaction can turn to nursing process for direction.

FOUNDING A GROUP

A common rationale for group work is that it allows more individuals to be helped with less expenditure of professional time and energy. This rationale is fallacious in several respects. Loomis (1979) stated that group leadership is an enervating activity which taxes the cognitive and affective powers of a leader, and that one individual cannot effectively lead more than a few groups each day. Coleadership, re-cording, observation, and supervision are other factors which negate a group approach merely for pragmatic reasons. More importantly, emphasizing the practical aspects of group treatment overlooks the unique benefits obtainable through a positive group experience. Group work should not be regarded as a second-rate treatment but as a complex, demanding process capable of maintaining functional be-haviors and of producing therapeutic change when the group is well-grounded in theory and organized with care.

During preliminary planning, nurses must consider whether their personal and educational qualifications are equal to the task. Nurses are accustomed to working on health teams, to teaching families, and to interacting with groups of patients who share the same clinical facilities. Even in these relatively unstructured situations nurses must possess a degree of self-awareness and some knowledge of group dynamics in order to be effective. If the proposed group involves psychotherapy, the group leader should meet the standards of the American Nurses' Association, which state that intensive psychotherapeutic groups should be led by nurses with graduate preparation in psychiatric-mental health nursing (Lego, 1978). Thus the question must be asked: Is the nurse planning a group equipped by temperament, experiences, and education to lead that particular group? It is not enough to determine which clients are suitable for membership in which group. The quali-fications of the nurse-leader must also be assessed, given the variables of expertise, available supervision, group composition, and group objec-tives. Having acknowledged that a nurse is ready to assume respon-sibility for a particular group, the health-care system sponsoring the group is likely to be supportive of organizational and other essential activities.

Assessing Needs and Resources

Assessing the needs of a target population often precipitates the wish to organize a group, but this single assessment must be greatly ex-panded. Before deciding that a group is needed, the health status of the target population should be assessed in relation to existing re-sources of individuals, of families, of the health-care system, and of the community at large. The nurse needs to consider population needs which are not being met in order to solicit support for group intervention. If there is no widely perceived need there may be no real demand for service, and no acceptance from the health-care system or the target population for the proposed group. Moreover, the health-care system itself may be unwilling to sponsor group work as a means for providing care.

A comprehensive assessment by the nurse may reveal numerous outstanding needs in the target population, some of which are already being met.   Further assessment may be indicated in order to set priorities, to determine who is affected and to what extent, and whether current health programs are adequate.   Occasionally the comprehensive assessment of needs and the survey of existing resources may result in referrals rather than in the organization of a new group. Duplication of service is a frequent hazard in health-care work which may be avoided by assessment of both needs and resources.

The attitude of health-care agencies toward group work should be included in the assessment, since an external system which is not generally supportive of a group may preclude a positive group experience. Conversely, an external system which is generally supportive cannot guarantee, but certainly can enhance, the probability of success (Loomis, 1979). An appraisal of the attitudes and policies of the external or suprasystem surrounding the group may be accomplished by asking the following questions.

- What treatment modality is given priority by the external system?
- Do persons in administrative positions of the external system advocate group intervention?
- What type of group interventions are likely to be anticipated by prospective group members? What type of interventions are likely to be considered appropriate and effective by the external system?
- Is there disparity between what the prospective leader considers therapeutic and what members and the external system are likely to accept?
- What group outcomes are expected by the external system and the larger community?

Planning the Group

There is no substitute for preliminary assessment and planning. It is advisable to assess and plan for the group long before the first prospective member is interviewed. Experienced group practitioners stress the importance of preparatory work and concur that the success of any group is related to pregroup activities carried out by the leader or leaders (Marram, 1978; Yalom, 1975). Early in the planning phase the question of coleadership must be addressed. This is an important consideration; a full discussion of advantages and disadvantages of coleadership is included in Chapter 9. A theoretical framework must be selected and criteria for group membership must be formulated during the preparatory period. Selecting a theoretical framework is a major decision, since the chosen framework reciprocally influences leadership functions and group objectives. Following these early decisions the persons being considered for the group are interviewed, and its members selected and prepared for the experience. During this last activity the group contract is established.

Selecting a Theoretical Framework

Even before member selection criteria are defined, consideration of an appropriate theoretical framework begins. The leader who initiates a group experience not supported by a theoretical framework risks using deliberative interventions in a haphazard fashion. Not only is there danger of overlooking important group phenomena but there is also danger of employing interventions which are inconsistent or unpredictable.

When adopting a theoretical framework for a group, the leader must sometimes forego personal preferences in order to consider multiple factors. There is no one theoretical framework which is suitable for all groups, but there are a number of frameworks from which to choose. Many group leaders follow their own inclinations or argue for eclecticism, but this should be tempered by the exigencies of the total situation. In an account of a group composed of prison inmates, the leaders reluctantly discarded their wish for a gestalt-existential framework in favor of a reality-therapy group. The leaders concluded that in a correctional institution a theoretical framework which stressed responsibility, decision making, and realism would cause relatively little anxiety and would be more productive for the members (Janosik, 1977).

In choosing a theoretical framework the following points should be considered.

- Criteria for member selection and group composition.
- Characteristics of the external system in which the group meets.
- Anticipated duration of the group and frequency of meetings.
- Experience and competence of the leader or leaders.
- Belief of the leader or leaders in the merits of the selected framework.

Determining Membership Criteria

Group practitioners have learned from educators that objectives should be presented in behavioral or empirical terms so that leaders and members have congruent expectations. Setting specific, reachable goals helps members to understand what the group is all about, and encourages them to engage in goal-directed activities (Cleghorn and Levin, 1973). In addition to assuaging the fears of members, clearly stated objectives are essential to any evaluation of group success or failure. Before establishing membership criteria for the group the leader must formulate tentative objectives, define them operationally, and introduce them into the selection and preparation of group members. In the absence of group objectives the leader cannot determine the suitability of prospective members for the group.

When moving into the selection and preparation of specific members these questions might be employed with good effect.

- What specific needs does this client have? Can these needs best be met in a group situation?
- Can the client tolerate the levels of emotion likely to be generated by the group experience?
- Will the client be able to share his or her concerns with the group?·
- What has the experience of the client been with primary, secondary, and reference groups in the past?
- Is there evidence of ability to accept group norms and subscribe to a group contract?

Several authorities on group work (Marram, 1979; Yalom, 1975) have dealt with the issue of heterogeneity versus homogeneity in groups, but rigid guidelines have not been suggested. It is thought that some homogeneity is necessary in order for members to be able to relate to each other, but it is also claimed that some heterogeneity in the group helps members to learn from one another. Whitaker and Lieberman (1964) proposed that change occurs among group members after an experience of incongruity or dissonance. If one accepts this premise, heterogeneous group composition could promote greater change in the attitudes, behavior, and knowledge of members, since incongruity and dissonance presumably would be higher in heterogeneous groups.

According to Yalom (1975) a salient curative factor is group cohesion. This term refers to the extent to which members feel they belong in the group. When promoting group cohesion through member selection, the *Noah's Ark principle* may be advocated. This principle states that the isolation of group members may be prevented when every member has a *compeer*, or companion, who is similar in some respects. Age, sex, and developmental level are among the characteristics relevant in matching group members to reduce isolation. Examples of unfortunate selection include an all-male group with one female member, a group of middle-aged members and a lone adolescent, or a group of disabled retirees with one member gainfully employed. The critical characteristics chosen to carry out the Noah's Ark principle should be those most likely to influence progress toward group goals. In a sense, homogeneity within groups is an elusive myth. Even individuals with shared problems and shared characteristics are heterogeneous when it comes to their coping skills, antecedent experiences, and defensive maneuvers.

Particular characteristics or behaviors have been identified as *facilitators* or *inhibitors* of group progress. In the context or psychotherapy groups, Yalom (1975) advised that individuals with disruptive behavior patterns be excluded from membership. Among those excluded were persons with brain damage, paranoia, suicide ideation, narcissistic behavior, hypochondriasis, addictions, acute psychosis, and marked sociopathy. This exclusionary list seems excessive if applied in arbitrary or automatic ways. While it is true that not every client can adjust to every group, there are few individuals who cannot benefit from a group experience tailored to their needs. Important considerations include the potential value to the individual from the group experience, and the capacity of the individual to contribute to the group. The attractiveness of the group to prospective members and their willingness to commit themselves to the group contract should be part of the criteria for membership.

Group Contract

Negotiation of the group contract is a crucial aspect of selecting and preparing members. The negotiations require close collaboration between prospective members and the leader in establishing the contract. Ultimately the therapeutic contract should be shared with appropriate members of the health-care system in which the group will meet. Sharing general information regarding the group contract is not a breach of confidentiality and helps insure an accepting climate for the group within the agency or health system. Provisions of the group contract should be articulated within the agency so that the goals and scope of the group are understood. Group members should be asked to indicate their understanding and acceptance of the collaborative agreement negotiated by leader and members. Discrepancy between leader and member expectations is an impediment to a rewarding group experience. It is true that members often entertain unrealistic expectations, but an unequivocal group contract reduces confusion and promotes consensual validation.

Group Size

The size of a group may vary according to the availability of members, the urgency of their needs, and their interpersonal strengths and weaknesses. Group goals constitute another variable affecting group size. Although there is little agreement on an optimal size for small groups there is consensus on the optimal *range* of group size: five to fifteen members is the ideal number, depending largely on the amount of interpersonal participation sought. Based on clinical observation and experience with groups, there is agreement that groups with fewer than five members or more than ten members are unlikely to engage in maximal therapeutic exchange. Obviously the size of a group is a more critical variable for groups whose major goals require extensive interpersonal exchange between members. Affective learning in groups may be inhibited by the presence of more than ten members, whereas cognitive and psychomotor learning may proceed without detriment. Groups with more than ten members tend to form subgroups that reassure the subgroup members but impair group-oriented transactions and interventions (Loomis, 1979). Additional research of a systematic nature is needed to identify ideal group size for specific kinds of groups.

IMPLEMENTING THE PLAN

Selection of Members

Following the assessment and planning phases, the leader begins to implement the plan. Methods used to select members vary with the type of group being organized. Yalom (1975) suggested that a screening interview with each prospective member is useful in selecting and preparing clients. The screening interview, while beneficial in choosing therapy group members, may not be needed for other types of groups. An alternative method, which may elicit more valid information, consists of observing prospective members in a group situation similar to the one which will be encountered in the actual group. Observing prospective members as they engage in social interaction may yield more accurate information than would be obtained in a screening interview with the leader or leaders.

Questions directed to a prospective group member or behaviors to be assessed are determined by objectives established for the group. If mastering knowledge, changing behavior, or learning a skill is a major goal for group members, it would be helpful to note the present accomplishments of the individual. This could be done by asking specific questions or by requesting a demonstration of skills or behaviors already present. Prospective members might be asked in an interview or in a group situation to complete a questionnaire appraising their own skills or behaviors. During this entire process the group leader tries to decide whether a group experience will be helpful for a given person, or which of several possible group experiences would be most rewarding.

The selection activities enable leaders and prospective members to share information about each other and the nature of the group. It is not unusual for prospective members to question leaders closely. Members frequently inquire about the qualifications and experience of the leader. Such questions may appear challenging to the leader, but should be answered truthfully and respectfully. Details concerning the time and location of the group meeting, the duration of the group, and whether the group will be closed or open to new members are disclosed at this point. Before asking a candidate to join the group a mutual appraisal should take place, with leaders encouraging prospective members to ask questions that would clarify expectations and alleviate fears concerning the group experience.

Preparation of Members

The group contract is presented to prospective members during these proceedings and may be described as a device which helps leaders and members understand their expectations of each other. Although group contracts may vary in detail, they are substantively alike. Generally, they are statements made by participants concerning what they are willing to attempt to adhere to for the duration of the group experience. It may be necessary at this time for leaders to translate the group goals into terms which accommodate members' perceptions of their own needs (Marram, 1978).

The length and frequency of meetings are affected by the nature and goals of the group. A psychotherapy group might meet once or twice a week for a one-hour session, while a didactic group for newly diagnosed diabetics might meet for thirty minutes a day over a period of several weeks. The surroundings in which the group meets should be accessible and as comfortable as possible. Except in unavoidable circumstances, the leaders should always meet the group in the same place at the times stipulated in the group contract.

When prospective members are interviewed privately, there is reluctance on the part of some leaders to discuss or describe other members who will be in the group. It is natural, however, for prospective members to wonder about the others joining the group, and there is no ethical objection to disclosing the number of persons expected in the group or to discuss its composition in general terms (Yalom, 1975).

EVALUATING GROUP PROGRESS

Evaluation of the group's progress is an ongoing activity which provides the leader with information about the developmental progress of the group as a whole and the progress of the individual member toward personal goals. Evaluating the progress of the group and of individual members permits the leaders to make assumptions about the effectiveness of their interventions. In evaluating group progress the original objectives are a reference point. Evaluation is more accurate if the objectives have been expressed in behavioral terms, and if adequate records have been kept of group development and of changes discerned in individual members.

Outcome Criteria

Group goals, if realistically set and operationally defined, can be the basis for establishing outcome criteria. The degree to which each member meets stated objectives may be measured in part by the member's adherence to the provisions of the group contract. The progress of the group as a whole may be evaluated in terms of the state of its development. Having previously selected a theoretical framework on which to base the group, the leader may apply concepts of the framework in evaluating progress. (See earlier chapters on group development issues and the usefulness of theoretical frameworks.)

Evaluation by Observation

Evaluation by observation calls attention to the presence or absence of predetermined cognitive or behavioral changes. This includes changes observed within the group, along with evidence of the transfer of acquired knowledge, behaviors, or skills to situations and relationships outside the group (Yalom, 1975). An illustration of transferred knowledge might be a member getting a job, or losing ten pounds, or reporting normal blood pressure.

Many health-care professionals who have developed impressive observational skills may find these skills diminished when they assume the position of group leader. Because of the multiplicity of data which a group leader must process while attending to the needs of the group, it is sometimes helpful to have a coleader whose chief task is to observe and record group interactions. If a recorder-observer sits in the room with the group, the presence of this person must be explained to group members when the contract is being negotiated. Among others, Johnson (1963) recommended that the recorder-observer be in the same meeting room as the group and the leader. Less intrusive methods of observing and recording data include the use of one-way mirrors or electronic recording equipment. All observation methods, no matter how unobtrusive, should be disclosed to prospective members during the contract negotiations and their consent given to the observation. If group sessions are recorded electronically, it is advisable to obtain the signed consent of group members. An observer is especially valuable to a group leader if there is opportunity for the two to review the group session immediately afterwards, while events are still recent. Immediate feedback enables the leader to validate or modify perceptions of group events.

Supervision Supervision of a group concentrates on leader interventions as these affect the group's progress. Obviously the supervisor should be clinically astute and theoretically sophisticated. A supervisor can be expected to offer both criticism and endorsement of the various interventions of group leaders, as well as comments on the relationship between coleaders.

Recording Records should be made of all contacts between group leaders and group members. Written or electronic documentation of group phenomena and of member outcomes is needed to provide a base for conceptual material (Gardner, 1979). For example, audiovisual taping of group sessions can be used to demonstrate deliberative interventions and testify to the consequences of interventions. Electronic documentation of group events can be used as a reference point for leaders organizing future groups. Regardless of the methods used, the record should document group events for a number of reasons, including the need for ongoing evaluation of group and individual progress and evaluation of the impact of leader interventions. Recording is an activity which helps leaders to sort out overwhelming amounts of information, and assists them in comprehending ambiguous events and relationships within the group.

The following Clinical Example shows how the nursing process was used as a guide for organizing a group.

CLINICAL EXAMPLE: ORGANIZING A REORIENTATION GROUP FOR ELDERLY CLIENTS

Assessing Needs and Resources

Terri Whalen worked as a nurse administrator in a minimum care facility for the elderly. She noted that many persons over the age of seventy became disoriented after admission even though they were not seriously impaired by the physical infirmities which accompany aging. Many of them were aware of being confused and this caused them additional anxiety, which heightened their confusion. Some adjusted after a short time, but all suffered distress initially. For a few of the clients the period of disorientation was prolonged and marked the beginning of a downward course. Terri observed that although the nursing staff took care of the routine needs of clients, there was no systematic attempt to reorient newly admitted clients who were confused. In addition, Terri saw that newly admitted clients tended to stay apart from established cliques in the facility, and that they avoided interacting with other new-. ly admitted persons. In assessing staff needs Terri discovered that many nurses felt guilty about not being able to help confused patients to a greater extent. When polled by Terri, the majority of staff members said that a reorientation group would be helpful. Several nurses indicated a desire to learn more about reorientation techniques and volunteered to participate as coleaders.

Planning the Group

The unhappiness of new clients and the frustrations of personnel, who had little time to spend with confused clients caused Terri to proceed with plans for a reorientation group. She hoped that when newly admitted patients met other individuals with similar feelings of loss and confusion, there would be mutual caring and support. Since all clients in the facility were under the care of personal physicians, attending physicians were informed of the group project. A handout describing the format and goals of the group was distributed to physicians and families of newly admitted clients. Routine approval was obtained for all eligible clients to participate in the group for one month following admission.

A committee of staff members chaired by Terri formulated behavioral objectives for persons attending the reorientation group.

- All newly admitted clients were expected to attend the daily sessions of the group for a period of one month.

- The purpose of the reorientation group was to acquaint new members with the care facility in order to make them feel more comfortable.
- Members attending the group were expected to know the following information:
  - Their own name, the date, day of the week, and the name of the care facility.
  - The location of their own room, the dining room, the day room, and the nurses' station.
  - The times that meals were served and medications given.
  - The location of the calendar of weekly events held in the care facility.
  - The name of the nurse or paraprofessional primarily responsible for meeting their needs.
  - The first names of the persons living in the rooms directly adjoining their own.

Implementing the Plan

A decision was made to use a coleader arrangement composed of a primary and secondary group leader. In leading the group sessions Terri functioned as both socioemotional and task leader. Because she was present at every session, she was considered senior leader by the members. The secondary leader changed each week, but was always a permanent member of the nursing staff. This arrangement did not prove disruptive to the group, since Terri's presence provided continuity. Indeed, many members chose to interpret the group to the secondary leader, imitatively using reorienting techniques. Coffee and cake were served at the end of every meeting.

Records were kept on the progress of individual members, including a brief anecdotal account of the behavior of each member. A checklist of group objectives was also used. This was a quick way of recording the current status of members, along with any improvement or regression.

A group record or log of significant events during a session was kept by the secondary leader. The amount of group interaction and the affective level of the group as a whole were mentioned. Evidence of friction and/or subgrouping was noted. The log described interventions which were helpful or inhibiting to the group. At staff meetings a report of group and individual progress was included on the agenda, and the log was available to interested staff members.

Evaluating the Group

Several methods were used to evaluate the effectiveness of the group. The individual progress of each member could be quickly determined by looking at the checklist of group objectives. The anecdotal summary provided additional information of a more impressionistic nature. Group progress as a whole could be measured to an extent by reading the group log. The log utilized some theoretical concepts such as curative group factors (Yalom, 1975). Group cohesion was thought to be present, but was not a major factor because of the open-ended, short-term nature of the group. Cohesion, however, seemed to be a factor which was transferred to unstructured activities in the care facility. Newly admitted members became more comfortable with one another and began to spend time together outside the group sessions. Among the major curative factors present in the group were interpersonal learning and instillation of hope.

A serendipitious outcome of the reorientation group was the interest it generated among staff members. When it became apparent that some clients required more than one month of group support, staff members suggested a second group be started. The second group would be called a socialization group and would be open to clients who had completed the reorientation group but wished or needed a longer group experience. Two members of the nursing staff agreed to begin reading about socialization groups with the idea of organizing a second group. Another unexpected outcome of the reorientation group was the interest it generated in using reorientation techniques routinely, as staff members became more knowledgeable and more convinced of the efficacy of the techniques. Among the evaluation procedures used for the reorientation group were the following:

- Checklist of group objectives and anecdotal summary for each member.
- Log of group development and group phenomena recorded by the secondary leader.
- Brief postgroup conference between primary and secondary leaders following each session.
- Inclusion of a report on group and individual progress on the agenda of scheduled staff meetings.

SUMMARY

Before undertaking a group, a comprehensive assessment of the health needs of a target population was recommended. The importance of obtaining support and acceptance from key personnel in the health-care system was discussed.

Among other criteria for group membership, homogeneity and heterogeneity were compared. Use of the Noah's Ark principle was advocated as a way of reducing feelings of isolation among group members. The advisability of establishing behavioral group objectives was suggested in order to facilitate the evaluation of group outcomes. Observation, supervision, and recording of group phenomena were considered essential to implementing and evaluating the group experience.

A Clinical Example was given which used the nursing process as a guide for organizing a group.

REFERENCES

Cleghorn, J.M., and S. Levin. "Training Family Therapists by Setting Objectives." *American Journal of Orthopsychiatry* 43 (4), April 1973, pages 439–446.

Gardner, K.G. "Small Groups and Their Therapeutic Force." In *Principles and Practice of Psychiatric Nursing*, G.W. Stuart and S. Sundeen, Eds. St. Louis: C.V. Mosby, 1979.

Janosik, E.H. "Reachable and Teachable: Report on a Prison Alcoholism Group." *Journal of Mental Health and Psychiatric Nursing* Vol. 15, No. 4, April 1977, pages 24–29.

———— , and J.R. Miller. "Theories of Family Development." In *Family Health Care*, D.P. Hymovich and M.W. Barnard, Eds. Vol. 1. New York: McGraw-Hill, 1979.

Lego, S. "Group Dynamic Theory and Application." In *Comprehensive Psychiatric Nursing*, J. Haber et al., Eds. New York: McGraw-Hill, 1978.

Johnson, J.A. *Group Therapy: A Practical Approach.* New York: McGraw-Hill, 1963.

Kellerman, H. *Group Psychotherapy and Personality: Intersecting Structures.* New York: Grune and Stratton, 1979.

Loomis, M.E. *Group Process for Nurses.* St. Louis: C.V. Mosby, 1979.

Marram, G. *The Group Approach in Nursing Practice.* St. Louis: C.V. Mosby, 1978.

Shaw, M.E. *Group Dynamics: The Psychology of Small Group Behavior.* New York: McGraw-Hill, 1971.

Whitaker, D.S., and M.A. Lieberman. *Psychotherapy Through the Group Process.* New York: Atherton Press, 1964.

Yalom, I.D. *The Theory and Practice of Group Psychotherapy.* New York: Basic Books, 1975.

8

Group Dynamics: Membership Role Enactment

Lenore Bolling Phipps

Any group eventually becomes a dynamic configuration of roles and role enactment. Role enactment in small groups is the interaction of individual members which reflects group process and creates a structure of roles. These roles may either enhance group development or inhibit its growth. No role is enacted in a vacuum but is related to intrapsychic, interpersonal, and external group forces which shape its form. An individual brings to a group personal needs and expectations which may be conscious or unconscious, but which influence relationships with other members. Conversely, a member's behavior is also a function of his or her relationship to others in the group. Assuming a role in a group provides an individual with an identity within the group (Marram, 1978). "Who am I?" and "Whom will I be in this group?" become real issues and are reactions to the group and to one's own self-perception. That role then solidifies within the context of the group. Thus, role enactment is not a simple event but is determined by multiple factors in a complex and dynamic process.

The purpose of this chapter is to describe various role-enactment concepts and link them to group structure, development, and salient pendular issues.

ROLE COMPONENTS

A *role* describes a set of behavioral expectations shared by members concerning the occupant of a position in the group (Hare, 1976). Role is a part the occupant plays during the life of a group or at some point in time. It may be assigned (determined by others), assumed (taken to satisfy individual needs), ascribed (determined by endowed characteristics, such as age or gender), or achieved (accomplished on the basis of ability). Regardless of the manner in which a role takes shape, the important point is that role defines and regulates behavior (Sampson and Marthas, 1977). Implicit in the concept of role are three vital elements: *expectation, perception,* and *enactment.*

Expectation

Expectations are the specifications or criteria by which individuals define their own and others' responsibilities, and they extend to attitudes, values, and behaviors. In other words, they are what group members anticipate will be done by a member occupying that role, and what the role occupant expects from others as the role is enacted. This implies that certain role behaviors will be approved while others will be prohibited (Hare, 1976). At times, role expectations are not met because the occupant is either unwilling or unable to meet group expectations, or because the occupant is unwilling or unable to accommodate confusing or incompatible roles (Fisher, 1972).

Perception

The second component, role perception, describes how the role occupant believes the role should be enacted. Perception may be influenced by many variables: motivation, primary-group experiences with significant others, culture, and self-image. Self-image influences the ease with which the individual shifts from one role to another. If one's identity is poorly developed, role transition is difficult. In this way self-image may limit or expand role behavior (Bonner, 1959). Consider, for example, the initial problems of the newly graduated nurse making the transition from student to staff nurse. Residual role expectations based on student experience continue for a time to shape the self-image of the new graduate nurse. Role perception also may be influenced by one's status and power in the group. The higher the status level, the greater the inclination to assume additional power. Expansion of a role often results from feelings of power and confidence. The wish to enact higher level roles may be fostered when role occupants are permitted a greater degree of latitude in the manner in which the role is enacted.

Enactment

The last component, role enactment (role performance) is the observable verbal and nonverbal behavior of a role occupant. Whereas role expectation is often implicit, and role perception is often covert, role enactment refers to tangible and explicit behavior. This behavior, expressed in the form of action and communication patterns, enables observers to identify the roles which group members assume. Assessment and analysis of role enactment is facilitated by tools such as Bale's (1953) Interactional Process Analysis, sociometry, and other research techniques, some of which are described in Chapters 17 and 18.

Role enactment is a function of the personal characteristics of the role occupant and of the intricate pattern of member interrelationships at a particular point in time. Individuals vary in their ability to enact a given role. The degree of harmony between the individual occupant and the role is termed *role fit*. Personal characteristics and motivation influence role fit, as does the phase of group development at which the role is assumed. Early in the group's life the first individual to occupy a role has greater flexibility in creating that role to fit personal needs, facilitating role fit. Conversely, role fit is more difficult for the person who follows a previously successful role occupant but wishes to alter the role enactment (Hare, 1976).

Roles tend to be reciprocal, so that the privileges of one role become the duties of another. This interrelationship means that role enactment must be congruent with group expectations in order to enhance group productivity.

Human beings feel secure when they can reasonably predict how others will behave. If a member's role enactment is not congruent with expectations, the effect on the group is confusion and diminished productivity. If the member whose role performance is incongruent is also the leader, the effect may demoralize the members, cause conflict, and may even bring about the dissolution of the group. Another example of incongruency between individual role performance and group expectation is that of the *deviant* member who enacts a nonacceptable role by rejecting group norms (Bonner, 1959). The deviant member is subject to considerable group attention and pressure to conform to its norms. The deviant role develops later in group life, after norms have begun to be established. The deviant role ultimately serves to crystallize group norms and to limit boundaries of group membership. (The deviant role will be discussed later in this chapter.)

ROLE CONFLICT

Considering the complex, multidimensional nature of group roles, it is not unusual for role expectations, perceptions, and performances to be discordant. The greater the discord between any of these elements, the greater opportunity exists for role conflict and group dysfunction. When the enacted role diverges from the expected role, either the role is changed or the occupant is removed, or removes her- or himself (Shaw, 1971). Contradictions or ambiguities in role expectations tend to make the individual role occupant more guarded, self-conscious, and self-critical of role behavior in general.

Role conflict includes any clash of expectations originating from either interpersonal or intrapsychic sources. Intense or prolonged interpersonal role conflict often affects the self-images of the members. Inability to satisfy another's expectations is projected and linked to the assumption that the behavior of the other person is uncertain or unreliable. This double failure of expectations engenders feelings of tension, isolation, and low self-esteem. One of the ways chosen to cope with this dilemma is for one or both of the participants to seek out others and establish new alliances. In this manner subgroups, in the form of supportive minigroups, arise which permit intimacy and sharing in an esteem-building and isolation-reducing environment (Starr, 1977). Intrapsychic role conflict is precipitated by attempts to enact more than one role at a time. Social role conflict is a societal conflict usually fought internally, on the battleground of the individual's mind.

Intrapsychic role conflict, which has the greatest impact, is concerned with personal identity and is generated when distinctions between a former role and an emerging role are not clear. An example of this is found in the conflict that many women in today's society experience as they are pulled between their traditional expectations and their newly encouraged self-expectations. Guilt about career versus personal life commitments is compounded by their concerns about their effectiveness and competency in managing their time (Nevill, 1975).

Role conflict may assume a variety of forms, among which are *role collision, role incompatibility, role confusion,* and *role transition.*

Role Collision When the roles of two members overlap, with both members assuming the rights and duties for a single task, role collision occurs. This commonly happens among parents in primary and secondary groups. Often, role collision may be alleviated through clarification of role responsibilities.

Role Incompatibility This conflict involves one member who occupies two or more roles, each of which entails opposing expectations and conflicting loyalties. This occurs when a peer member temporarily fills the role of leader or supervisor. Role incompatibility is typical in the operations of one-parent families in which a mother or father is caught between the role expectations of being a parent and of being an employee. The solution to role incompatibility requires temporary disengagement from one role and focus on the other. The individual must learn to set aside time and energy for only one role at a time.

Role Confusion Incompatible or inconsistent expectations about the appropriate behavior for a role may precipitate this conflict. Roles which are ambiguous or subject to frequent changes run a high risk for role confusion (Hare, 1976). The ensuing confusion may be intrapsychic or interpersonal, but the result, inevitably, is tension and uncertainty.

Role Transition This occurs when one occupant gives up one role for another. It may be a conscious, deliberate action — such as choosing to change a job, surroundings, or marriage — or it may be the result of a developmental event, such as the altered role of parents as children mature and separate from the family. In many durable, informal groups, members undergo role transition as various group roles are passed from one member to another. For example, the role of group leader may be occupied sequentially by several members. There is usually a degree of anxiety related to role transition, as the occupant learns new behaviors and adjusts to new expectations.

Structural Role Conflict

There is another type of role conflict which is a function not of individual personality but of the nature of the group. Structural role conflict is intrinsic to the patterned arrangement of group positions and interactions, with the result that any occupant of a particular role experiences tension and anxiety. Understanding that the source of the conflict is related to the structural characteristics of the group rather than to personal ones can reduce tension and anxiety. Beyond that, structural role conflict may require a major change in the communication and power aspects of the larger system (Sampson and Marthas, 1977).

Role conflict is a clash of expectations. It may result from the incompatibility of realistic time demands and simultaneous role enactments, or from the incompatibility between a role occupant and the expectations of others about that role. Regardless of the cause, role conflict is problematic, especially in situations which are ambiguous or transitional.

GROUP STRUCTURES

When several persons relate to one another in a group, various individual differences appear. Some members relate actively, others are more passive; the active members are those who influence the group. These differences contribute to a pattern of *positions* as group structure forms. A position refers to one's standing in relation to others, or to one's place in the group's social system relative to power, leadership, and attractiveness. Each member occupies one or more positions in the group. The position is evaluated by the occupant and by other group members according to the perceived prestige of that position to the group. Evaluation by the group members designates the status of a position. Some positions may have equivalent status, but most are arranged in a hierarchical structural manner. High status positions are those which are most powerful, most respected, and have the greatest communication potential. Conversely, low status positions are the least powerful, least respected, and least satisfying (Shaw, 1971). Status is a vertical dimension in the ranking of group members. It may be ascribed by society's values, which are external to the group, or it may be achieved. Achieved status is attained by individuals or is conferred by internal group values (Anderson and Carter, 1978). Status develops by group consensus, and affects role enactment and degree of influence. It is not a static dimension but is subject to change. Changes in status often emerge from alterations in group goals or roles, and from the addition or loss of group members (Kreigh and Perko, 1979).

Every group has multiple structures and numerous positions within these structures. A member may occupy one or more positions and thus be expected to enact the behaviors of several positions. Whenever a task group exists there is a tendency to divide the activities and responsibilities among the members. As this process of distribution of function and differentiation of parts is stabilized, the group becomes structured in several ways. Four typical group structures emerge: *communication, sociometric, locomotion,* and *power* (Cartwright and Zander, 1953). Identification of the patterns formed by these structures permits the identification of individual positions and roles relative to a particular structure.

Communication

This structure reflects the rules, policies, and status, and determines the type, frequency, and level of participation. Members who occupy a powerful central position have the highest frequency of communication directed to them as compared with peripheral members.

Sociometric

This structure provides data on the degree to which group members are liked. Interaction links reflect member's choices which define central, isolated, and clustered members. This structure also determines how well a person is able to satisfy personal needs for affection and acceptance; when such needs are not gratified for isolated or peripheral members, they are likely to leave the group.

Locomotion

How the group moves toward its goal and the feasibility of changing positions within the group are determined by this structure. The degree to which members may shift roles and gain satisfaction has a marked influence on the morale of the group.

Power

The power structure influences the amount of autonomy, freedom, and activity of group members. It can be identified by determining the power differential between two or more positions in a group. Attributed power is a rank-ordered group consensus pertaining to the relative influence of members. Group members tend to perceive correctly other members' behavioral clues which represent their attributed power positions. The reactions of members are influenced by perceived power differential between themselves and more powerful members. Behavior toward members with high attributed power tends to be less directive and more deferential. Power-related behavior is also more likely to be initiated by others as an attempt to gain additional influence or acceptance. Members who perceive that they have greater influence tend to use power in direct proportion to the amount of power they believe they have. In an atmosphere of group competition for power, those members who already have power are more unlikely to share it (Lippitt et al., 1953).

Power is a commodity in any group. It may be distributed in order to achieve group goals, or it may be hoarded by one or more members. The group with marked inequity in the distribution of power tends to become problematic, thereby affecting the morale and productivity of the members. Members who believe they have little influence within the group are less inclined to commit themselves to group goal behaviors (Wilson and Kneisl, 1979).

Sources of Power Shaw (1971) identified several sources of power: *attraction, reward, coerciveness, legitimacy,* and *expertise.* A person is considered to have attraction power when other group members emulate that person's behavior. An individual with reward power is one who can provide positive rewards and remove negative effects. A person with coercive power is able to mediate punishment for proscribed behavior. Legitimate power is earned as a result of group consensus that power is deserved by specific members or by the positions they hold in the group. Power acquired through expertise is bestowed on persons perceived to have greater resources, skills, or knowledge. The effects of possessing power vary, depending on the source of power at a particular time and the need of the group for that type of power. Identification of group power structure may be made by answering the following questions:

- Whose decision carries the most weight?
- Who is listened to the most?
- Who receives the most attention from others?
- Who receives the least attention from others?   (Sampson and Marthas, 1977).

Within the various group structures, positions may have different consequences for individual members. Not all positions are equally attractive; for example, power and sociometric positions may be regarded differently. The attractiveness differential attached to group positions frequently motivates members to change positions within the group, or to leave the group when attempts to change positions fail. The desire to change or maintain a position influences the member's behavior. The drive to preserve or alter one's position may be countered by restraining forces of group norms or by the desire of other members for power, attention, or locomotion. The degree of satisfaction or frustration inherent in changing a position has a marked impact upon a member's morale, productivity, and mental health (Cartwright and Zander, 1953).

Group structure delineates patterned arrangements of roles which emerge as a function of group process in order to insure the stability, consistency, and viability of group life. Role structure often overlaps power, communication, and sociometric structures. The remainder of this chapter deals with the development of roles which are productive for the life of the group (role *differentiation*) and those which may be counterproductive (role *specialization*).

ROLE STRUCTURE DEVELOPMENT

Numerous theorists have proposed rationales that explain why roles develop in a small group. For a time, groups were viewed as the sum of the dynamics of the individuals. In other words, roles were believed to develop as a result of individual members' traits or needs. This premise was supported by the observation that members assume roles based on their childhood experiences combined with their current needs. Attention was upon the members' inclination to re-enact familiar roles, such as leader or scapegoat. Further observation of groups indicated that roles also developed as a function of group need. Every group requires a division of labor and needs individuals to fill those positions. Bales (1953) noted that all groups must develop role structures in order to deal with external tasks (group goals) and internal tasks (group maintenance). These two prominent functions of any group precipitated the emergence of two major divisions of roles: goal-focused and socioemotional-focused. By identifying the type of communication used by a member, observers could determine the particular functional role. Bales described a set of communication patterns which exemplified goal-directed versus socioemotional-directed functions. Although the occupants of these roles may vary, these two major functions must be accomplished and roles must develop to meet them during the groups' existence. For any group, both task and maintenance functions must be adequately served.

In small, informal groups without an assigned leader, the individual who initiates most of the ideas and begins to organize the group becomes the first task specialist and emerging leader. Eventually these administrative efforts begin to frustrate the immediate socioemotional needs of members, and another role develops, that of the socioemotional specialist whose function is to relieve tension and task pressure. This second emerging leader becomes the member who is most liked. Generally, two separate and distinct leaders emerge. The role differentiation of leaders appears to vary according to the extent that task functions prove costly or unrewarding. When the socioemotional needs of most members are met, and when commitment to the task is high, there may be a single leader who contributes to task issues as well as serves as the socioemotional specialist. In groups whose members have minimal or moderate commitment to task accomplishment, two-leader role differentiation is more likely, with the task leader ranked high on productivity but low on popularity. It appears that, when group task commitment is high, general leadership, popularity, and task specialization blend together, and separate socioemotional specialization is not necessary. When group task commitment is low, leadership and popularity are unlikely to merge, and separate socioemotional specialization becomes necessary for group viability. This suggests that a group leader spend time in task definition in order to enhance individual and group task commitment (Gustafson, 1973).

Egocentric Roles

Benne and Sheats (1948) elaborated on Bales' two-dimensional model of role classification and development, and added a third category of roles. These are identified not as group roles but as individual roles, which were considered counterproductive (Bonner, 1959). Benne and Sheats postulated that group behavior is a function of group development, and that task and maintenance roles are distributed and shared among members. Task roles are essentially administrative behaviors, and, depending upon the particular need of the group, any one of the task roles may become a position of leadership. Maintenance roles are behaviors concerned with the members as a group, and therefore encourage participation and interaction which maintain and enhance group relationships (Marram, 1978). The third category is composed of individual roles, or egocentric behaviors, which express aggression or seek action on personal matters at the expense of the group. Such behaviors are irrelevant to the group task and to group maintenance. These role occupants are not participants in the group purpose but act against the group. Bonner (1959) argued that these were not role enactments but were simple forms of intergroup conflict. Table 8-1 provides a descriptive compilation of group functional roles and individual roles.

From another perspective, the process of role development was perceived as a function of the interaction between individual needs and group processes (Bogdanoff and Elbaum, 1978). Whitaker and

Table 8-1   GROUP AND INDIVIDUAL FUNCTIONAL ROLES

Task Roles

Initiation	defines problem, proposes solution, mobilizes group toward problem-solving
Elaboration	illustrates ideas, predicts, and plans
Information and Opinion Seeker	requests data, opinions, ideas related to problem
Information and Opinion Giver	brings own experiences, opinions, and suggestions regarding group goals and values
Coordinator	clarifies ideas, offers suggestions to demonstrate relationships between them; harmonizes activities of members
Evaluator	measures group decisions and achievements against group standards and goals
Energizer	stimulates group to perform at a higher level
Orienter	summarizes discussion; raises questions regarding group's direction
Liaison	performs bridging function between group and external authorities; communicates group needs and concerns

Maintenance Roles

Encourager	accepts ideas with understanding, approval, and praise
Diplomat	mediates group conflicts and relieves tension; is sensitive and tactful
Process Observer	reflects observation of group process back to group
Communication Facilitator	uses skillful communication to enhance consensual validation; encourages other members to participate
Follower	passive member; frequently an audience in decision-making situations

Egocentric Roles

Aggressor	expresses behavior which reduces others' status and contributions; attacks the group, or its task
Blocker	uses resistive, negative behavior; returns to issues which have been rejected or discarded previously
Playboy	is aloof; displays lack of concern and involvement through "horseplay" or other irrelevant behavior
Monopolizer	assumes responsibility for maintaining communication; dominates group, creating group hostility
Recognition Seeker	attempts to gain admiration and attention by boasting of accomplishments, dressing flamboyantly, arriving late

Source: Compiled from Bales, 1953; Benne and Sheats, 1948; Kreigh and Perko, 1979

Lieberman's theory of focal conflict described in Chapter 6 provided one example of this approach.

Role Differentiation

As a group matures, it becomes more interdependent, complex, and integrated, which contributes to role distribution. Task and maintenance functions are shared among members, between leaders, and among leaders and members. As roles become differentiated, different patterns of group members' behavior can be identified. In other words, role differentiation is the result of the evolution of the group and follows the development of norms. Roles become differentiated during the control or second phase of group development, after the group has dealt with issues of inclusion (Shutz, 1966). The *gate keeper* of the group plays a decisive role in determining who may gain entry. This concept of a gate keeper member is very important and must be kept in mind when delivering health care to families. The family member who acts as gate keeper must be identified if one is to gain access to family groups in order to influence the change process.

Role development is a result of conscious and unconscious psychological elements. This formulation asserts that roles express idiosyncratic needs and also perform necessary psychological functions for groups, such as tension release and group maintenance (Gibbard, 1974).

Bridging Members The recurrent, or pendular developmental model introduced in Chapter 2 described the polarity of groups on a continuum with instrumental (task) behaviors allowing the group to adapt to the external environment shown at one extreme, and expressive (maintenance) behaviors related to internal integration of the group shown at the other. The group is described as swinging in a pendular fashion between the two poles, seeking to meet task and maintenance needs, but rejecting the extreme instrumental pole as too rigid and the extreme expressive pole as too isolated from external supplies (Anderson and Carter, 1978). The role structure which develops within the group influences and is influenced by the group's pendular motion. Differentiation of roles in this model reflects the attempt to resolve the contest between expressive versus instrumental needs. In a similar way the Bennis and Shepard model (Gibbard, 1974) related role development to group development and to the two major issues of power distribution and member interrelationships. These two issues are resolved sequentially through the development of role specialists, or *bridging* members who are the least conflicted about authority and intimacy and can facilitate compromise within the group. Bales and Slater (Gibbard, 1974) envisaged role development as an *evolutionary tree* with a developmental process branching according to functional divisions. In this explanation roles emerge at specific times and function during those periods. Role specialists symbolize major choices which confront the group during its development (Dunphy, 1974). As the group interacts with these role specialists it is able to resolve its major conflicts and issues. The scheme presented by Bogdanoff and Elbaum (1973) later in this chapter provides an example of this concept of role development.

ROLE SPECIALIZATION: CAUSES AND CONSEQUENCES

The conflicts and issues which arise during any group's lifetime create disequilibrium for individual members and for the group as a whole. This disequilibrium then becomes a catalyst for the development of role specialization. Specialized roles emerge and serve to restore intrapsychic and intragroup equilibrium. Therefore role specialization is, in part, a restorative effort to deal with conflict, authority, intimacy, or task issues. Role specialization, however, may inhibit an individual's potential to grow and may limit the individual's ability to assume other roles or experience other behaviors. The force of group pressure together with the individual's characteristic style of relating may lead to interpersonal entrapment, or *role lock*. The role specialist does not see alternative ways of relating and remains in a fixed position, such as that of scapegoat, isolate, or monopolizer. Role specialization phenomena affects all members of the group. The group unconsciously uses projection as a defense mechanism, and divides itself into actors (role specialists) and audience. Group emotion is projected to role specialists who become actors dramatizing the group conflict while the audience disclaims involvement but participates vicariously. In this way the conflict can be compressed into a small arena for resolution. Role specialists serve a dual purpose: they symbolize and express group conflicts, and facilitate their resolution (Gibbard, 1974).

Types of Specialization

A few types of specialized roles occur with such frequency that their labels have become part of our vocabulary. Scapegoat, clown, and deviant describe roles commonly found in everyday life. For group practitioners who must deal with these behaviors, however, their enactment constitutes a real challenge. It is helpful, then, to understand the intrapsychic and interpersonal group dynamics which cause these roles to be imbedded in group life.

The Deviant The deviant of the group can appear only after the group norms are established and the group has decided what is and what is not acceptable. The deviant behavior tests boundaries and norms by exhibiting actions which are not tolerated. In return, the group uses communication as a mechanism to exert power and to insure conformity by responding to the deviant with increasing frequency. If the deviant continues enacting this role, the frequency of directed interaction reaches a peak and declines at a rapid rate (Schacter, 1973). Then the group figuratively casts out the deviant member, diminishes communication with the deviant, and tries to ignore rather than seek to understand or change behavior. Members confirm the exclusion among themselves, sometimes with knowing glances or smiles. Any member whose demeanor or appearance differs from the majority may be a candidate for the role of deviant. Although behavioral expression of deviant members may vary from silence to agitation, the deviant is always an isolated member. If a deviant member continues in the role, the effect upon the deviant is loneliness, lowered self-esteem, and dissatisfaction with the group experience (Yalom, 1975). Isolation may be both the cause and effect of deviancy. The individual with limited communication and limited attractiveness for others occupies a lower sociometric status position in the group. These elements often propel the person into the role of deviant; ultimately, the deviant may terminate prematurely (Festinger et al., 1953). Prevention of deviant behavior has implications for the group selection process. Using a Noah's Ark principle of choosing group members is advocated as one way of avoiding this dilemma. Another suggested method is using the curative factor of universality (Yalom, 1975) to bind the group together so that isolated members are not permitted to develop into deviant members.

The Scapegoat The scapegoat role has been historically significant as a target of aggression in both group and social phenomena. Scapegoating provides an outlet for aggression that does not threaten the unity, stability, and integrity of the group. The scapegoat represents the group's anxiety concerning its own inadequacy, and the scapegoat's futile reactions sustains the role. Through a process of group denial, displacement, and projection, the group unites in a cohesive way against the scapegoat who now represents impotence in the face of authority (Dunphy, 1974). The vulnerability of the scapegoat binds the group together, providing a common purpose and increased sense of intimacy. The target member chosen for the aggression is incapable of retaliation, while the group avoids guilt through rationalization of its action. Blame, censure, and condemnation of the scapegoat provide a vehicle for aggression. Often the group uses a triad arrangement in its attack, with the attacker, the scapegoat, and the group audience forming the three points of the triangle. The degree to which the scapegoat provokes attack, invites aggression, or offers defense influences the amount of direct aggression. Greater provocation and minimal defense are likely to unleash greater hostility. Although the scapegoat helps the group release its anxiety, guilt, tension, and hostility, the price paid by that role is increased isolation and lowered self-esteem. When scapegoating occurs, the leader's task is to help the group heighten its awareness of unconscious feelings of frustration and inadequacy, and to encourage a supportive atmosphere in order to prevent the exclusion or isolation of the scapegoat (Toker, 1972). Scapegoating is a dramatic expression of a group's endeavor to deny its own imperfection and to exploit an individual member. It is indicative of a dysfunctional group, and its occurrence impedes the group's productive efforts (Stafford, 1977).

The Humorist The humorist occupies a position on the edge of the group. This member is able to challenge opinions and to present possibly unacceptable ideas disguised as humor. Comedy may be used to provide an escape from despair or a special insight into tragedy. Generally, groups with humorist role-specialists are more productive, and its activities are more satisfying. Humor may assume different styles and cause different effects: sarcasm is a powerful but unpopular style of humor; clowning is a popular but powerless style (Hare, 1976). Humor serves paradoxical purposes; it has the potential to elevate and diminish, to isolate and bind, to give pleasure or pain, and to defend or attack. It has been identified as the honest element in communication (Grotjohn, 1971), as an element which assists sanity and balance, and as a contagious social gesture (Hatlan, 1962). Laughter is born from the precarious nature of the human condition and from the realization that humankind is at the same time infinitely grand and infinitely wretched. Laughter often has a corrective quality. Ridicule can function to maintain group norms when an idea which is "laughed at" becomes an object which is isolated or excluded. Laughter may serve an inclusive, binding purpose, forging a bond of empathy or alleviating a common fear. The idea rather than the individual is isolated, while the group members are included in the universal experience of laughter. Humor is sometimes a double-edged sword which cuts as well as cures. It has significant implications for group interventions, since humor can also be employed to lower group productivity by permitting avoidance of the task. Wit and humor may constitute an attack as well as a defense for individual members. Humor and laughter are tools for harnessing curative factors for binding and healing, but they must be used with care. The actions of the humorist, who serves an important function for the group, may need regulation if humorous communication is thought to mask anxiety, or if it is used as a form of avoidance to deflect the group from real issues.

The Silent Member   The silent member enacts a role which is relatively safe. There are numerous motivational causes for remaining silent during group interactions. These include fears of self-disclosure, of failure to meet self-demands for perfection, of attack by another member, and of unleashing one's own aggression. Prolonged silence may also constitute a form of covert punishment for the group. Group members often react to silent members by ignoring them or becoming frustrated by their apparent lack of participation in the group. The silent-role specialist experiences the safety of uninvolvement, but pays the price of isolation and diminished self-worth. Yalom (1975) suggests that the leader use an approach which acknowledges the silent member, consider the cause for silence, and comment on the nonverbal behavior, perhaps by stating that all members may not be quite ready to speak. An alternative approach is to ask for other member's reactions to the silence, and then request that the silent member validate or refute their comments. When dealing with a silent member one must realize that silence is not tantamount to indifference.

The preceding examples of role specialization present a real challenge to group leaders undertaking task and maintenance functions of the group. In addition, leaders must deal with two variations of role specialization — *role lock* and *pairing.*

ROLE LOCK AND INTERVENTION STRATEGY

Role development is a continuous process throughout the life of the group. The process is productive as long as roles are fluid, flexible, and growth-promoting, but may become nonproductive if roles become fixed and rigid. This latter phenomenon is termed *role lock* and results from the interaction of group issues at a particular stage of development with dynamics of individual members. A group can be said to act much like a vacuum cleaner which draws certain members into available role spaces. Available roles which seem to serve group needs may not necessarily enhance group development but instead may impede it. Role lock is an example of such an impediment.

Role lock develops as a compromise solution to a focal or group conflict resulting from interaction between disturbing and reactive issues. Focal conflict (as noted in an earlier chapter) is shared conflict caused by a wish and a fear of consequences if the wish is fulfilled. A focal conflict may precipitate various roles and role locks as a way of dealing with unresolved group conflict. The forces of disturbing wishes and reactive fears create a group atmosphere which sets the stage for role specialization. Individuals with characteristics which fit a certain specialized role are then drawn into that position. The person selected for the role has either unconsciously collaborated with the selection process or helped to create the current group atmosphere which asks that the role be filled. Table 8-2 describes various types of role locks and behaviors characteristic of specific disturbing and reactive issues.

The management of role-lock situations calls for a two-pronged approach. First an approach is made toward members occupying the role-lock position and then toward the group system which encourages and perpetuates the process. It is not necessary to use these approaches simultaneously, since the intervention chosen depends on the group's reaction to the role lock. If the group ignores or avoids the issue and its own contribution, the interventions should be arrived at by increasing the group's cognitive awareness of the process; identifying the disturbing and reactive issues; and attending to the role-enactment behaviors of the individual. Such statements as, "You are doing the group's work" or "Why does the group allow this to continue?" or "Perhaps we are afraid to get involved in working out our feelings," are helpful.

The most common reaction of the group is cognitive awareness that a member is occupying a role, but this is accompanied by lack of awareness by the group of its collision in locking a member in place. Effective management of this situation requires recognition of the dual nature of role lock and use of interventions which clarify the components of this phenomenon.

In dealing with problems attendant on role specialization, one must realize that the stage of group development influences the

Table 8–2   ROLE LOCKS, BEHAVIOR CHARACTERISTICS, AND RELATED ISSUES

Role Lock	Behaviors	Disturbing Issue	Reactive Issue
Mistruster	Rejects trust, elicits hostility and attack from others, which confirms distrust; group uses mistrust to avoid the task	Disclosure	Concealment
Truster	Shows excessive or premature self-disclosure which threatens members by denying their need to mistrust for a time; may become group deviant	Disclosure	Need for self-esteem
Professional patient or scapegoat	Acts as self-styled expert and perfectionist who tries to undermine the leader; may become disruptive by causing the group to question its competency; may become scapegoat as group hostility mounts	Expertise	Domination vs. submission
Monopolizer or scapegoat	Functions as competitive, attention-seeking member whose excessive talking reactivates old group conflicts with family of origin; members feel victimized and show resentment which increases the anxiety and compulsive behavior of the monopolizer	Control	Domination vs. submission
Performer	Competes for love and acceptance; is seductive "scene-stealer" who generates interest and vicarious experiences for passive members	Authenticity	Sincerity vs. deception
Rescuer	Performs as oversupportive rescuer who fears conflict and uses an altruistic shield; initial group reaction is positive, but later group is exasperated; group may then attack or ignore the "do-gooder"	Caring	Help vs. hurt
Warrior	Displays overt anger and transmits group anger to the leader; initially group is intrigued; later the group may be terrorized or intimidated	Violence	War vs. peace
Victim	Assumes victim role, internalizes anger and blames fate; initially encouraged by rescue fantasy of members; rejection of suggestions causes group to become hostile, thus causing another bad experience for the victim	Fatalism	Good luck vs. bad luck
Isolate	Assumes passive, dependent, isolated role and is fearful of self-display; at first is ignored by group; later group becomes curious or hostile— isolate becomes a target for hostility or protection from the group	Alienation	Involvement vs. separation

Source: After Bogdanoff and Elbaum, 1978; and Yalom, 1975

emergence of role specialization.   In addition, individual dynamics determine who occupies certain roles, and group focal conflict defines which roles develop (Bogdanoff and Elbaum, 1978).

PAIRING AND SUBGROUPING

Another problematic area in group life is the establishment of pairing and subgrouping, both of which often work at cross-purposes to task and maintenance functions.   Role pairing may be described as a mutual attraction of two group members, or, more specifically, as the joined support of two or more members in a maneuver to avoid task accomplishment (Kaplan and Sadock, 1971).   Pairing may occur early in group development if the dyad has had a previous relationship.   Pairing or subgrouping often occurs during periods of intragroup conflict.   The group is fragmented into smaller subgroups in an effort to increase the security and satisfaction of members.   These pairs or subgroups compete with other subgroups or with the leader. In psychotherapeutic groups this pairing may be constructive if the pair is able to explore the unconscious reasons for their attraction to each other.   It is therapeutic for members of the pair to recognize that each has chosen the other in order to fill unconscious needs for dependency, intimacy, or power.   Pairing is destructive when it remains unexplored or when the pairing excludes interaction with other members (Lego, 1978).

Cliques and Cabals

Pairing and subgrouping occur as attempts to meet security needs by means of a coalition.   These needs may be conscious or unconscious and may vary in intent.   Two types of subgroup coalitions which differ in intent are *cliques* and *cabals*.   A clique has a socioemotional orientation and serves as a protection for otherwise powerless members who may see themselves as partial failures in the group as a whole.   The clique is a compensatory subgroup which provides reassurance, and is characterized by withdrawal from the central group.   A cabal, on the other hand, has a power-seeking orientation and holds the promise of seizing control by those not in power.   Unlike the clique, the cabal is a subgroup of secure members who join together with the intent to wield power by changing rules, policies, or procedures (Bales, 1953).

Types of Pairing

According to Mills (1967) role pairing serves a defensive and tension-reducing purpose for members.   Among the types of pairing patterns are: *lovers, enemies, friends*, and *collaborators*. Lovers are an intertwined dyad, the partners fusing together to achieve self-completion and gratification. Each half of the pair lacks a sense of self-definition, therefore any independent move is perceived as a form of rejection. Through exclusive mutual admiration, cooperation, and sharing the pair resists intrusion by other group members. Because membership in the dyad excludes the assumption of other roles, it leads to stagnation for dyad members and for the group as a whole. Enemies are members who are protagonists or rivals, whose contest with each other provides vicarious pleasure for the group, enabling the group to avoid work. Each member loses identity in the struggle, and the potential to assume other roles is reduced. Two types of pairing which serve task accomplishment are the pairing of friends and collaborators. Friendship pairing is based on mutual respect, which may be tested by disappointment, conflict, or work, but which encourages growth and individuality. The pairing of friends often introduces a marked generative capacity for the group. Collaborators are members who are able to work together to pursue a joint goal as a way of reducing group tension, but who are not committed to intimacy or mutual satisfaction. The boundaries between friends and between collaborators are more permissible than those between lovers and enemies. This allows a wider variety of experience with other group members, and a greater development of interpersonal skills. Kadis et al. (1965) identified another type of dysfunctional pairing: the *passive-dominant* dyad. In this form of pairing each member enables the other to maintain a growth-inhibiting pattern of placating and aggression. This reciprocal interaction exploits both members, limiting their opportunities for other role enactment.

Bion (1959) provided a theoretical rationale for the development of pairing phenomenon within his basic-assumption framework. The development of pairing may be understood in terms of the group's collective anxiety regarding separation versus engulfment, and how this anxiety is expressed over time. Pairing occurs later in group life, following flight-fight and dependency assumptions, and is generally considered a more advanced way of handling anxiety. It surfaces after the group revolt, when the group has lost some of its dependency on the leader, but is still subject to conflicted fears of engulfment and estrangement. Following revolt, pairing is a kind of reunification process which protects the group from recent fighting and from possible dissolution (Sampson and Marthas, 1977). Characteristically, the group turns toward two members in the hope that they will protect group identity and survival. This couple symbolizes intimacy and sexuality as a defense against dependency or aggression (Kernberg, 1978).

Expressions of hopefulness and expectations are typical thematic material at this time and may be used as evidence that a pairing basic-assumption group exists. Manifest content themes proclaim the "unborn leader" in the form of a person or idea which members hope will protect the group from hatred or despair. These hopeful expectations provide the stimulus for the eager and attentive focus of the other members on the paired interaction of the symbolic rescuer (Bion, 1959).

CLINICAL EXAMPLE: ANALYSIS OF ROLE DEVELOPMENT IN A MENTAL HEALTH GROUP

A supportive group for single parents met one evening a week at a community mental health center. It was a closed, three-month, time-limited group consisting of seven members who were either widowed or divorced. Selection criteria for the group included: referral by a staff member of the mental health center; male or female parent with at least one child under eighteen years old living at home. One primary task was to begin to redirect their lives in an independent manner. An additional task was to share the concerns of single parenthood. The group was led by Bill, a psychiatric nurse. During the first few meetings the group members were cautiously polite with one another, frequently expressing sympathetic remarks. The group's most recently widowed member was Debbie, a twenty-three-year old secretary who was struggling with the demands of raising two toddlers, managing a household, and working part-time. She was a shy, timid woman who seldom initiated comments during the meetings. Debbie usually sat next to Marcia, a middle-aged, attractive divorceé whose only son was about to graduate from high school and enter the navy. Marcia seemed to take Debbie under her wing, like a fledgling sparrow, protecting her from making decisions by patting her hand and telling her, "You have plenty of time to think about that. You have your whole life ahead of you." Marica also began transporting Debbie to and from the meetings, as "it is a good way for Debbie to save money." By the second month, group members began ignoring Debbie, perhaps annoyed by her lack of participation, using the rationalization that Marcia would tend to Debbie's needs. About the same time Bill was taken ill suddenly and another staff member, Jack, agreed to fill in as group leader. The group received the news of the change of leadership with little comment, although Harry, a salesman, suggested that he would be happy to fill the role of therapist if Jack would split the fee. This comment was met with smiles and laughter, as if the members knew they could rely on Harry to provide a joke. For the following two weeks attendence was erratic and the group seemed unable to attend to its tasks. Conversation was superficial and socially focused. Marcia, as the most verbal and assertive member, began to assume increasing command of the group, suggesting that the group plan a party to celebrate Bill's return the following week. Jack seemed unable or unwilling to direct the sessions to focus on group goals. When Bill did return, he apologized for his inability to prepare them for his absence and began to explore what it had meant to the group to have had yet another loss imposed on them at a time when they were struggling to deal with their marital losses. Marcia replied that she was relieved to see him return, as "the other leader, 'what's his name,' really couldn't understand us."

The following roles are evident in this example. Debbie, the passive, silent member, quickly became the isolate, although she did pair with the more assertive Marcia. Marcia assumed the role of rescuer, or Helpful Hannah, both for Debbie and the group as a whole. She changed her role into one of assumed leadership — when the group's dependency needs for a caring, helping role emerged — during Bill's absence. The disturbing issue focused on the group's fear for safety precipitated by the loss of its assigned leader. The group's anger was denied (lack of comment regarding Bill's initial absence) and then displaced on the substitute leader, a less threatening and ineffective person (Jack as scapegoat). Harry, the group humorist, attempted to alleviate the member's fears, by jokingly offering himself as leader. Debbie's individual needs for protection were expressed in her passivity and acceptance of Marcia's attention, which then cast her into the role of silent member and isolate. In a reciprocal way, Marcia was able to deny her forthcoming loss of motherhood role by providing surrogate mothering for Debbie. Neither one was able to escape the role lock, and, as a pair, were unable to contribute to the group's task function of sharing parenthood concerns and initiating a more independent life-style.

SUMMARY

This chapter described various role enactment concepts including role components, role conflict, and role structure development. Role structure was linked to other group structures (communication, sociometric, locomotion, and power) and to group pendular issues within the life cycle of the group. Finally, the causes, consequences, and types of role specialization phenomena were discussed.

REFERENCES

Anderson, R.E., and J. Carter. *Human Behavior in the Social Environment, A Social Systems Approach*. 2nd ed. Chicago: Aldine, 1978.

Bales, R.F. "A Theoretical Framework for Interaction Process Analysis." In *Group Dynamics, Research and Theory*, D. Cartwright and A. Zander, Eds. Evanston, IL.: Row, Peterson, 1953.

Benne, K.D., and P. Sheats. "Functional Roles of Group Members." *Journal of Social Issues* Vol. 4, No. 2, 1948, pages 41–49.

Bion, W.R. *Experiences in Groups*. New York: Basic Books, 1959.

Bogdanoff, M.A., and P.L. Elbaum. "Role Lock: Dealing with Monopolizers, Mistrusters, Isolates, Helpful Hannahs, and Other Assorted Characters in Psychotherapy." *International Journal of Group Psychotherapy* Vol. 28, No. 2, 1978, pages 247–262.

Bonner, H. *Group Dynamics, Principles and Applications*. New York: Ronald Press, 1959.

Cartwright, D., and A. Zander, Eds. *Group Dynamics Research and Theory*. Evanston, IL.: Row, Peterson, 1953.

Dunphy, D.C. "Phases, Roles, and Myths in Self-Analytic Groups." In *Analysis of Groups*, G.S. Gibbard, J.J. Hartman, and R.D. Mann, Eds. San Francisco: Jossey-Bass, 1974.

Festinger, L.; S. Schacter; and K. Back. "The Operation of Group Standards." In *Group Dynamics, Research and Theory*, D. Cartwright and A. Zander, Eds. Evanston, IL.: Row, Peterson, 1953.

Fisher, L., and R.C. Warren. "The Concept of Role Assignment in Family Therapy." *International Journal of Group Psychotherapy* Vol. 22, No. 1, 1972, pages 60–76.

Gibbard, G.S. "Individuation, Fusion and Role Specialization." In *Analysis of Groups*, G.S. Gibbard, J.J. Hartman, and R.D. Mann, Eds. San Francisco: Jossey-Bass, 1974.

Grotjohn, M. "Laughter in Group Psychotherapy." *International Journal of Group Psychotherapy* Vol. 21, No. 2, 1971, pages 234–238.

Gustafson, D.P. "Task Commitment and Role Differentiation." *Human Relations* Vol. 26, No. 5, 1973, pages 667–679.

Hare, A.P. *Handbook of Small Group Research*. 2nd ed. New York: Free Press, 1976.

Hatlan, T. *Orientation to Theater*. New York: Appleton-Century-Crofts, 1962.

Kadis, A.L.; J.D. Krasner; C. Winick; and S.H. Foulkes. *A Practicum of Group Psychotherapy*. New York: Hoeber Medical Division, Harper & Row, 1965.

Kaplan, H.L., and B.J. Sadock, Eds. *Comprehensive Group Psychotherapy*. Baltimore: Williams and Wilkins, 1971.

Kernberg, O.F. "Leadership and Organizational Functioning: Organizational Regression." *International Journal of Group Psychotherapy* Vol. 28, No. 1, 1978, pages 3–25.

Kreigh, H.Z., and J.E. Perko. *Psychiatric and Mental Health Nursing: A Commitment to Care and Concern*. Reston, VA.: Reston Publishing, 1979.

Lego, S. "Group Dynamic Theory and Application." In *Comprehensive Psychiatric Nursing*, J. Haber et al., Eds. New York: McGraw-Hill, 1978.

Lippitt, R.; N. Polansky; F. Redl; and S. Rosen. "The Dynamics of Power." In *Group Dynamics, Research and Theory*, D. Cartwright and A. Zander, Eds. Evanston, IL.: Row, Peterson, 1953.

Marram, G.D. *The Group Approach in Nursing Practice.* 2nd ed. St. Louis: C.V. Mosby, 1978.

Mills, T.M. *The Sociology of Small Groups.* Englewood Cliffs, N.J.: Prentice-Hall, 1967.

Nevill, D., and S. Damico. "Role Conflict in Women as a Function of Marital Status." *Human Relations* Vol. 28, No. 5, 1975, pages 487–498.

Sampson, E.E., and M.S. Marthas. *Group Process for the Health Professions.* New York: Wiley, 1977.

Schacter, S. "Deviation, Rejection, and Communication." In *Interpersonal Behavior in Small Groups,* R.J. Ofshe, Ed. Englewood Cliffs, N.J.: Prentice-Hall, 1973.

Shaw, M.E. *Group Dynamics: The Psychology of Small Group Behavior.* New York: McGraw-Hill, 1971.

Shutz, W. *Interpersonal Underworld.* Palo Alto, CA.: Science and Behavior Books, 1966.

Stafford, L.L. "Scapegoating." *American Journal of Nursing* Vol. 77, No. 3, 1977, pages 406–409.

Starr, P.D. "Marginality, Role Conflict, and Status Inconsistency as Forms of Stressful Interaction." *Human Relations* Vol. 30, No. 10, 1977, pages 949–961.

Toker, E. "The Scapegoat as an Essential Group Phenomenon." *International Journal of Group Psychotherapy* Vol. 22, No. 3, 1972, pages 320–332.

Wilson, H.S., and C.R. Kneisl. *Psychiatric Nursing.* Menlo Park, CA.: Addison-Wesley, 1979.

Yalom, I.D. *The Theory and Practice of Group Psychotherapy.* 2nd ed. New York: Basic Books, 1975.

9

Group Dynamics: Leadership Roles and Functions

Lenore Bolling Phipps

Leadership is an issue in all groups and a phenomenon that has long intrigued group observers. Leadership style has inspired and intimidated countless groups regardless of their composition or form. Implicit in the term *leader* is its dialectic counterpart *follower,* and the interaction between leader and follower is crucial in group dynamics. One cannot lead without followers; one cannot follow without a leader. This interrelationship may assume many forms, change over time, enhance or impair group productivity, and meet or negate the group's needs.

It is the purpose of this chapter to explore the dynamic interplay between leader and follower by identifying the concepts, functions, and styles of authority relations; discussing coleadership; and examining problematic areas inherent in the leadership role.

ESTABLISHING A LEADER

As indicated in Chapter 5, during the first stage of group development members seek a leader who is willing to counter feelings of insecurity and dependency. In immature groups the members give up a measure of autonomy and separateness in their search for the protection and direction of a leader. Not until the members join together in the group "revolt" do they attempt to retrieve some of their power from the leader and begin to take more responsibility for the group's direction.

The term "leader" has diverse connotations. The leader may be the person with the greatest influence or highest sociometric ranking or someone who achieves, through performance or attributes, the function of guiding the group toward its goal. The leader may be designated or assigned to the leadership role by an external authority. In some instances leadership may not reside with a single individual but be distributed among all or several members who influence the group's performance at any given time (Shaw, 1971). In this case leadership is defined by the enactment of leader functions or behaviors.

An accepted view of leadership in terms of small group dynamics depends on the nature and distribution of functions or behaviors within a group rather than on any specific person. In one group the designated leader may retain or dominate leadership functions while in another the members may perform the majority of leadership functions. The perspective of distributed rather than centralized leadership provides a more encompassing and less restrictive view of leadership functions (Sampson and Marthas, 1977).

In general, effective leadership harnesses total group resources thereby utilizing group members in the enactment of leadership functions. Mills (1967) referred to leadership as an executive process in which the executive role is assumed by persons who accept responsibility for the group and strive to increase its potential. According to Mills, this executive process is distributed among the group members. Entry into this executive system is determined by a set of intellectual, moral, affective, and behavioral orientations, and is monitored by constant feedback which supports the group's normative values. Further discussion of the executive level of group interactions is found in Chapter 5.

CONCEPTS OF LEADERSHIP

Group leadership is a complex interaction among various factors affecting the group: orientation, composition, expectations, needs, tasks, and setting. Changing any one of these factors precipitates the need for a complementary and responsive leadership adaptation. For example, if resistance to the task threatens a group, members will often seek or respond to firm, structured leadership. If the leader does not help the group find a solution which diminishes resistance, members tend to replace the ineffectual leader with a new one (Hamblin, 1973).

What actually determines leadership? The emergent leader is one who embodies group norms, is aware of group needs and weaknesses, and is capable of facilitating positive group movement. Group norms are evident in two areas of group life: task and socioemotional functions. Usually two leaders emerge to meet these needs. The task leader usually appears first and is followed by the emergence of the socioemotional leader. These differentiated leaders are necessary for group productivity and cohesion (Lego, 1978). Task and socioemotional leadership functions are often distributed among the members. If a group does not produce a socioemotional leader, a scapegoat may be selected to help the group discharge emotional tensions (Hare, 1976). (For a discussion of scapegoat role enactment see Chapter 8.)

Leaders tend to be seen as possessing more favorable traits than do members, although those traits are not perceived as extreme enough to be deviant. The member who does most of the talking during sessions or makes most of the decisions often becomes the leader, unless the talking and decision making aggravates other members. In any communication network the person who receives the greatest number of messages tends to be regarded as the leader. The more one person attempts to influence others, the greater the chances of that person successfully assuming a leadership role. Power, influence, and consistency are factors which shape assumed leadership. The more influence someone has, the greater is that person's ability to direct others and to resist being directed. Conversely, persons with less influence react toward others with greater deference and with more nondirective approaches (Hare, 1976).

Authoritarian versus Egalitarian Leaders

Two basic leadership styles have been identified: *authoritarian* and *egalitarian*. Authoritarian leaders tend to be status-conscious, self-oriented, egocentric, and aggressive. Emergent leaders, when contrasted with designated leaders, tend to be more aggressive and authoritarian, perhaps because dominating behaviors are necessary to establish and to maintain nondesignated leadership. Once a member has assumed the nondesignated leadership role it is difficult to reverse that position.

Egalitarian leaders tend to be group-oriented, goal-oriented tension-reducers who are more able to share leadership when necessary. The traits of individuals who become leaders are related to the needs of the small group as determined by the group's composition of members and culture. The nature of leadership and leader characteristics vary depending upon the nature and characteristics of the group (Hare, 1976).

Effective leadership requires flexibility, sensitivity, and ability to discharge or relinquish responsibilities when conditions change. Situational demands within the group and external expectations influence the type of leadership qualities which are needed for effective group work (Cartwright and Zander, 1953). As group size and distance between members increase, the distribution of power, prestige, or skills in the group tends to become unequal. The member with the greatest power, prestige, or required skills often becomes the leader (Hare, 1976).

Although a single individual may become the controlling member, other central figures are discernible as personifications of object identification, drive identification, or ego supports. The potential of central figures to direct group members accelerates if these individuals also are designated leaders. The central figure may become for other members either a loved or feared object of identification, perceived by them as an *ego ideal,* or as a *tyrant.* Drive objects of aggression or love may be represented by the group scapegoat or the group idol. The central figure who embodies ego supports may assume the role of the *organizer,* who reduces guilt, the *hero,* the *seducer,* or the *good example,* who activates defenses against instinctual drives. The traits and functions of persons who become leaders, as well as the attributes of critical group figures, are related to the overall needs of the group (Hare, 1976).

LEADERSHIP FUNCTIONS

For the neophyte group leader, establishing and maintaining an effective therapeutic group may be an awesome responsibility. Leadership functions and interventions presented in this section are intended to serve as guidelines in that challenging endeavor.

Every designated leader has the responsibility for creating and maintaining the group as a whole, while helping to build a culture which enhances accomplishment of the group's goals and attends to the individual member's needs. Through leadership style and orientation, the designated leader influences the potential of the group.

At the same time the group leader is maintaining a dual orientation. Through participant observation the leader remains both within and outside of the group boundary. This dual orientation is necessary to monitor group dynamics and development objectively.

Mills (1967) in discussing the leader's role and responsibility asked three core questions: What is the group's purpose? What psychosocial processes are essential to accomplish the group's purpose? What is needed to enhance those processes, in terms of resources, style, and feedback?

The Primary Task

Determining and adhering to the group's purpose is a primary task for the leader. This primary task influences decisions regarding creation, time, preparation, frequency, and length of the meetings in addition to type of member activity, style of leadership, member selection criteria, group expectations, and procedural rules. For example, if the stated purpose of the group is to increase assertiveness, the group will likely be short term, structured, and somewhat didactic, and the members will be expected to role-play behaviors within the group. Leader interventions will focus largely on individual performance. If, on the other hand, the purpose of an interpersonal group is to increase the insight of its members, the group will tend to be long term and relatively unstructured. The cognitive, affective, and behavioral styles of the members will be channeled toward self-awareness and alternative interpersonal behaviors. Leader interventions in an interpersonal, insight-oriented psychotherapy group tend to focus upon the group as a whole in a context of here-and-now issues in the group.

Once the group's purpose has been determined and delineated, the groundwork of building and maintaining a social system can begin. Early attrition of members has the potential to sabotage a fledgling group. The need for thorough preparation to familiarize members with the orientation and contractual obligations cannot be overemphasized. Anxiety levels of members and leaders are often high during the initial phase of the group. Therefore, providing information, correcting misperceptions, and guaranteeing safety and nonjudgmental acceptance are essential in regulating the anxiety of members and leaders.

Establishing Norms

Sustaining the psychosocial processes essential to a group's purpose is accomplished by leader functions which help build the group's culture. Because the group itself is a change agent (Yalom, 1975), the leader must endeavor to establish norms which encourage interpersonal relatedness. Participation, careful self-disclosure, nonjudgmental acceptance, rules concerning feedback, and receptivity to change are norms which precede a positive group experience. Norms are created fairly early in group life and, in the first stage of the group, the leader is in an influential position to determine norms. The position of the leader in shaping norms is unique in two respects: first, the leader is the technical expert who exerts influence by virtue of status and specialized skill or knowledge, and, second, the leader is considered the model participant who sets an example of honest, spontaneous responsiveness, and nonjudgmental acceptance. The leader may deliberately choose to join the group, thereby reducing the distance between leader and members through the use of self-disclosure and status denial (Yalom, 1975).

In addition to helping set norms for the group, the leader must be aware of current needs of the group at a particular stage of development. This includes awareness of dependency and inclusive issues in the formative stage of the group; recognition of conflict, independency, and intimacy issues in the working phase; and awareness of separation issues during the termination stage.

While contributing to the group culture by encouraging cohesion through various means, such as the use of curative factors (Yalom, 1975), the leader also begins to transfer some responsibility for the group to the group members. This does not mean, however, that the leader relinquishes overall responsibility. By facilitating member-to-member interaction, eliciting feedback, and communicating to members confidence in the group's capacity to accomplish the task the leader integrates the group members into a cohesive, working, reality-oriented unit (Mann, 1967).

Marram (1978) distinguished between leadership functions and leadership interventions. Leadership functions are those which are not relinquished to group members. They include responsibility for facilitating cohesion, providing for a safe environment, monitoring growth, and enhancing individuals' growth. Interventions refer to specific behaviors or actions which facilitate the group's goal, and may be shared with the group. Thus, group members may enact leadership interventions but not leadership functions, since those lie within the realm of the leader's responsibility.

Monitoring Process and Content

One of the more complex functions of the leader is monitoring process and content, which represent the warp and woof of group interaction and form the fabric or pattern of the group. It is the leader's responsibility to recognize the relationship between content and process, for it is the content of group interaction which provides clues to understanding the process (Lego, 1978). Monitoring group process requires cognitive and affective recognition of the group field and those factors which influence the occurrence or nonoccurrence of events. Monitoring group events should include: observation of overt and covert behavior; informational decoding of verbal and non-verbal behavior; inference of messages that link individual members to the group system; and formulation and testing of analysis of behaviors (Mills, 1967). In other words, the leader must identify what is occurring in the group and how and why it is occurring, and he or she must be able to do something about it.

Monitoring Skills Monitoring group interaction requires complex skills in which perception, cognition, and interpersonal abilities are used to provide ongoing feedback to the group. It involves leaders' ability to analyze their own participation, as well as the members' participation, with detachment and objectivity, and to sensitively assess and comment on members' verbal and nonverbal interactions. The goal of monitoring is to provide reflective feedback regarding behavior, to enable the group to examine its own transactions, and to integrate group events and experiences within the context of here-and-now reality.

Feedback may take various forms, including:

- Specific descriptions of behaviors.
- Description of the effects of behavior on leader or members.
- Requests to have views consensually validated.
- Interaction of problem-solving efforts regarding direction and alternatives.

The timing of interventions is critical and requires an accurate assessment of group readiness to accept feedback. A general rule for leaders is to wait until anxiety is replaced by trust and cohesion before risking confrontation or interpretation. Clarification, reflection, and support are intervention techniques which may be attempted earlier in the development of the groups.

Monitoring Problems There are other problematic features inherent in attempts to monitor or process group material. One problem is that it is difficult to interact and observe performance at the same time. This means that observations of others may be immediate and reflexive while perceptions of self can only be made reflectively. Processing group interaction runs counter to social norms, is not considered "polite," and is often denied. One way to counter this is to encourage members to offer feedback regarding the leader's behavior. It is not unusual, however, for leaders to fear that such commentary may threaten their appearance of strength, competence, or sagacity (Sampson and Marthas, 1977).

Leadership requires attention to individual member's needs, to the group as a whole, and to cognitive and affective understanding of the experience of group participation (Kanter, 1976). Effective leadership includes the development of an empathic relationship with group members. Self-awareness, perceptiveness, and empathy are helped by a wide range of life experiences, by exposure to diverse cultures, and by the ability to tolerate ambiguity. It is apparent from this discussion that group leadership skills are extremely comprehensive (MacLennan, 1975).

AUTHORITY RELATIONSHIPS

Authority relationships are an example of the interplay between members and the leader. The emotional needs of the group as a whole, as opposed to the leader's intrapsychic needs, may be noted in five different types of authority interactions: *dependent/nurturant, insurgent/coercive, bureaucratic, idealistic,* and *democratic* (Mills, 1967).

Underlying those types of authority relationships are various dynamic issues. The need to be cared for is evident in the dependent/ nurturant relationship, in which members give up individuality in order to guarantee the leader's provision of security. This dependent/nurturant stance is frequently accompanied by repressed anger and jealously among the members who fear depletion of the leader's resources. The insurgent/coercive relationship between leader and members is typical of the common need to control aggression, since both leader and members perceive the other as the aggressor. This type of authority precipitates mutual guardedness and constraint, and results in the coalescing of members in the face of frequent checks on their loyalty by the leader. This divisive group relationship has limited task effectiveness, for the energy of the group is diverted to constraining aggressive influences. The need to avoid failure is seen in bureaucratic leader-member relationships in which the common need of leader and members is to avoid making mistakes. Multiple rules and procedures are used to guard against the possibility of failure. The leader is perceived as a symbol of safety and righteousness, and the members demand explicit rules in order to avoid all risks. The leader tries to protect the group from error and deviance by using excessive organization, formality, regulation, indoctrination, and diminished emotional relatedness. Group need to accomplish an ideal is evident in the fourth type of authority relationship in which the group forms to pursue a nonnegotiable, sacred ideal. Members identify with one another and with the leader in the attempt to attain the ideal. The last type of authority relationship, the democratic group, differs from the others in that the thrust is not for self-protection but for generativity, and the impetus is to create a group in which leader and members relate as partners.

The role of leader and the role of members are often interchangeable; leadership of the group is differentiated, distributed, and transitory. The democratic group accepts a sense of responsibility for its own growth, providing a climate which deals with relationships both cognitively and emotionally.

Intrapsychic Influences Variation in authority relationships may also originate in the leader's philosophy. Personal beliefs influence a leader's style, and because initial power rests with the leader, philosophical beliefs of the leader may influence the members. As in a self-fulfilling prophecy, the leader's beliefs may be validated by the group's behavior. Leader expectations are absorbed by the members and enacted in the group. For example, if the leader distrusts others, believes that people basically dislike work and need to be controlled by a powerful, strong leader, the resulting leadership style is likely to be authoritarian. On the other hand, if the leader believes that most people enjoy work and are capable of initiative and autonomy, the leadership style is likely to be problem-solving and democratic (Sampson and Marthas, 1977).

The connection between leadership style and member reactions in authority relationships has been the subject of considerable research in the fields of management psychology and group sociology. Different leadership styles appear to engender different respective patterns of group interaction.

Leadership Styles

Three styles of leadership have been identified by White and Lippitt (1953): *autocratic, democratic,* and *laissez-faire* — all of which have been studied in terms of productivity and morale. Autocratic leadership has been found to increase productivity and decrease morale, as compared with democratic leadership. Hostility, aggression, and scapegoating were found to be significantly greater in autocratic as opposed to democratic groups. Laissez-faire leadership resulted in the least productivity and lowest morale. Democratic leadership, which delegates authority and distributes leadership, was found to increase group cohesion and stimulate groups to develop their own direction and resources beyond the leader's capacity (Lego, 1978).

While the benefits of a democratic style of leadership appear to be overwhelming, flexibility in leadership style is advisable. One style of leadership may be more appropriate than another to a particular task or situation. Most leaders tend to adhere rigidly to one style and to disregard the need for flexibility.

In some situations a more directive, autocratic approach is necessary and appropriate, such as:

- When the group is in jeopardy of dissolving and an immediate decision is necessary to maintain the integrity and viability of the group.
- When the task is highly structured with limited alternatives for action (Sampson and Marthas, 1977).
- When members expect a strong, central leader, and leadership sharing is negatively valued.
- When members' support for and acceptance of authoritarianism is substantial.

An illustration of the smallest autocratic relationship is seen in the health interview between clinician and patient, where it has been shown that progress toward health has been associated with approaches which are directive and interpretive (Hare, 1976).

Situations appropriate for democratic leadership include:

- Those in which there are multiple alternatives to the task.
- Those in which no single, clear issue is available.
- Those in which ethical issues are involved (Sampson and Marthas, 1977).
- Those in which there is a need to change attitudes or opinions.

Democratic or participatory leadership is an effective technique for influencing and changing opinion, and enhancing member satisfaction with decisions. This apparently occurs because each member has an opportunity to express opinions and to contribute to the decision, thus giving a sense of ownership for the group's decision (Hare, 1976). A comparison of the characteristics and results of the three types of leader styles are shown in Tables 9-1 and 9-2.

Multigoal Leadership Sampson and Marthas (1977) suggest that it is difficult to pursue opposing leadership goals simultaneously. Task leadership, with its emphasis on goal accomplishment, requires a directive approach. Task issues tend to center on the division of labor, to encourage a hierarchy, and to emphasize differences. Socio-emotional leadership, with its emphasis on cohesiveness and member satisfaction, allows for a more democratic approach. Socioemotional issues accentuate similarity, universality, mutual respect, and equal status. Few persons are able to serve both needs equally, since it is difficult to push members toward equality and inequality at the same time.

Communication Networks

Another facet of leadership style involves the type of communication network which is developed. Kadis et al. (1965) identified four types of networks present in therapeutic groups, all of which have corresponding influences on the development of the group. *Vertical* communication flows directly from leader to member, but allows minimal return of feedback, thus precipitating leader-centered interaction with marked control over member-to-member interactions. *Triangular* communication is a variant of the foregoing in which the leader remains the pivot of activity, although member-to-member interaction continues. *Horizontal* communication is an authority-denying structure with reciprocal therapeutic results for the group. *Circular* communication is group-centered interaction in which the leader expects the group to possess inherent maturational and curative abilities; leadership and participation are distributed among members, thus enhancing their equality and interdependence.

Negative Results of Leadership Style   A classic study of encounter-group casualties related to leadership style (Yalom and Lieberman, 1972) revealed that some leadership styles precipitated persistent, severe psychological dysfunction. Intrusive, aggressive confrontation of members by an authoritarian and charismatic leader was correlated with the highest number of member casualties. It appeared that leaders with these characteristics sought immediate evidence of members' growth and therefore increased the pressure on members to change quickly. For vulnerable members, the combination

Table 9-1 COMPARISON OF THE CHARACTERISTICS OF THREE LEADERSHIP STYLES

Democratic	Autocratic	Laissez-Faire
Member-oriented	Leader-oriented	Diffuse orientation
Problem-solving approach	Persuasive approach	Style drifts and changes
Facilitates participation	Members have limited access to information	Few clear goals
Group evaluates its process and progress by means of extensive feedback and extensive activity.	Control by a central leadership figure	Little evaluation of process
Leader guides group	Limited tolerance of diversity	Minimal feedback
Requires more skill and self-confidence of leader	Limited feedback	Increased confusion
Leader uses a more complex approach	Leadership retained by one or two designated persons	Decreased effectiveness
Diversity is a resource to be tapped		Leadership neither centralized nor distributed
Leadership distributed among multiple persons		

Source: After White and Lippitt, 1953; Shaw, 1971; Sampson and Marthas, 1977; and Lego, 1978.

Table 9–2 COMPARISON OF THE RESULTS OF THREE LEADERSHIP STYLES

Democratic	Autocratic	Laissez-Faire
Increased member participation	Highest productivity level	Decreased morale
Increased member enthusiasm	Consistent surveillance required	Decreased cohesiveness
Increased member commitment	Decreased morale, cohesiveness	Decreased productivity
Increased productivity, but less than autocratic	Decreased innovation	Increased scapegoating
Increased cohesiveness, morale	Repressed aggression leads to scapegoating, resentment, passive-aggressive, acting out behaviors	Decreased learning of leadership skills
Increased initiative	Increased dependency	Decreased quality of work
Leadership skills learned by members	Decreased individuality	Increased requests for information
Self-corrective feedback maximizes member's potential	Conversations restricted and related to task	Decreased cooperation
	Increased uniformity	Increased emotional dissatisfaction

Source: After White and Lippitt, 1953; Shaw, 1971; Sampson and Marthas, 1977; and Lego, 1978.

of intrusiveness and controlling entrapment was sufficient to precipitate psychological dysfunction. The four basic leadership tactics which emerged from the study were 1) emotional stimulation and confrontation; 2) caring and support; 3) meaning attribution or cognitive explanations of meaning; and 4) executive or managerial structuring of the group. Group leaders who were found to bring about the most positive results were those who provided high-caring and high-meaning attribution with only moderate amounts of executive structure and confrontation (Lieberman et al., 1973).

Loomis (1979) suggested that the four different leader functions identified in that study may be applicable in matching leadership styles to various specific types of groups. Table 9-3 presents types of groups that might respond well to an emphasis on a particular leadership function.

COLEADERSHIP

Coleadership provides an alternative pattern of leadership for small groups. It is an arrangement which is demanding and complicated, but, if successfully negotiated, coleadership can enrich the group and strengthen the endeavors of the leaders.

Coleadership Patterns

Three patterns of coleadership have been documented. The first is the *leader-recorder* model, in which the leader discharges the planning and direction of the group while the recorder collects data and participates nonverbally in the group. In the second arrangement the *junior-senior* model is used in training leaders, based on the assumption

Table 9–3   STYLE OF LEADERSHIP AND TYPE OF GROUPS

Leader Style	Type of Group
High in caring	Support
High in executive function	Task
High in caring and executive function	Socialization
High in meaning attribution and executive function	Behavior change
High in emotional stimulation and meaning attribution	Sensitivity group
Moderate in emotional stimulation, moderate in executive, high in caring, high in meaning-attribution	Psychotherapy

that the senior person is more qualified in skills and knowledge. This arrangement is usually not reversible, even when the junior member demonstrates growth and ability. The arrangement gives the senior person responsibility for goal identification, planning, and implementation of interventions. Both the leader-recorder model and the junior-senior model are examples of status differential and may frequently increase tension for the junior member trainees.

The third model is an *egalitarian* arrangement in which coleaders share responsibility for goal direction, planning, and interventions. This coleadership model allows more freedom within the leadership role, but considerable effort is required to make it work effectively. It is a relationship which needs a foundation of mutual respect, openness, and shared responsibility (Marram, 1978). The quality and nature of the egalitarian model can strongly influence group effectiveness, particularly if the leaders model equality between males and females, or between juniors and seniors.

There are at least five activities during which coleaders can and should interact: 1) screening and preparatory procedures for potential group members; 2) planning and implementing the group meetings; 3) postsessions immediately following the meeting during which a critique and catharsis of the session takes place; 4) supervision sessions; and 5) organizational or social contacts related to the group. The nature and frequency of these interactions clarifies, and provides insight into, the nature of the coleadership relationship (McGee and Schuman, 1970).

Pros and Cons of Coleadership

There are advantages and disadvantages to coleadership arrangements. Numerous advantages have been identified in the literature (Rosenbaum, 1971; Yalom, 1975; Hellwig and Memmoh, 1978; Dick et al., 1980). Some advantages pertain to psychotherapy group work, but are relevant to many other types of groups as well. Data collection regarding content and process is facilitated through increased observation, validation, and feedback.

Mutual cognitive and emotional support is made accessible by coleadership because the variety of interventions and tactics is enriched by the work of two leaders. Mutual support lowers leader anxiety and strengthens leader stability against group pressure or attack. Coleadership also expands energy levels and leadership powers by permitting the use of the combined techniques of support and confrontation. Group continuity, in the event of sickness or vacation of one of the leaders, is more secure. Another advantage, particularly for psychotherapy groups, is the more realistic simulation of family interaction, the intensified transference phenomena of authority and gender relationships as well as sibling rivalry. In this sense coleadership enables members to identify with various models in the group who symbolize early healthy or dysfunctional figures in the family of origin.

The disadvantages of coleadership have been cited in the literature (McGee and Schuman, 1970; Rosenbaum, 1971; Dick et al., 1980). Coleadership is not an easy technique but is an arrangement which requires maturity, mutual respect, temperamental compatibility, and trust. It provides fertile ground for the development of rivalry and power struggles. Other disadvantages include: higher operating costs (two salaries instead of one), increased time consumption, and increased complexity.

Personality Factors

As much care should be exercised in the matching of coleaders as in the selection of group members. Perhaps greater care is required in selecting a coleader, for the quality of the coleader interaction is of utmost importance. Related personality factors in coleader interaction may be divided into three categories: *extrinsic, characterologic,* and *dynamic* factors.

Extrinsic personality factors relate to age, sex, race, discipline, and physical appearance, which provide the external "set" for initial transference reactions between group members and the coleaders, and for predictions of later transferences evoked in the course of the group's development. Characterologic personality factors of group coleaders are evident in the degree of verbal and nonverbal activity, affect, self-disclosure, timing, and cognitive style. These factors have the potential either to increase antagonism between coleaders or to become the key to effective group functioning. Dynamic factors include defensive patterns, understanding, self-esteem, and competition for dominance or affection. These factors are essentially out of conscious awareness and not clearly available for scrutiny, unless intraleader conflict occurs which would make dynamic personality factors clearly evident (Davis and Lohr, 1971).

Four Stages of Development

Dick et al. (1980) emphasized the need to recognize and manage the strengths and limitations of each coleader. A four-stage sequence was presented in the coleader relationship: *formulation, development, stabilization,* and *refreshment.* The first stage includes intrapsychic issues of confidence, performance anxiety, and personal-identity struggles; and also structural issues of treatment philosophies, strategies, tactics, and personality styles. The energy required for these issues depletes the level available for therapeutic interactions with patients and, therefore, causes coleadership to be less effective than in later stages. Formulation effort is difficult and arduous, necessitating sharing of thoughts, feelings, and strategies between sessions. In all stages the comfort and rate of progress is related to partner agreement regarding therapeutic orientation, style, resources, and corresponding activity levels.

Development The second stage involves interpersonal support of symbiotic needs, with each leader collecting data about the other's strengths and limitations while monitoring his or her own functioning in the group. Generally, each leader knows what to expect from the other. They begin to support each other, using the other's strengths and making allowances for deficits. One leader may be more supportive, confrontive, creative, affective, or cognitive than the other. One leader may elect to deal with leader-group interactions while the other may attend to individual member issues. It is in this manner of dividing and sharing functions that a complementary coleadership relationship develops.

Stabilization The third stage is a period of mutual trust. With major energy flowing between leaders and members, less energy is required for the leaders' intrapsychic or interpersonal concerns. The coleaders attend to their therapeutic tasks in an increasingly effective manner. There is evidence of growing confidence in oneself and in the other leader. Ability to anticipate mutual tactics and strategy improves, with less urgent need for supervision as the coleaders learn to monitor each other. At this stage the two leaders are both economically and therapeutically effective, although variations in group or individual issues may precipitate temporary regression of the leaders to less complementary work.

Refreshment The last stage is a period of effortless coleadership, with marked satisfaction, creativity, and fresh perspectives emanating from personal and professional experience. At this point coleadership and group work are vehicles for increased cognitive and affective change. The coleadership relationship has moved beyond mere technique.

PROBLEMATIC ISSUES

Some issues occur with such frequency in small groups that they may be anticipated by group leaders. Three problematic issues to be explored in this section deal with managing the following issues: *volume of data; fears and security operations* of neophyte group leaders; *and* group *conflict.*

Volume of Data

The volume of data generated within the context of one group meeting is enormous, considering the possibilities of individual material, member-member interactions, group versus leader issues, and stage of development phenomena. Not only does the sheer volume of data often exceed the processing abilities of the leader, allowing only a small portion to be analyzed, but unconscious resistance to processing certain data prevents many feelings, beliefs, and taboos from being recognized. The result is that only a fraction of what occurs in a group is brought to awareness and acted upon by the leader(s). Because the task is so awesome, numerous dysfunctional responses may be consciously or unconsciously maintained. The leader may deter the group from its original purpose by manipulating the group into pseudo-issues, by blocking action, obscuring genuine issues, postponing decisions, suppressing material, advocating a simplistic version, or by subjectively justifying a response by virtue of the leader's authority or position (Mills, 1967).

Fears and Security Operations

The second problematic issue relates to the fears and security operations of the leader. Some of the common fears include: exposure of incompetence and the need to maintain a professional image to impress the group, coleader, or supervisor; loss of control of the group, especially during periods of intense expression of hostility or acting-out behavior; exposure of self as sharing the same human frailties as the group members; and encountering group disintegration through the attrition of members. Like most individuals, group leaders are prone to project their own fears and needs on to members (Sampson and Marthas, 1977). Their desire for approval, power, and competency may lie beyond their awareness or, hopefully, may become integrated into their objective self-awareness. For the inexperienced group leader the burden of dealing with group pressures, managing group cohesiveness, enacting the leader's role, and understanding group phenomena may seem overwhelming (Yalom, 1966). Utilizing cognitive and affective understanding of group dynamics and identifying leader countertransference by means of adequate supervision may provide a workable solution to the dilemma of the fledgling leader.

Conflict

Managing group conflict is an asset to the group if used in a problem-solving manner which attempts to negotiate a compromise. Managing group conflict becomes a liability if it is denied or concealed rather than expressed. When denied, it often finds its expression in the group through passive-aggressive behavior, overt hostility, or the development of subgroups. Conflict is an inevitable stage of group development and its constructive use is growth-promoting for the group. If disagreement is construed as disloyalty, group effectiveness diminishes and reduces objective feedback. The leader must identify conflicts which are destructive to group life, such as covert power struggles, hidden agendas, or loyalty issues which have external sources. After identifying destructive conflicts the leader may intervene early to avoid escalation or acknowledge the conflict and continue with the task at hand. A possible sequence of interventions includes: identification of the conflict, reflection of the behavior and feelings, and eventual confrontation.

Constructive conflicts often arise from members who are invested in the group, but disagree with certain policies or procedures. The resolution of constructive conflicts involves checking support and validation of the legitimacy of the conflict, identification of commonalities and opposing positions related to the conflict, and, finally, negotiation of an acceptable compromise. Successful conflict resolution is feasible when members are able to tolerate disagreements and deal with them in a climate of accommodation and trust. It is not possible to eliminate conflicts from group life but it is possible to use conflict as a catalytic resource (Sampson and Marthas, 1977).

CLINICAL EXAMPLE: DISPUTED ISSUES IN COLEADERSHIP

Carol Roberts, the nursing staff development coordinator at a general hospital, initiated an assertiveness training group in response to requests from staff nurses. She had decided that she would like to colead the group and invited Howard Stewart, a respected team leader of an inpatient unit, to join her as a coleader. Carol believed that Howard would augment her skills and validate her perceptions of the group. Because of Howard's experience as a team leader, Carol was sure that he would reinforce the group's attention to the stated goal of assertiveness training.

Both leaders had prior experience leading patient groups and health team groups. Each approached the task with enthusiasm and confidence. A joint decision was made by the coleaders to limit the group to eight members and to meet for one-and-a-half hours a week for ten weeks. The majority of group members were female staff members. The first two group sessions were primarily didactic and proceeded according to plan, utilizing role-playing and group exercises. In the second and third sessions the group began to follow Howard into discussions of individual needs and concerns, and to disengage when Carol introduced exercises in assertive behavior. Before long Carol began to experience frustration and to reveal her impatience with Howard's tendencies to promote un- structured "rap" sessions and group avoidance of assertive training. In addition, Howard used interventions with group members which focused on socioemotional issues and distributed leadership among various members. This was contrary to Carol's expectations and she felt that she was losing control of group leadership and goals. Her sense of powerlessness reduced her self-confidence and level of participation. She attributed the group's obvious affection for Howard as evidence of male-female attraction and to cultural stereotypes of male aggres- sion and female passivity.

Carol realized that assertiveness training is based on a structured format, and wished to use exercises which followed a specific sequence. She believed that the relatively unstructured climate fostered by her coleader converted the assertiveness training meetings into group ther- apy sessions. She attributed the conflict between Howard and herself to his violation of the group contract, and considered his tactics detri- mental to group development. After several frustrating sessions, Carol proposed to Howard that they set aside a time to discuss the progress of the group and clarify its focus.

They decided to meet informally on neutral ground (in the hospital coffee shop) in order to share their perceptions of the group. Carol commented that "we seem to be pulling and tugging in opposite direc- tions rather than working together at leading the group." This brought a nod of agreement from her coleader. Howard then voiced his own frustration at the lack of member participation in assertiveness training and expressed his wish to meet the socioemotional needs of individual members by encouraging honest, open discussion of various issues. He also expressed commitment to the distribution of leadership among the group members. It was apparent from the discussion that both leaders were feeling a loss of power because of their unresolved disagreement and were experiencing threats to their competency. When confronted by Carol, Howard admitted attempting to deal with the disagreement by covertly changing the contract and discarding principles of assertive- ness training in favor of his preference for psychotherapy. Carol told him that she was uncomfortable with the group's direction, but ad- mitted that she had taken his acceptance of assertiveness training for granted. The need for each leader to clarify and validate the manner in which executive roles would be enacted had not been included in early discussions. Other disputed issues included the degree to which leadership would be distributed, the level of structure required to meet the goal of assertive training, and the divergent commitment of the leaders to the group contract. The different expectations, dynamic characteristics, and security operations of the coleaders altered the group interactions and negatively affected group development.

Both Howard and Carol found their open discussion helpful. Indifference of the members to assertiveness training stemmed chiefly from the incongruent messages transmitted by the two leaders. Carol and Howard realized the hazards of using the group as an arena for their own differences. They decided that it was essential to participate in ongoing pre- and post-session discussions in order to compare group progress and clarify disputed issues before they became detrimental to group progress. Commitment of both leaders to the contracted goals was reinforced. At the same time Carol was persuaded of the benefit of dealing with members' socioemotional needs and of leadership distribution. She became more willing to delegate responsibility for the assertiveness exercises among the group members.

SUMMARY

The phenomenon of leadership, which occurs in all groups, was explored as an interaction between the leaders and group members. Leadership characteristics and functions were identified, along with various styles of authority relationships and their effects on group success or failure. Finally, issues of coleadership and problematic events were discussed in detail. Advantages and disadvantages of coleadership were discussed and types of coleadership outlined. Constructive versus destructive conflict issues were compared, and several approaches to conflict resolution were suggested.

REFERENCES

Cartwright, C., and A. Zander, Eds. *Group Dynamics Research and Theory*. Evanston, IL.: Row, Peterson, 1953.

Davis, F.B., and N.E. Lohr. "Special Problems with the Use of Co-therapists in Group Psychotherapy." *International Journal of Group Psychotherapy* Vol. 21, No. 2, 1971, pages 143–158.

Dick, B.; K. Lesseer; and J. Whiteside. "A Developmental Framework for Cotherapy." *International Journal of Group Psychotherapy* Vol. 30, No. 3, 1980, pages 273–285.

Hamblin, R.L. "Leadership and Crises." In *Interpersonal Behavior in Small Groups*, R.J. Ofshe, Ed. Englewood Cliffs, N.J.: Prentice-Hall, 1973.

Hare, P.A. *Handbook of Small Group Research.* 2nd ed. New York: Free Press, 1976.

Hellwig, K., and R.S. Memmoh. "Partners in Therapy: Using the Co-therapist Relationship in a Group." *Journal of Psychiatric Nursing* Vol. 16, No. 4, 1978, pages 42–44.

Kadis, A.L.; J.D. Drasner; C. Winick; and S.H. Foulkes. *A Practicum of Group Psychotherapy.* New York: Hoeber Medical Division, Harper & Row, 1965.

Kanter, S.S. "The Therapist's Leadership in Psychoanalytically Oriented Group Psychotherapy." *International Journal of Group Psychotherapy* Vol. 30, No. 2, 1976, pages 139–147.

Lego, S. "Group Dynamic Theory and Application." In *Comprehensive Psychiatric Nursing,* J. Haber et al., Eds. New York: McGraw-Hill, 1978.

Lieberman, M.A.; I.D. Yalom; and M.B. Miles. "Encounter: The Leader Makes the Difference." *Psychology Today* Vol. 6, No. 10, 1973, pages 69–76.

Loomis, M.E. *Group Process for Nurses.* St. Louis: C.V. Mosby, 1979.

MacLennan, B.W. "The Personalities of Group Leaders: Implications for Selection and Training." *International Journal of Group Psychotherapy* Vol. 25, No. 2, 1975, pages 177–183.

Mann, R. *Interpersonal Styles and Group Development.* New York: Wiley, 1967.

Marram, G.W. *The Group Approach in Nursing Practice.* 2nd ed. St. Louis: C.V. Mosby, 1978.

McGee, T.F., and B.N. Schuman. "The Nature of the Co-therapy Relationship." *International Journal of Group Psychotherapy* Vol. 20, No. 1, 1970, pages 25–36.

Mills, T.M. *The Sociology of Small Groups.* Englewood Cliffs, N.J.: Prentice-Hall, 1967.

Rosenbaum, M. "Co-therapy." In *Comprehensive Group Psychotherapy,* H.I. Kaplan and B.J. Sadock, Eds. Baltimore: Williams and Wilkins, 1971.

Sampson, E.E., and M.S. Marthas. *Group Process for the Health Professions.* New York: Wiley, 1977.

Shaw, M.E. *Group Dynamics: The Psychology of Small Group Behavior.* New York: McGraw-Hill, 1971.

White, R., and R. Lippitt. "Leader Behavior and Member Reaction in Three Social Climates." In *Group Dynamics Research and Theory,* D. Cartwright and A. Zander, Eds. Evanston, IL.: Row, Peterson, 1953.

Yalom, I.D. "Problems of Neophyte Group Therapists." *Journal of Social Psychology* Vol. 12, No. 1, 1966, pages 52–59.

――――, and M.A. Lieberman. "A Study of Encounter Group Casualties." In *Progress in Group and Family Therapy,* C.J. Sager and H. Kaplan, Eds. New York: Brunner-Mazel, 1972.

――――. *The Theory and Practice of Group Psychotherapy.* New York: Basic Books, 1975.

PART THREE

Special Population Groups

10

Working Together in Health-Care Teams

Madeline H. Schmitt

The "team" has become the standard answer for the question of what to do about the fragmentation of modern medical care brought about by the increasing specialization of professionals in the field. The word "team" conjures up notions of people working together in some fashion. Yet there are many ways of working together, and it is in the specifics of *how* people work together in *teams* that misunderstandings arise.

For nurses and physicians the concept of health-care team often means different things. The physician may conjure up an image of a team as a group whose members are extensions of him- or herself and whom the physician leads. The physician views medicine as a mulitifaceted, all-encompassing domain of health and illness knowledge and treatment, whose exploration and application require an increasingly numerous array of assistants with the physician retaining the position of leader of the team (Lewis, 1968). For nurses, health-care occupations (social worker, dietitian, and so forth) involve knowledge and treatments not encompassed by the physician's approach. "Teams" are viewed as vehicles for the application of that knowledge to patient care. According to this view, the leader of the team should be an individual member whose special expertise is central to the problem at hand and whose leadership position helps other team members interact in ways that maximize the application of diverse skills to the problem (Aradine and Hansen, 1970; Leininger, 1971). It follows that the physician need not always be the "natural" leader of all health-care teams.

In this chapter several aspects of the discrepant perceptions of physicians and nurses are examined which help in understanding why physicians and nurses may reach an impasse when trying to utilize the team approach to health-care delivery. To clarify the discrepant perceptions of physicians and nurses, various meanings of the concept of "team," and the developing relationships between the professions of medicine and nursing are examined.

EARLY MEANINGS OF THE WORD "TEAM"

An historical overview of the evolution in meanings of the word "team" is available in *The Oxford English Dictionary* (1961). An old meaning referred to two or more animals harnessed to perform some sort of work together, a team of horses or oxen. The person who drove the horses was known as a "teamster." Thus, in the past "team" meant a grouping based on *likeness*, as might be true of horses whose similar size and strength were important to their ability to work together. Moreover, like units may carry out *joint action* which could not be accomplished alone, or might be less efficiently accomplished alone. In short, through combining *similar* efforts the goal was obtained.

In the 1800s the idea of working together was applied to efforts in industry and sports. The discovery was made that some activities could be accomplished more easily by a specialized division of labor. As a result, the concept of "team" took on the meaning of a grouping comprised of *different* parts working together to achieve the goal.

HISTORICAL OVERVIEW

The first reference to "team" in medical care appeared in an article by Barker (1922). It was suggested that the growth of "teamwork" in medical practice was the direct result of increasing *specialization*, which itself was the result of "the organization of modern science and the application of experimental method to the development of technic" (p. 774). Specialization resulted in the differential distribution of knowledge and skills among medical practitoners; the practice of referral between general practitioners and specialists evolved as a means of bringing the best medical knowledge to bear on patient problems. Among the dangers seen in the growth of specialization were improper self-referral by patients, lack of cooperation between the general practitioner and the specialist, and peculiar dangers to which specialists might succumb (such as "excessive aggressiveness," "self-interest," and "materialism"). Key problems isolated by Barker were potential lack of coordination of specialists' and general practitioners' efforts and lack of integration of the diverse medical findings. "It is the 'knitting together of specialists' into a well-coordinated producing mechanism that group practice of the better sort or team-work in practice has to find its place" (p. 776). Barker envisaged three new specialists who would be required to make teamwork effective: a specialist in team organization, another specialist in team management, and a third specialist in the integration of the diagnostic data collected by team members.

The type of team referred to differs from the earlier concept of team in an important respect. Barker described various physician members of the team as being *differentiated* from each other by their *special* training and *unique* contributions to the overall effort to provide care for the patient. Although the physicians on Barker's team were "alike" in the sense that they were all physicians, they were also different. Getting them to work together was not a mechanical matter but required new skills. It required the vision of a person or persons who could see how the different parts worked together. The physicians were not completely specialized, since all had the same basic medical education and were generally committed to viewing the patient from similar frames of reference. Thus, there was a basic ability to communicate, but there was also fear among some of them that the specialists would usurp the role of the general practitioners and offer the patient generalized care as well as specialized services.

The Status of Nursing

It is important to note the status of nursing vis-a -vis medicine during this important transitional period. Until the beginning of the twentieth century hospitals were places where individuals mostly received nursing care. During the early part of this century reforms in medicine led to expanded use of hospitals for medical education. Expansion of medical technology for diagnosis and treatment led physicians to centralize a great deal of complicated diagnostic and treatment activity in hospitals. As a result, hospitals became an excellent context for rapid expansion of physician income. Historical study of this period (Ashley, 1976) documented the exploitation of student nurses as cheap and obedient laborers in the staffing of hospitals. In return for uniforms, room, and board, along with a minimal education given when it did not interfere with hospital staffing needs, students worked up to a hundred and five hours a week, often under extremely stressful conditions. Attempts to include nurses in labor laws aimed at improving working conditions were strongly opposed by the medical profession and even by some nurse leaders. Efforts to improve the level of nursing education lacked support within the ranks of nursing, and serious nurse educators were ridiculed by members of the medical profession. One outstanding exception, however, was Richard Olding Beard, who assisted in founding the first university-based school of nursing at the University of Minnesota. Separate licensure for nurses was opposed; large numbers of graduate nurses were unemployed, and diploma mills for nurses proliferated as each hospital recruited its own unending supply of student labor. It was not until the 1950s that all states had nurse licensure laws! One might summarize this period by saying that although nurses and physicians worked in the same facilities, there was no pretense that they coordinated or integrated their efforts through teamwork. Medicine was rapidly becoming more complex, while the development of nursing was contained by internal and external forces.

There has been a proliferation of medically-oriented occupations to meet the demands for sophisticated laboratory studies and other services required by specialized medical practice. Typically, education for these occupations remained under the control of organized medicine since the primary purpose of such occupations is to facilitate the work of physicians by preparing others to act as surrogates in carrying out routine procedures and common diagnostic tests.

Multidisciplinary Teams

References to *multidisciplinary* teams — those teams whose members represented more than one discipline (not just medicine) — began to appear in the 1940s, particularly in the field of rehabilitation. In this speciality the complexity of responding to rehabilitation problems resulted from the awareness of the impact of the disability on the whole person. Social, psychological, and vocational adjustments, as well as physical rehabilitation, had to be considered. Such tasks extended well beyond the scope of the physician's specialized training. Physical therapists, prosthetic specialists, vocational counselors, social workers, and others were organized into a multidisciplinary team (Margolin, 1969). Since the 1950s multidisciplinary teams have been used in the management of chronic illness, and the team approach to chronic illness has been linked with the goal of comprehensive health care (Katz, Papsidero, and Halstead, 1973).

THE CURRENT STATUS OF TEAMWORK

The next advance of teamwork in medical care occurred in the 1970s. During the War on Poverty substantial amounts of federal money became available to support the development of neighborhood health centers.   Because these centers were initially established in poor, underserved areas, there was recognition that success in treating illness and teaching preventive health practices depended on measures beyond the circumscribed focus of medicine. Nurses, social workers, dietitians, indigenous health workers, and physicians were brought together and expected to coordinate and integrate their multiple specialized skills and services (Banta and Fox, 1972; Brunetto and Birk, 1972).   Major difficulties were encountered and relevant literature of this period is filled with reports of failures. Some insight about the failures is gained from the writing of organization and management experts who were called in to unravel some of the problems of health-care teams (Wise, Beckhard, Rubin, and Kyte, 1974).

Types of Teams

At least three different kinds of team are referred to in current literature. The *unidisciplinary* team has a relatively narrow disciplinary focus.   The *multidisciplinary* team involves specialists of different disciplines who work primarily in a parallel or sequential manner to contribute their disciplinary skills to the resolution of a problem. And the *interdisciplinary* team involves the interaction of various disciplines around an agreed-upon goal to be achieved only through a complex integration or synthesis of various disciplinary perspectives. This requires that participants have knowledge of the observational categories and key concepts of various disciplines (Petrie, 1976; Woollcott, 1979).*

Confusion about the concept of team is created in the literature as writers shift from a unidisciplinary to a multidisciplinary to an interdisciplinary focus. Concurrent with shifts in focus, goals identified for teams subtly shift from *medical care* to *comprehensive medical care* to *health care*. Medical care often requires diversified teams of specialists and assistants for implementation. Comprehensive medical care, concerned with the whole person, requires different disciplinary contributions.   Health care, which is concerned with health more than illness, requires a reformulation of the contributions of the disciplines to this broader, more ambiguous goal.

*The literature sometimes refers to multidisciplinary or interdisciplinary teams within medicine. This reflects the complexity of disciplinary knowledge and the specialization process that has occurred within the field.

The Role of Nursing

Nursing has a complex history in relation to these various meanings of "team." Contained in many ways until the early 1950s, nursing changed significantly from the submissive occupation it had previously been. The movement of nursing education from hospitals into colleges and universities greatly increased the proportion of time students spent in the classroom, which led to broader general knowledge and firmer grounding in the physical sciences. The demand for teachers and later for nurse "specialists," who developed expertise in the nursing of patients receiving complicated diagnostic testing, surgery, or drug therapy, led to the growth of graduate education in nursing. And, importantly, federal financing beginning in the 1950s contributed to the expansion of educational programs, research training for nurses, and research projects by nurses. All these activities represented for nurses the opportunity for a better understanding of medicine and fostered the development of a knowledge base within their own profession.

THE CURRENT STATUS OF NURSING

In the 1970s the expansion of nursing's capabilities included some of the traditional diagnostic and treatment skills of physicians. The development of roles like that of the nurse practitioner demanded new working relationships between physicians and nurses, and raised questions on both sides about the nature of those relationships. Are such nurses "physician extenders" or "physician assistants"? Are they multidisciplinary contributors to comprehensive medical care, or are they interdisciplinary contributors to the development of new *kinds* of knowledge in health and illness? Nursing started relatively late, compared with medicine, to articulate the profession's independent formulation of knowledge for and about nursing practice.

Identity Ambiguity

With nursing moving in the direction of an autonomous profession, tensions implicit in nurse-physician relationships have become manifest. Central to this is the delineation of the nurse's identity. On the one hand the nurse acts as the physician's substitute in the performance of direct medical-care activities for the patient, on the other hand the nurse provides services to patients that reflect nursing's independent contribution to the well-being of individuals and families. In hospitals the provision of *nursing* care to patients simultaneously undergoing *medical* treatment highlights the overlap between medicine and nursing. Nurses are responsible, under nurse practice acts, for the nursing care rendered: maintenance of nutrition, skin care, mobility, safety, prevention of infection, and so on. They are also responsible for independent assessment of the medical-care activities they are charged with carrying out, such as administering medicines and monitoring physiological changes requiring medical intervention. Thus, nurses are interpreting medical factors as well as practicing nursing.

This unusual interoccupational situation creates interpersonal complexities; examples of these are given in a classic article by Stein (1968). The ambiguity in nurses' identity and in their potential contributions to medical and health care has contributed to controversy within nursing and medicine about nurses' "expanded role" and relationships between nurses and the physicians (Greenlaw, 1980).

Nursing's Future Role

Most references to "teamwork" between physicians and nurses (or physicians and other health-care providers) do not define the concept "team," leaving the definition of the relationship to the reader. One might suggest that there are advantages for both physicians and nurses in perpetuating this ambiguity. Physicians have traditionally relied on nurses, and most nurses are still employed to assist physicians in the delivery of medical care. Nurses have only recently begun to develop knowledge bases of their own profession and are relatively inarticulate, among themselves and with others, about the role of nursing. Except in unusual instances where both physicians and nurses have clear visions of and competence in their own fields, openness to adventure, and a mutual willingness to learn the observational categories and key concepts of the others' discipline (Petrie, 1976), expectations for successful *interdisciplinary* teams seem doomed to disappointment at present. Given the history of both professions, a more viable model for the present seems to be the *multidisciplinary* team with nurses accepting the burden of intellectual proof for the contributions of nursing and physicians accepting the burden of acknowledging the observational categories and key concepts of nursing.

The evolution of the various kinds of teams is summarized in Table 10-1. As illustrated in this table, two types of differentiation occurred historically. The first was among physicians themselves, who were likely to establish working relationships with one another so as to utilize the full range of medical knowledge on a patient's behalf. The second was the differentiation of technicians employed

Table 10–1   THE GROWTH OF TEAMS IN MEDICAL AND HEALTH CARE

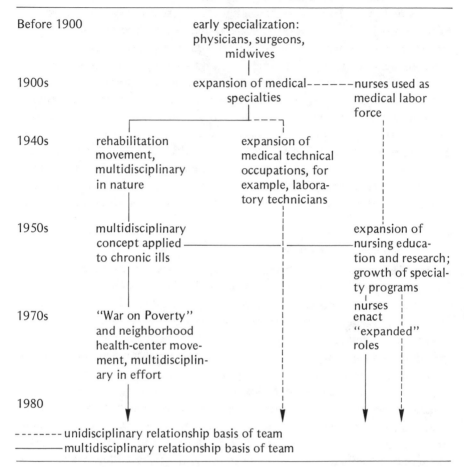

-------- unidisciplinary relationship basis of team
———— multidisciplinary relationship basis of team

by the hospital with whom the physician was not likely to establish direct working relationships. Nurses employed by large institutions to assist the physician in the delivery of medical treatments were also unlikely to experience a direct working relationship with the physician. This is a concept of "team" as merely an increase in the number of persons performing similar tasks to get the job done, all the while being led by the "head" of the team.

Since the 1950s, when nursing's professional autonomy began, an increasing number of nurses have held membership in multidisciplinary teams as professionals with separate disciplinary contributions to make. An example of this in the area of chronic institutional care and rehabilitation nursing is the creation of Loeb Center at Montefiore Hospital in New York City, where patients referred by physicians are admitted to a nursing care facility for multidisciplinary care under nursing direction. More recently nurses have had an active involvement in the multidisciplinary neighborhood health-center movement.

As can be seen in the table, the confusion around the nurse's role in team care stems from the nurse's dual position on the team — an assistant to the physician, and an independent contributor of nursing skills. The nurse's future role as an interdisciplinary team member in the development of *health* care will depend on issues still unresolved within and between professions.

Developing a Working Definition of "Team"

Any working definition of teams useful in specific situations must focus on a single entity. Certain minimum characteristics must be identified so that one can say when there is a team in existence and when there is not (Londey, 1978). First, teams are small groups with boundaries. They are comprised of *particular, selected* individuals. Teams also have specific *goals* and may be disbanded after achieving these goals. Though teams do not have to be assembled physically in order to act, team members are often involved in *face-to-face interaction* for at least part of their activities. In the absence of face-to-face interaction, a *communication structure* of some kind is necessary.

Teams are *organized* with an overall structure for getting the work done. The structure includes role assignments to do the work, role expectations about how it will be done, and a communication structure that enables the members of the team to relate to one another. Many details of the preceding discussion focus on similarities or differences between team roles. In some teams members have similar skills and may substitute for one another. In other teams members' roles are highly differentiated on the basis of unique experience or expertise.

The communication structure may be of a *coordinating* type, where the key problem for successful team effort involves proper sequencing and timing of the actions of team members, or it may be *collaborative* or problem-solving in nature, where the key problem is analytic. Collaborative communication is appropriate when the nature of the work or the way to accomplish the work is uncertain, requiring the creative participation and synthesis of the various perspectives of team members. Most typically, teams that operate in health-care settings must create structures that permit activities of coordination and collaboration. Communication structures should include feedback mechanisms that examine the degree of effectiveness of the team in all aspects of its work.

The leader is the person most influential in the team's activities. Allocation of leadership responsibilities is an activity of crucial importance to the success of the team's efforts. Ideally, the leadership role is given to the team member able to contribute most to the team's current efforts. In this decentralized structure, leadership changes as the goals of the team change. More often, however, a leader is chosen by criteria other than expertise and the position is "frozen" for the life of the group. This kind of centralized leadership can work against the success of the team when it blocks the contributions of other "expert" team members in problem solving.

Teams may accomplish their goals through many kinds of actions. Probably the bulk of team activities in medical settings is performed by individual members not acting alone but as agents of the team. Teams can be said to act as a unit only when some or most of the team members act together in roles within the team structure (Londey, 1978). For example, carrying out activities like coordination and collaboration are unified team efforts.

THE DYNAMICS OF MULTIDISCIPLINARY TEAMS

The most frequently offered advantages of team care are (1) avoidance of duplication and fragmentation, (2) development of a more comprehensive data base, (3) better identification of health problems, and (4) development of more comprehensive health plans. These advantages accrue through the team's communication, collaboration, and coordination of expertise represented among team members. Many status attributes of individual members are thought to affect the ability of the team to utilize the expert potential. Such attributes as sex, age, and occupational ranking have been shown to affect participation, leadership, communication, and decision-making in many kinds of small groups in both natural and laboratory situations.

Torrance (1954) found that military rank, age, and formal education were positively associated with participation, leadership, and influence in a study of three-man teams. In situations where participation and leadership of the low status member were needed to meet survival goals, the teams were not able to change their communication pattern to utilize the expertise. Strodtbeck, James, and Hawkins (1957), in a study of juries, found that being male and having a higher occupational rank were associated with higher participation, leadership, and influence in the jury group. Two early studies in medical settings showed similar patterns. Caudill (1958) found that in a psychiatric ward's multidisciplinary meetings the various members' degree of participation in discussions about patients was directly related to formal occupational rank. It was also found that group recognition of a member's expressed concern for a patient was directly related to formal status of the member expressing the concern. Thus, the concerns communicated by physicians were attended to more frequently than those of nurses. The concerns of senior physicians were concerns attended to more frequently than those of junior physicians. Wessen (1966) found in a general hospital ward that communication across disciplinary lines flowed primarily in one direction, from the higher status physicians to the lower status nurses. More recently, Wise (1974), who had expected to create teams to facilitate multidisciplinary problem-solving, found team members exhibiting interaction patterns more typical of status dominance by physicians. He reported that physician communication in these teams often consisted of giving orders.

High Status Influence

Small group laboratory researchers like Bales (1951, 1953) originally thought that interaction patterns reflecting differences in participation and leadership in task groups emerged on the basis of distribution of expertise related to the task. Others have confirmed the findings of naturalistic studies that high status on a wide variety of characteristics places members possessing them in positions of influence (Berger, Cohen, and Zelditch, 1973). Some researchers have tried to control the emergence of influence based on status characteristics. In a laboratory study of small problem-solving groups where participation in the group was controlled artificially by "taking turns," more influence was attributed to members with good solutions (Richardson, Dugan, Gray, and Mayhew, 1973). In another laboratory study where low status members were said to possess certain "expert" characteristics, their influence increased (Freese, 1974). These studies suggest that it is possible to structure task group interactions in ways that will encourage the utilization of expertise, but without such specific changes it is likely that the group will be dominated by the high status members, who may or may not possess the expertise relevant to the problem at hand.

Team Care for Diabetics   In the only study linking these laboratory and naturalistic study findings in small task groups to multidisciplinary medical care teams, Feiger and Schmitt (1979) analyzed interaction patterns and patient care outcomes in four teams each consisting of a physician, two nurses, and a dietitian. These teams cared for half of the diabetic population in a residential facility for the chronically ill. The other half of the population, who received usual institutional care, served as a control group. Each team met initially to review comprehensive data on each patient and to set health-care goals that were unanimously agreed on. Each team reviewed the progress of their patients once a month and progress was formally measured on all patients at six-month intervals. The researchers (whose hypotheses were unknown to the team members) believed that the patients receiving team care would fare better than those in the control group, and that, among the teams, better patient progress would be associated with team interaction patterns that reflected collegiality or more equal participation of the team members. The first hypothesis, that patients treated with team care would do better than the control group, was supported with statistically significant results after one year. Among the teams, participation patterns resembled the high status dominance patterns of previous studies — physicians held the positions of influence. There was considerable variation in the participation patterns reflecting this dominance, however. The team scoring highest on collegiality had a physician member who displayed the broadest range of concerns about his patients and who seemed concerned about eliciting the opinions of other team members. He used his influential position to draw them out. The team scoring lowest on collegiality had a physician member who rejected his influential position by withdrawing from team interaction. The nurses directed a great deal of attention to him to try to force him to behave like "a leader." The other two teams displayed traditional status-differentiated dominance patterns to varying degrees. Most important, the more collegial (multidisciplinary) the interaction patterns, the more positive were the patient outcomes.

Low Status Team Members

The other side of the principle that high status members tend to dominate team interaction regardless of expertise is the principle that lower status members tend to conform to the influence of the high status member. Conformity behavior has not been systematically studied in multidisciplinary medical-care teams, but existing studies of conformity in small task group situations in the laboratory are helpful in making inferences about the reactions of lower status members. These reactions have implications for the quality of scientific and ethical patient care decisions made in team situations, and, therefore, patient care outcomes.

In the laboratory studies attributing expertise to high status members, it is apparent that this attribution is of a generalizing nature;

high status members are assumed to be expert in almost any domain asked about. Lower status members engage in a process of devaluing their own opinions and concerns, declining to offer them, and accepting the opinions of the high status member. The latter's opinions may be infused with a scientific aura. In a famous study by Milgram (1974) students were asked to inflict electric shock as part of a "learning" experiment under the direction of a psychologist. Most of the subjects ignored verbal cries and pleas from the hidden victim (a confederate of the experimenter) as increasing amounts of voltage were delivered under instructions from the psychologist. Importantly, the subjects' willingness to administer the shocks decreased as the experimenter and his authority were more distant from the subject or as the immediacy of the victim was greater. A majority of subjects were willing to act in potentially dangerous, harmful ways toward others because the high status member was "cloaked in science." Subjects assumed that the experimenter "knew what he was doing" and that, because of his position he "would not do anything that could possibly be harmful."

The suppression of misgivings and disagreement with the high status member occurs not only in a climate of blanket acceptance of expertise but also in a climate of intense liking and loyalty. Janis's study of *group think* (1972) examined the tendency for task groups to increase their sense of togetherness by ignoring private misgivings and negative information about their group performance. They took pride in being a "good" group, avoiding conflict, and suppressing doubts about group decisions.

Nurses, because of the split in their professional identity — between being the good assistant and the autonomous professional — may experience ambivalent reactions in situations where the authority of physicians in specific health-care situations is not matched by their expertise. They may resist the authority in indirect ways as some subjects in Milgram's experiment did, or they may be susceptible to the suppression of misgivings out of loyalty and affection for the leader. Both forms of response to authority conflicts, which avoid direct confrontation with the problem, may be assumed to have negative effects on the ability of the team to work effectively. The dynamics between members who are engaged in conflicts around authority push the team out of work-group mode of functioning and into the basic-assumption modes described by Bion and discussed earlier in this book.

There are many current analyses of the dysfunctional results of medicine's narrow focus on causes and treatments of disease. Critics point to the lack of regard for the whole person, and to the under-valuing of the contributions of the consumer and other health profes-sionals (other than physicians) to the understanding of disease and promotion of health. Simultaneously, other health professions such as nursing, social work, and dietetics are moving toward more substan-tial description and research within their own disciplines. Physicians may respond to the challenges either by continuing to see other health professions as extensions of themselves, as disciplines developing domains of knowledge ultimately to be claimed by physicians as part of medicine, thereby resisting any recognition of multidisciplinarity outside the profession; or physicians may recognize the opportunity to use their influence to foster the development and inclusion of these other health-care disciplines. Indeed, the relatively few studies of medical-care teams suggest that physicians necessarily display these different reactions in *team actions* since their very nature implies the involvement of more than one team member. Only a decision-making process that actively sought the opinions and ultimate consensus of all of the team members would be a *team decision*. These somewhat abstract ideas can be illustrated and linked to issues raised earlier in the chapter by presenting an example.

CLINICAL EXAMPLE: HEALTH TEAMWORK IN A HOSPITAL

Mr. B., seventy-two years old, had been hospitalized following a massive myocardial infarction. He was very ill during the acute phase of hospital-ization and had twice been placed in intensive care. Part of his treat-ment involved pacemaker insertion. He had had an ileostomy performed for a persistent gastrointestinal disorder several years previously.

After a long period, Mr. B.'s cardiac condition was stabilized, and, theoretically, he should have been showing gradual improvement. In-stead, he was wasting away. He refused to eat, "I can't eat this hospital food. Either something has to be done or I shall just curl up and die." He refused to walk or perform self-care activities. His hospital equip-ment for his ileostomy leaked badly. All day he lay curled in a fetal posi-tion, facing away from the door to his room; he pretended to be asleep when people entered the room. In conversation, he asked people to leave him alone and let him die. His wife was very attentive, but in despair over his deterioration. She asked the doctors and nurses to leave him alone and let him die in peace. Nurses and physicians caring for him were very frustrated. By their own admission they avoided his room. He was a frustrating focus of conversation in the weekly "inter-disciplinary team meetings." The intern in charge requested psychiatric consultation. The psychiatrist who visited wrote a note on the chart indicating "no pathology." He noted that Mr. B.'s depression was situationally appropriate and he offered no suggestions for care. The head nurse requested assistance from a nurse consultant who had a broad range of skills in nursing-care problems. The nurse consultant became a part of the multidisciplinary team and obtained information about the situation from chart review and talking with the medical and nursing staff. The intern reacted with encouragement to the consultant's involvement in the case, stating that he "knew Mr. B. needs that kind of attention" but that the intern didn't have the "time or energy" to give it.

In discussion with the patient and his wife, the nurse consultant found that Mr. B. was a retired highway supervisor who had a great love of the outdoors. Their only son had been killed in an automobile accident three years earlier. Mr. B. had returned to work following his son's death, often working seventy to eighty hours a week. His wife said Mr. B. and his son had been very close; that Mr. B. had never gotten over his son's death; and that she thought his need to work was his way of forgetting about the tragedy. Mr. B. spontaneously talked about his son's death, and his behavior indicated a prolonged grieving process. He talked fondly of neighborhood children who had given him consolation and stated how much he missed seeing the children during his hospitalization.

Several aspects of his hospital care were distressing to Mr. B. He had no clear idea of how limited his future daily activities might be as a result of his cardiac condition. He was terribly upset about the leaking ileostomy equipment. He said his own mail-order equipment had always worked very well, but the hospital personnel would not let him bring it from home. (The nursing and medical staff had assumed that it could not be as good as the new equipment they had provided.) Mr. B. did not understand the new equipment and had to rely heavily on nursing care for its management. Finally, he was very upset about the hospital food. His adjustment to his ileostomy had involved a long-term modification of his eating habits. He ate frequent small meals. Because his appetite was capricious, his wife kept small amounts of a great variety of foods at home that could be prepared quickly. The whole approach to meals in the hospital violated his long-term adjustment.

The nurse consultant reported back to the team the patient's nursing problems:

1. Extreme malnourishment with no individualized attention to nutritional intake.
2. Poor ileostomy functioning with no individualized attention to ileostomy care.
3. Inadequate information about the implications of his cardiac condition for daily living.

4. Isolation from sources of personal support: neighborhood children, cronies, and his wife (by virtue of her acceptance with his deterioration and wish to die).
5. Unresolved grief over the lost son, which was intensified by his current sense of helplessness.

A nursing-care plan was devised by the consultant in collaboration with the primary nurse. The team concurred with the planned nursing actions:

1. Obtain assistance from an enterostomal therapist.
2. Obtain Mr. B.'s own ileostomy equipment from home for his use.
3. Ask his wife to bring food from home which suits Mr. B.'s tastes to supplement the hospital menu.
4. Ask assistance from the dietitian in individualizing the hospital menu as much as possible.
5. Institute small, frequent feedings.
6. Request a cardiovascular nurse specialist to teach Mr. B. about his disease and daily living limitations.
7. Institute regular supportive visiting by the consultant with Mr. B. and his wife to interrupt Mr. B.'s withdrawal, to encourage resolution of grieving, and to focus attention on parts of his life that remain motivational forces for the future, such as enjoying the outdoors, children, wife, and so forth.

This plan was implemented by nurses caring for Mr. B. Feedback on the patient's progress was provided to all professionals involved in his care at the unit's weekly "interdisciplinary team meetings." Eventually he recovered enough to be discharged to his home under the care of his local physician. About six months later the nurse consultant received a note from his wife indicating he was doing extremely well at home. The note was shared with the team.

We can identify the presence of three interconnected teams involved in the care of Mr. B. by focusing on the changes in goals for his care over time, and on the team members who contributed to the accomplishment of each set of goals. In the acute phase of hospitalization the priority was on the stabilization of his medical condition. Two interconnected teams can be identified during this period: the team of attending physician who admitted the patient, the resident, the intern, and the nurses on the medical unit; and, the team of attending physician, the resident, the intern, and the nurses in the intensive care unit. During the acute phase the team expanded its resources by involving medical specialists in the diagnosis and stabilization of Mr. B.'s coronary problems, associated medical problems, and psychological status. Medical goals predominated during this phase.

During the convalescent phase the team became multidisciplinary by involving the dietitian, enterostomal therapist, the nurse consultant, and others in the recovery process. This multidisciplinary team was operative during the weekly "interdisciplinary team meetings" which encompassed all the team members and disciplines involved in Mr. B.'s care. The members from a variety of disciplines were active in both coordinating and problem-solving.

During the acute phase of Mr. B.'s care, nursing actions strongly reflected the emphasis on medical assistance activities: carrying out medical orders and monitoring physiological status. Medical activities and goals had priority over nursing activities and goals. Marked by the involvement of the nursing consultant, the convalescent phase of care emphasized nursing's separate contribution to and responsibility for comprehensive medical care. The multidisciplinary teams organized around nursing goals were quite different in membership and roles from the specialist team organized around medical goals during the acute phase of illness. The patient and his wife were included as team members. Nursing activities and goals had priority over medical activities and goals. This is *not* to say that nursing was unimportant in the earlier phases or medicine unimportant in the later ones, but, rather, that it is a matter of evolving emphasis, goals, and leadership.

The care of Mr. B. over time involved complex coordination of various professional actions by varying team-member combinations involving clear shifts in leadership. The underlying elements of team structure for communication included the occasions on which team members met face-to-face and communicated in writing. The communication structure was built into hospital procedures for charting, rounds, reports, "team" meetings, and so forth. Care was organized around the general goal of returning Mr. B. to a state of homeostasis. More specific goals relating to the expertise of various disciplines provided the basis for the multiple "teams" that sprang up around Mr. B.'s care. The specific, selected members were chosen through hospital procedures for assigning the intern, resident, and nurses to the patient. Mr. B.'s attending physician, however, was the "leader" of the team. His attitude towards the involvement of members of the team(s) in various roles, because of his influential position, determined the range of expertise that was brought to bear on Mr. B.'s problems.

This clinical example not only demonstrates what good multidisciplinary team action can consist of, but also illustrates some serious constraints on such actions. At all times specific goals were clearly articulated, the responsibilities of members in accomplishing those goals were explicit, and ongoing assessment was evaluated when the goals had been met. Over time new goals emerged, and the nature of the responsibilities of members changed. The guiding principle was to place the leadership (responsibility for recognition of problems, identification of goals, and planning for accomplishment of these goals) on the team member(s) whose expertise was most relevant to the current situation.

A critical shift in leadership occurred when medical members of the team relinquished leadership to nursing members, whose expertise was the most relevant for the latter phases of Mr. B.'s illness. The example also suggests resistance on the part of the intern and the nurses in recognizing the nurses' expertise. The intern would admit only to "lack of time and energy" rather than lack of expertise, and the behavior of the staff nurses was more oriented toward medical goals than nursing goals until their skills were activated by the nurse consultant.

SUMMARY

Ultimately, good teamwork in medical care and health care depends on resolution of the dynamics problems *and* the demonstration of expertise in the task at hand. The building of expertise and the resolution of the dynamics problems are general professional and interprofessional issues which need to be approached on an institutional level. As long as the social structure of health-care systems overvalues medicine and undervalues other disciplines, status dynamics will continue to impede the full development, testing, and potential impact of team care on patient welfare. Teams, as individual small task groups, will need to continue to create ad hoc solutions to those problems which cannot be generalized beyond the specific experience. On the other hand, premature legislation of requirements for "team" modes of care delivery in various parts of our health-care systems will not replace the need for the development of disciplinary expertise by those asserting a right to a place on the multidisciplinary team.

REFERENCES

Aradine, C.R., and M.F. Hansen. "Interdisciplinary Teamwork in Family Health Care." *Nursing Clinics of North America* 5, June 1970, pages 211–222.

Ashley, J. *Hospitals, Paternalism and the Role of the Nurse.* New York: Teachers College Press, 1976.

Bales, R.F. "The Equilibrium Problem in Small Groups." In *Working Papers in the Theory of Action*, T. Parsons, E. Shils, and R.F. Bales, Eds. Glencoe, IL.: Free Press, 1951, pages 111–116.

———— ; F. Strodtbeck; T. Mills; and M. Roseborough. "The Channels of Communication in Small Groups." *American Sociological Review* 16, 1951, pages 461–468.

Bales, R.F. "A Theoretical Framework for Interaction Process Analysis." In *Group Dynamics, Research and Theory*, D. Cartwright and A. Zander, Eds. Evanston, IL.: Row, Peterson, 1953.

Banta, H.D., and R.C. Fox. "Role Strains of a Health Care Team in a Poverty Community." *Social Science and Medicine* 6, 1972, pages 697–722.

Barker, L.F. "The Specialist and the General Practitioner." *Journal of the American Medical Association* 78, March 18, 1922, pages 773-779.

Berger, J.; B.P. Cohen; and M. Zelditch. "Status Characteristics and Social Interaction." In *Interpersonal Behavior in Small Groups*, R. Ofshe, Ed. Englewood Cliffs, N.J.: Prentice-Hall, 1973, pages 194-216.

Brunetto, E., and P. Birk. "The Primary Care Nurse — The Generalist in a Structured Health Care Team." *American Journal of Public Health* 62, June 1972, pages 785-794.

Caudill, W.A. *The Psychiatric Hospital as a Small Society.* Cambridge, MA.: Harvard University Press, 1958.

Feiger, S.M., and M.H. Schmitt. "Collegiality in Interdisciplinary Health Teams: Its Measurement and Its Effects." *Social Science and Medicine* 13A, March 1979, pages 217-229.

Freese, L. "Conditions for Status Equality in Informal Task Groups." *Sociometry* 37, 1974, pages 174-188.

Greenlaw, J.L. "Winners and Losers: Physician Assistant Medication Orders." *Nursing Law and Ethics* 1, 1980, pages 6-7.

Janis, I.L. *Victims of Group Think.* Boston: Houghton Mifflin, 1972.

Katz, S.; J. Papsidero; and L. Halstead. "Team Care and Chronic Illness: A Framework for Teaching Comprehensive Health Care." In *Teaching of Chronic Illness and Aging*, D.W. Clark and T.F. Williams, Eds. Department of Health, Education, and Welfare (NIH) 75-876, 1973, Chapter 5, pages 45-61.

Leininger, M. "This I Believe About Interdisciplinary Health Education for the Future." *Nursing Outlook* 19, 1971, pages 787-791.

Lewis, C.E. "The Physician as a Care Team Leader." *Group Practice* 17, 1968, pages 20-24.

Londey, D. "On the Action of Teams." *Inquiry* 21, Summer 1978, pages 213-218.

Margolin, R.J. "Rationale for Teamwork." *Rehabilitation Record* 10, March/April 1969, pages 32-35.

Milgram, S. "Obedience and Disobedience to Authority." In *Conceptions of Social Life*, W.A. Gamson and A. Modigliani, Eds. Boston: Little Brown, 1974.

The Oxford English Dictionary. James Augustus Henry Murray, Ed. Vol. 7 Oxford: Clarendon Press, 1961, pages 129-130.

Petrie, H.A. "Do You See What I See? The Epistemology of Interdisciplinary Inquiry." *Journal of Aesthetic Education* 10, 1976, pages 29-43.

Richardson, J.T.; J.R. Dugan; L.N. Gray; and B.H. Mayhew. "Expert Power: A Behavioral Interpretation." *Sociometry* 26, 1973, pages 302-324.

Stein, L.I. "The Doctor-Nurse Game." *American Journal of Nursing* 68, January 1968, pages 101-105.

Strodtbeck, F.L.; R.M. James; and C. Hawkins. "Social Status in Jury Deliberations." *American Sociological Review* 22, 1957, pages 713-719.

Torrance, E.P. *Some Consequences of Power Differences in Decision Making in Permanent and Temporary Three Man Groups.* Research Studies Washington State College, 22, 1954, pages 130-140.

Wessen, A.F. "Hospital Ideology and Communication Between Ward Personnel." In *Medical Care*, W.R. Scott and E. Volkhart, Eds. New York: Wiley, 1966.

Wise, H. "Making Health Teams Work." *American Journal of Diseases of Children* 127, 1974, pages 537–542.

———— ; R. Beckhard; I. Rubin; and A.L. Kyte. *Making Health Teams Work.* Cambridge: Ballinger, 1974.

Woollcott, P. "Interdisciplinarity." *Bulletin of the Menninger Clinic* 43, March 1979, pages 161–170.

11

Group Work with Couples and Families

Joan E. Bowers

Family and marital approaches to health care have been available since pioneer work in the early 1950s of Ackerman (1958), Jackson (1961), and Bowen (1961), among others. Theoretical orientations to family therapy have been categorized as psychodynamic, interactional, behavioral, structural, communications-based, and systems-based (Jones, 1980). Theoretical orientations to marital therapy have been categorized as psychodynamic, systems-based, and behavioral (Jacobson and Margolin, 1979). Although these treatment modalities originated in work with pathological families and couples, the approaches have proved valid for family and marital problems which represent other than acute or chronic psychiatric disorders.

In recent years concepts of family therapy have been applied to a variety of situations ranging from school behavior problems to alcohol or drug abuse by a family member. More recently, mental health professionals have begun to utilize *anticipatory guidance* with families who are approaching developmental transitions. Some examples of the latter include expectant parents' classes, group counseling for parents of adolescents, and group support for families with a handicapped child.

Marital therapy emanated from the experience of therapists working with individuals having conflicted marital relationships. Papanek (1971) described six therapy configurations available to therapist and client ranging from dyadic therapy to married couples' group therapy, in which the group is composed of several couples treated by one or two therapists. During the 1970s marriage encounter groups, in which couples met together with lay leaders for intensive weekend experiences to renew and enrich the marital relationship, were popular (Calvo, 1975; Doherty et al., 1978). Some of these methods are discussed in this chapter, with primary emphasis on family problems which lend themselves to group intervention.

NUCLEAR FAMILY THERAPY

In this chapter the focus is on the clinical problems likely to be encountered by a general practitioner using a family or marital approach.

The identified patient in psychiatric and nonpsychiatric family dysfunctions is often a symptom bearer who represents the family's need for help and indicates the existence of conflicts within the family system. The family with a problem adolescent, for example, not only has difficulty with that particular member but may also be struggling with uncertainty about how to survive without this "buffer" person in the home (Langner and Kaplan, 1968). Whether or not such abstruse conflicts, estrangements, and fears are part of the family system, the emergence of an identified patient within the family is not a singular event. The incidence of a problem within the family causes all members to be affected by it, even if they are not active participants in the development and maintenance of the problem. It follows, then, that involvement of the entire family in the change process is the most expedient mechanism by which to effect a solution of the problem.

Dealing with Transitional Problems

Unlike families of psychiatric patients, families who are in developmental transition or those dealing with a member who is having physical problems may not realize that this constitutes a family problem. Even when the burden is apparent to all members, they may remain unwilling to participate in formal therapy which focuses on family dysfunction. If the intervention process is presented as family therapy, with the problem immediately identified as belonging to the family, the usual response will be resistance. If, instead of labeling the family, the health professional accepts the problem as belonging to the patient but requiring the support and involvement of the family if change is to be effected, the response is likely to be positive. This intervention cannot be a superficial, manipulative maneuver, however. The thrust of the therapeutic work must be on the management of the presenting problem by the family system. This is necessary if the family is to remain involved. For example, the child who is overweight cannot alone be expected to make the behavioral and attitudinal changes required to avoid gaining weight or to lose weight, if that is a goal. It may be that in the family the mother and child are enmeshed with each other. This would be shown by lack of limit-setting or overconcern for the child. If this were the case, the mother would need education and support in order to modify the over-involvement. Changes in family behavior regarding limit-setting can begin with food management, since that is a goal which has priority in the family. As therapy progresses, limit-setting issues can be broadened to include the mother's too-ready access to the child and the child's egocentric, demanding behavior. Sibling involvement in such an approach can be enlisted as well. The older sibling who insists on rich desserts may need to change this behavior so as not to torment the overweight child. Conflict within the family or between the marital couple can be incorporated as conflicts relate to the presenting problem. As with more traditional family therapy, caution is advised in dealing too early with those problems which may be construed by the family as divergent from the original contract (Bowers, 1980).

Time-Limited Problems

A similar model of problem-focused therapy can be adapted for families where the initial assessment indicates that the family is not seriously dysfunctional. As a rule, therapy is responsive to those issues in the family which can be directly related to the management of the presenting problem. As the family and the identified patient experience success through initial interventions, the therapist can begin to generalize interventions to include indirectly related issues while continuing to attend to the management of the presenting problem. When the problem is time-limited (a family in crisis because of an adolescent pregnancy), the resolution of the crisis may mean the termination of the therapy or a renegotiation of the therapeutic contract to work on family issues which emerged during the crisis event.

Multiple Family Therapy

Problem-focused therapy with families lends itself to multiple family therapy. Multiple family therapy as conducted with psychiatric patients and their families can often be used to advantage when patient selection is random and not based on specific diagnosis. McCuan-Rathbone and Pierce (1978) conducted this type of therapy with families in which child abuse and delinquency occurred multigenerationally.

Multiple family therapy is an approach which seeks neither development of insight nor basic personality change. Rather, the goals are improvement in family communication patterns, improved understanding of family functioning and dynamics, and some element of change in family functioning (Frager, 1978). These goals are achieved through various mechanisms including: use of families as cotherapists; competition among families in the group; delineation of the field of interaction (the individual member's behavior is seen as occurring within the context of the family); learning by analogy and through identification; learning through the identification constellation (the confrontation with identical patterns in the other families promotes attention); learning through modeling provided by the healthier family groups; and the amplification and modulation of signals (families translate for each other and for the therapist) (Benningfield, 1978).

Little research has been done on the outcome of multiple family therapy, but a number of authors have reported success based on clinical evaluations. Much of this success appears related to the available change mechanisms listed above and to the fact that multiple family work combines the advantages of family therapy and group therapy structure. The reader is referred to Benningfield (1978) and Frager (1978) for reviews of multiple family therapy approaches.

Network Therapy

Network therapy was described by Attneave (1969), Speck and Attneave (1971), and Rueveni (1979). In this approach, the extended family, including friends and neighbors, is called into sessions to work with the nuclear family around resolution of a problem. The network approach has been used in working with multiproblem families, communal groups composed of unrelated persons living in one household or complex of households, and clan or tribal problems such as those reported by Attneave (1969).

Despite the prevalence of nuclear family households in contemporary society, the exchange of communications, goods, and services among family members and across generations remains a potent force (Sussman, 1964). Exchange of goods and services is particularly important when the nuclear family is in crisis because of illness or in transition because of birth, death, or other social change. Regardless of the cause, when the nuclear family unit is in crisis it behooves the nurse to explore the availability of family resources and to encourage the extended family and social network to contribute problem-solving resources and skills. With geographic dislocation common in this country, the nurse may find that the nuclear family does not have ready access to their extended family or possess a well-developed social network support system. In these circumstances social agencies may be mobilized to provide the required supports.

Attneave (1969), and Speck and Attneave (1972) described therapy with native American extended family groups and provided examples of such intervention. In one example, a native American child was taken into another family because the biological mother was not capable of caring for the child. Another case example described work with a network which was deteriorating rapidly and which had already lost several significant members, including the grandfather who had headed the group. Losses had occurred through physical illness, murder, and suicide. The family came into therapy not because of the above incidents but because the newly designated leader was depressed, acutely suicidal, and deemed in need of psychiatric hospitalization. Attneave described various interventions *with the clan* which resulted in a regeneration of "the network's cooperative distribution of nurturing responsibilities" (1969, p. 206).

Regardless of whether the nuclear family is struggling alone with the crisis or whether the entire network/clan is faced with multiple crises, this approach to therapeutic intervention has claimed clinical success. With family treatment in general, little or no outcome research data have been reported to date.

MARITAL COUPLE TREATMENT

As mentioned in the introduction, marital couple therapy has been in existence for the last two to three decades. While there are at least three major approaches (*psychodynamic, systems,* and *behavioral*), only the psychodynamic approach has been reported as being used in the group setting to any extent (Jacobson and Margolin, 1979). Brownell (1978) reported a high degree of success in working with couples using behavioral approaches to weight management for one of the partners. Use of groups with a highly structured behavioral approach may be effective, but there is need to refer the couples to a group only after several sessions in which data is gathered and needs are assessed. Similar procedures were described by Blinder and Kirschenbaum (1967) in a report of a psychodynamic approach. The rationale for using individual conjoint sessions is based on the belief that each couple's problems are idiosyncratic. The therapist, therefore, needs to explore fully the communication problems and the neurotic components of the marital relationship before involving the couple in a group setting.

There appears to be considerable movement toward the use of behavioral approaches in marital couple therapy even by those practitioners who classify themselves as psychoanalytic or psychodynamic in their orientation. Gurman and Knudson (1978), however, criticized the strict or predominant use of behavioral approaches in marital therapy, asserting that it neglects the deeper, more neurotic components of the marital relationship. Behavior therapy does have the distinct advantage of lending itself readily to evaluation. Consequently there is more outcome research in the use of this behavior therapy than there is on more traditional approaches. For an extensive review of relevant literature, Jacobson and Margolin (1979) may be consulted.

Treating Sexual Dysfunction

Treatment approaches for sexual dysfunction have been classified as psychoanalytic, behavioral, and the "new" sex therapy. The latter includes the approaches of Masters and Johnson, and Kaplan (Fogel, 1979). When marital couples seek treatment, sexual dysfunction is frequently a component of their problem. Whether the marital relationship or the sexual dysfunction should be the primary focus of treatment will depend on several factors. These include the priority the couple expresses and the clinical judgment of the therapist regarding the advantages and disadvantages of treating the sexual dysfunction first. Adequate clinical judgment necessitates an assessment of the couple's state of alienation and their readiness to work on the sexual problem as well as the probability of a relatively straightforward resolution of the problem (Jacobson and Margolin, 1979).

The Masters and Johnson program for treatment of sexual dysfunction is widely acknowledged as the paradigm for behavioral sexual therapy currently in practice. Their requirement that the couple take a two-week leave to engage in this extensive program is sometimes unrealistic for couples needing help. As a result many sex therapists use components of the Masters and Johnson program which can be carried out in a more traditional out-patient setting (Messersmith, 1976; Fogel, 1979; Jacobson and Margolin, 1979). In addition there is need to view the sexual dysfunction as closely related to conflicts and problems occurring in the total marital relationship (Messersmith, 1976; Kaplan, 1974). This treatment philosophy mandates that the therapeutic process encompass both the sexual dysfunction and the relationship problems (Messersmith, 1976; Fogel, 1979; Jacobson and Margolin, 1979).

Maddock (1976) described an extensive program in sexual health which treated individuals and couples primarily in a group context.

This program utilized the processes of education and enrichment as a means of overcoming sexual distress which was believed to be based on distortion and misinformation. Sexual health-care programs are designed to relate to each of the following dimensions and beliefs about human sexual relationships: A healthy sexual relationship requires: shared sexual meanings and mutually acceptable behaviors; basic knowledge of self and the partner; certain behavioral skills; and shared desire for physical and emotional intimacy. Finally, group treatment has been used with individuals who manifest sexual dysfunction and who either do not have or cannot involve a partner in the treatment process (Barbach, 1974; Fogel, 1979; Zilbergeld, 1975).

Specific Family Problems

Killilea (1976) extensively reviewed the literature for descriptions of self-help and mutual-help organizations and groups. These groups have emerged in response to the need for contact and communication among people who are coping with similar life experiences which need to be made bearable. The format ranges from face-to-face encounters, written communications, hot lines, radio talk shows, and newspaper advice columns. A majority of the organizations are not led by professionals and are problem-oriented or situationally focused. Some of the characteristics of these mutual-support groups which have evolved over time include: members share a common experience; members offer each other help and support; recipients of help become transformed into dispensers of help; successful members help newcomers adopt a self-concept of normality; members offer information about problems and transitions; and members participate in constructive action toward shared goals (Killilea, 1976). Out of this consumer-developed movement and his own clinical experience, Caplan (1976) developed a paradigm for professional intervention with populations at high risk. It is this model, in large measure, which forms the basis for the problem-focused family group interventions described in the following sections of this chapter.

GROUP WORK WITH CHILD-ABUSING PARENTS

The study of child abuse has been approached from a variety of frameworks. Steele and Pollock (1974) wrote extensively of the psychiatric assessment and treatment of child-abusing parents. Gil (1970) emphasized the sociocultural patterning of abuse, and Martin (1976) approached the problem from a multidisciplinary framework.

While researchers have not been able to define a specific child-abusing personality, there is agreement that the following factors are shared by abusing parents: 1) a history of abuse by his or her own parents; 2) unrealistic expectations of the abused child; 3) a conflicted or stormy relationship between the parenting partners; 4) isolation of the family (Freu and Alden, 1978; Steele and Pollock, 1974; Helfer, 1977). In addition abusing parents manifested immaturity and poor self-image, poor impulse control, and limited capacity to express their own needs. Gil's findings (1970) about circumstances surrounding the documented abusive incidents in this national sample are relevant: mounting stress because of life circumstances was reported in fifty-nine percent of the cases; seventeen percent of the abusive incidents occurred when the child was left with a male caretaker or partner who was not the child's parent; and thirteen percent of abusers were intoxicated at the time of the abusive incident. On data analysis, there was strong correlation among these three factors.

Most frequently, child abuse is diagnosed in the hospital emergency service. Public health nurses, welfare caseworkers, and primary school teachers, because they have ready access to families and children, are also important case-finders. For a thorough treatment of assessment criteria the reader is referred to Sideleau (1978).

Intervention Models   Several intervention models have been proposed in the literature. Steele and Pollock (1974) described an individual, analytical, psychotherapeutic approach. Savino and Sanders (1973) described a multimethod approach which combined a self-help group approach with regular home visits and parenting classes in which behavior modification techniques were taught. Egan (1980) completed the study of an intervention model in which a group of abusing mothers were taught stress-management techniques. An intergenerational treatment approach in which a minimum of three family generations were involved in therapy was described by McCuan-Rathbone and Pierce (1978).

Reaching the Abusive Parents

Regardless of the intervention approach selected, abusing parents require special sensitivity if they are to profit from the experience. First and foremost, the professional needs to be aware of personal reactions such as the anger aroused by the abusive behavior. Being able to recognize the abused child within the abusing parent is one means of dealing with one's personal feelings. Dealing with one's own reactions is critical because the abusing parent is sensitive to rejection. In addition, contacts with police, community agencies, and other health professionals are inevitably stressful, thus raising the level of defensiveness. Flexibility on the part of the professional as well as a willingness to expand the bounds of the usual therapist-patient relationship are extremely important if abusive parents are to be treated successfully (Savino and Sanders, 1973; Steele and Pollock, 1974).

The group approach to intervention appears to be highly useful in working with abusive parents. As mentioned previously, social isolation is a major factor in the lives of these people. Group experience brings them in contact with others who are undergoing similar difficulties, and opens avenues for developing social and self-help skills. In order to allow the latter to occur, it is important that the group be open-ended (members come into the group as they are referred). This provides a framework in which older members can use their developing skills to help newer members benefit from group process. In turn, this gives the newcomers a feeling of "if they're making it, so can I."

This approach is similar to that described by Savino and Sanders (1973) in which the members are encouraged to share feelings of anger and frustration directed toward the community at large and toward individuals in particular who seem responsible for their predicament. It is not uncommon for child abusers to attribute their difficulties to their child's pediatrician, school teacher, or visiting nurse. Goals for the group beyond this preliminary ventilation phase are two-pronged: to explore the circumstances causing the abuse, and to understand developmental and parenting issues. The former involves exploration of their own histories of poor parenting, poor peer relationships, and poor social experiences. Because a majority of these parents have experienced stress prior to the abusive incident, active assistance in dealing with life stresses is a major aspect of the treatment process. Crisis intervention methods in the group setting, and having staff and other group members available to assist with utilizing community resources are effective measures.

Parenting Issues When individual parents have moved beyond defensiveness and into a trusting relationship with leaders and other group members, focus on parenting issues can begin. In the group this can be accomplished by talking about reasonable expectations for children at certain ages. This alone is insufficient and two other approaches are used in addition. Home visiting, whereby the nurse can discuss individual problems *and* model parenting skills is one. Another is the use of a group training approach in which parents are taught to use behavior modification and positive reinforcement. This could be provided through a format devised especially for a particular group of parents or the parents and their children may be referred to special preschool programs if these are available.

If a child has been removed from the home, one needs to assess family readiness for the return of the child. Guidelines for this assessment include the following questions:

- Can the parents support each other and ask help from others in the environment when a crisis occurs?
- Have they developed and demonstrated more realistic expectations of the child?
- Have they found sources of gratification in their own lives so that the child will not be expected to meet their needs (Krindler, 1976; Justice and Justice, 1978; Kempe and Helfer, 1972)?

Furthermore, when the child returns home, parents should continue in treatment in order to test out and consolidate new parenting skills. In those cases where alcohol abuse, an unstable marriage, or financial pressures are present, great care must be taken in advising that the abused child return to the home.

Guidelines similar to those mentioned above may be used to determine readiness to terminate therapy. In addition, actual improvement in the parent-child relationship should be assessed. Assessment should include the parent's ability to accept the child as an individual, to demonstrate age-appropriate expectations, to tolerate negative behavior, and to show affection without expecting a return of affection (Martin, 1976).

GROUPS FOR BATTERED WIVES

Wife battering, which has long been evident in society, has only recently gained attention as a problem of major proportions in our own culture. As a phenomenon, it cuts across socioeconomic class, religious affiliation, and geographical location. No group of women is exempt. Past efforts at describing the syndrome have concentrated on the characteristics of the victim as a precipitator, or at least as an active and willing participant in the abuse (Elbow, 1977; Symonds, 1979). Most of these explanations stemmed from the theory of masochism, an important part of Freud's theory of feminine psychology. More recently, it has been recognized as one more aspect of "blaming the victim" (Ryan, 1971).

In a recent article Symonds (1979) refuted masochism as an explanation for understanding violence against women and posited that violence-prone marriages may be divided into two groups: those in which the husband has a history of violence which precedes the marriage, and those in which violence is a form of communication used when all other attempts at communication fail. In the latter relationships violence makes both partners feel worse, not better (p. 171). It is these relationships which appear most often in private practice and family therapy; while not exceptional, they do not represent the majority of wife-battering cases.

It is the first group of wives, married to violence-prone husbands, who are more likely to seek a women's shelter and who are the subject of this discussion. These are women who have generally experienced intermittent but continuing acts of violence at the hands of their partners. Often violence begins during the courtship period or within the first year of marriage. Frequently these wives do not seek treatment for injuries sustained, and if treatment is sought, will not honestly report the cause. This is because of fear of further retaliation from the partner. The problem remains secret because physicians rarely investigate the cause of an injury beyond a perfunctory question or two. In a recent study, Petro, Quann, and Graham (1978) found that in its first six months of operation, a women's crisis center had only six of three hundred cases referred by physicians; all six cases were seen in the same hospital emergency service.

Psychological Reaction Patterns among Victims

In an effort to understand why these wives stay married to their violent husbands, Symonds (1979) turned to the literature dealing with victims of castastrophe (Spiegel, 1955) and found similarities between the two groups of victims in their psychological reaction patterns. The majority of catastrophe victims reacted either with panic, characterized by terror, or with apathy, characterized by emotional exhaustion. Furthermore, these victims later interpreted the catastrophe as justified punishment, resulting in feelings of guilt, unworthiness, and depression (Spiegel, 1955). This framework may be used to understand an abused wife's acceptance of guilt as deserved punishment, a frequent finding among these women. It is thought that when a woman has been severely beaten by her partner, the terror which she feels *infantilizes* her. Isolation and hopelessness are other feelings resulting from the violent partner's threats and from the wife's discovery that there is no one out there to help her. As apathetic and despairing as a prisoner of war, the wife may subsequently experience total submission to the "enemy," who is her violent partner (Symonds, 1979). Between abusive attacks her partner may be kind and apologetic for his abuse. Early attempts to find help, which met rejection, are abandoned, and the woman becomes more isolated, caught in a two-person world inhabited by herself and her violent partner. Never knowing when the next attack will occur, she exists in a constant state of dread and fear. Until these processes are interrupted, the battered woman generally cannot take constructive action for herself. The opportunity for escape is now more available through shelters and other services, both physically protective and psychologically supportive, that offer alternatives to victims of abuse.

Group work with battered wives has the advantages of providing a support group in which the woman can, perhaps for the first time, realize that she is not alone. This realization has several meanings, not the least of which is that there are many other women who have experienced and are experiencing similar traumas. Her isolation is also reduced because she now has the opportunity to share with sympathetic listeners her traumatic experiences. This supportive group network, led by health-care workers, is in a position to help with basic services such as financial advice, job counseling, and legal advice.

How the Group Works

Because a major offering of the group is peer support and crisis intervention, the access to the group should be open-ended, with new members accepted as they are referred or seek entry on their own initiative. In this way, older members in the group can function in supportive, cotherapy roles. Rounsaville (1978) found that those abused women who followed through on referral for counseling differed in several respects from those who did not. Those who followed through on referrals were women who had already taken serious steps to end the abusive relationship; who had demonstrated an ability to use public assistance to advantage; and who had shown less hesitation about using psychiatric services. These findings have important implications for working with women who may be entering the group through referral rather than individual initiative. Women who are referred to the group may join it, but they will need special attention and concern if they are to continue in the group long enough to derive benefit. First and foremost, neither the group leaders nor other members should encourage or urge the woman to leave her partner. Other people have probably attempted this strategy in the past, but to no avail. The abused wife will not leave her partner until she has developed enough self-confidence and trust of the community at large to be able to do so. Initially, she needs help in recognizing that she has alternatives. Elbow (1977) listed these alternatives: the woman can leave; she can continue in the relationship while hoping that her husband will change; or she can continue in the relationship while giving up hope that he will change. When women opt for the second or third alternative, they are encouraged to recognize that this is a conscious, deliberate choice. After becoming involved in counseling, during which self-esteem is fostered, the woman is more able to carry out plans to leave.

Because the battered wife, in her psychologically infantilized state, is often protective of her abusing partner, it is important that the group leaders not berate or deride him. It is important to acknowledge the woman's ambivalence by recognizing her pain in being abused by a man who at other times is kind, loving, and sensitive to her needs. If she has a history of attempts to leave him, this can be acknowledged as part of the same ambivalent pattern. If her ambivalence is not dealt with openly and with support, she may feel further alienated and misunderstood (Elbow, 1977).

Exploring Abuse Patterns Symonds (1979) has indicated the abused wife's acceptance of guilt and punishment. In dealing with this it is important that attention be given to exploring the patterns of abuse in individual cases. While avoiding any implication that the woman herself is to blame for the violence, she need not be told that she did not cause the abuse. With the goal of helping her master the situation, she should be encouraged to explore abuse patterns. Exploration may help develop the means to avoid further abuse and give her a sense of doing something positive for herself.

Facing Problems Realistically

Assessment of the woman's readiness to leave her partner is an important facet of treatment. Many women make enthusiastic plans prematurely, are overcome by ambivalence, and return to the partner, only to find that life with him continues in the same abusive way as before. During these vacillations the woman needs support for her efforts and encouragement to face her problems as realistically as possible. Indicators that the battered wife has approached a point of readiness to leave include: sensible and concrete planning — she has thought through some of the details of income, shelter, and legal service and has begun to make an investment in taking the step; concern for herself as a person, whereby she moves from wanting to "show him," to a position of recognizing the hazards to herself and her children; and acceptance of the reality that the abuse is a long-standing pattern and not merely isolated episodes. Thus her decision to leave hinges not on the abusive episodes but constitutes a well-planned action carried through in the nonabusive periods (Elbow, 1977).

As with several of the other groups discussed in this chapter, the major goal of group work with battered wives is *not* basic personality change. It is likely that a reasonable number of these women would benefit from treatment aimed at ameliorating neurotic patterns and improving ego functioning. These women should be informed of the professional's assessment of this need and be made aware of the community resources available to them.

Since the battered wives' group is open-ended, the members will at any given time be in different phases of progress. Because of vacillation caused by ambivalence which most of these women experience, the group itself goes through recurring phases of progression and regression, typified by the pendular life cycle model of groups. Experiencing these recurring phases gives the group members opportunity to see others face temporary setbacks and to function as role models for newer members in the group. In addition to these benefits, the group approach for helping the battered wife uses a pool of problem-solving resources to meet the basic survival needs which many of the women face.

CLINICAL EXAMPLE: GROUP INTERVENTION FOR A BATTERED WOMAN

Anne M., twenty-six years old and mother of an eight-year-old son, Billy, entered the battered women's group after being referred by the emergency room physician who treated her for contusions and lacerations sustained in a fall down her apartment steps. At that time Ms. M. was upset and readily admitted to the emergency room nurse that her partner had pushed her down the steps after threatening to strangle her during an argument. She was most upset by this episode because her son had attempted to intervene on her behalf and "shouldn't have to see these things."

Ms. M. had run away from a foster home at the age of sixteen with a man eight years her senior. She became pregnant after one year and continued to live with the baby's father for another three years. At that time she left him amicably ("I just didn't love him") and returned to the city where several family members lived. She met her current partner, Ed, through mutual friends and decided to move in with him because she "wanted out" of the house in which she and Billy were living. At the time of this decision she knew that Ed drank heavily, but did not foresee problems. Two years of living together proved her wrong: they argued constantly "over everything and anything" and he began pushing her around during the arguments. The physical abuse became more serious and she made the decision to leave him. He did not openly disagree with this decision but then became intoxicated on the day of the move and the episode which resulted in her referral to the group ensued. She denied suffering any physical abuse as a child or during the relationship with Billy's father. She did report a history of running away from home as an adolescent, which resulted in the foster home placement from which she also ran away.

After she implemented her decision to leave Ed and sever all contact with him, Ms. M. described herself as fearful and depressed. She was impatient with Billy and worried about being able to make it on her own. She had no job skills and had been employed only briefly as a waitress. Currently she was being assisted financially by relatives and had applied for a welfare grant. A major goal for her was to get a high school diploma and obtain vocational training in order to become more independent.

In the group she was praised for her ability to make a decision to leave Ed and stick with the decision. She was helped to explore options and was supported in her efforts in this direction. As she gained self-confidence she began to explore the similarities in the way she interacted with Ed and with her previous partner. While exploring these similarities, she also recognized that Ed's explosive temper and alcohol abuse were factors which tipped the balance and resulted in the abusive behavior. From this, she began to question her own behavior, which seemed directed at avoiding intimacy and closeness in her various relationships. By this time she had successfully completed a diploma equivalency program and was enrolled in the vocational training program of her choice. She was encouraged to consider psychotherapy to help with relationship problems which she had identified for herself and was given several community resources to contact when and if she decided to do this.

Despite individual differences among battered wives, Ms. M. represents important similarities to women described in the literature. She followed through on referral to the group mainly because she had already decided to leave the abusive relationship. She realistically assessed the escalating danger to herself and her child in leaving Ed. She felt uncertain of her ability to support herself and her child, and this made her more vulnerable and frightened. She demonstrated social resourcefulness, in being able to rally family support, and follow through on her own in applying for a welfare grant. Finally, her relationship pattern with her parents and the two men in her life bore many similarities which, through the group process, she began to explore. She recognized the possibility of being in need of further therapeutic work. A year after leaving the group she had completed vocational training, was employed, and had entered therapy through a local mental health center.

GROUP WORK WITH PARENTS OF HANDICAPPED CHILDREN

Because the range of physical and mental handicapping conditions which affect children is extensive, this section is addressed to some general considerations of parents' needs. Johnson (1979) listed the factors which influence a family's adaptation to a child with a disability: whether the disability is present at birth or is diagnosed at some later time; whether it is a life-threatening disability; whether the disability is permanently handicapping, as opposed to temporary and treatable; whether the disability will interfere substantially with daily routines; and whether the disability is outwardly observable. Generally, the family's adapation to a physically disabled child will be more difficult when the disability is life-threatening (congenital heart disease), potentially permanently handicapping (cerebral palsy), substantially interfering with daily routines (blindness or deafness), outwardly observable (spina bifida), and when the presence of the disability at birth interferes with successful bonding.

When a disabled child is born the entire family system is affected. The severity of the impact will be determined by the family's previous experience with the disability, the family's preparation for the possibility of a birth defect, and the severity of the disability. In addition, family patterns, such as the stability of the marital relationship, the presence of unimpaired children in the family, and the age of the parents, affect the family's adaptation to the disability. Economic and social resources of the family also influence their ability to cope. Finally, the family's experience with the health-care system can be a positive or negative influence in the ongoing process of adaptation.

The immediate event of disability in a child, either at birth or at some later time, is a crisis experience for the family. In addition, growth and development of the child and the family will entail sequential adaptations over time. For many families, the affective undercurrent is one of chronic sorrow.

The initial crisis event for the family can best be dealt with on an individual basis by health professionals who are sensitive, empathetic, and caring. Principles of crisis intervention and awareness of the grieving process are necessary components of the intervention during this phase. Parents should be helped to enter a group with other parents whose children have similar conditions such as cerebral palsy or juvenile-onset diabetes. The adjustment and adaptation process for families with disabled children has core similarities regardless of the handicapping condition. There are also basic problems which confront all such families and which are specific to the handicapping disability. A group of parents helping each other to deal with these problems and providing anticipatory guidance to parents of newly diagnosed children can be of inestimable help. Because need for help is ongoing, it is recommended that the group be open-ended, with new members entering as need arises.

Core Issues

Some of the core issues with which the group must deal may be considered in developmental terms. An initial task is the continuous work on resolution of the acute grieving process. Both parents should be encouraged to participate in the group, and adequate resolution is related to the strength of the marital relationship. Help from professionals and from group members in dealing with anger, guilt, and shame as reactions to the disability promotes the family's ability to deal with current and future problems. Reactions to the child, particularly one with an observable anomaly, by relatives, friends, and neighbors can be difficult for the family (Mercer, 1977). Coping with the health-care systems and the numerous professionals involved in the care of the child is also a draining task. Parents need help in determining what their family can reasonably manage while continuing to provide optimal care for their disabled child (Johnson, 1979). Advocacy, along with guidance, in using community resources can help the parents develop the skills to function as advocates for their child in the future.

Parents of disabled children need help in balancing overprotection and unduly high expectations if they are to help the disabled child to develop to the fullest potential (Waechter, 1975). Other children in the family encounter difficulties both within and outside of the family. If the disabled child requires a great deal of physical attention, siblings may feel neglected and react with behavioral problems. Parents need assistance in working out the distribution of their limited resources of time and money. Not to be overlooked are the parents' own needs, both as individuals and as a couple. Respite from constant attention to the disabled child may be difficult to arrange. In addition to making useful suggestions, group members often work out a system for relieving each other periodically to provide safe care for the child in the parents' absence. This is especially important when the child needs constant attention.

The Importance of Professional Advice

While parents often reach reasonable solutions to many of their special problems, they will continue to require expert guidance from the health professional. Well-meant but inaccurate advice from friends and relatives, or conflicting advice from various health-care professionals will need sorting out. Because this is an important aspect of the leader's role, the leader should be well acquainted with the disability, the problems expected, and the rehabilitative treatments in use. Additionally, liaison with primary health-care professionals and with representatives of community agencies can be of great importance.

It may be seen from the foregoing that a group such as this facilitates the adjustment of the parents and families through the use of group process. In the group, crisis intervention is available; problem-solving skills, a support network, and advocacy relationships are promoted. The group process is one of recurrent phases, based on its open-ended nature and on anticipation that recurrent adjustments will confront the group members throughout the life span of the group. It is suggested that the group be considered as a resource which the parents will utilize for an unspecified period of time, depending on the nature of the disability. As family strengths increase and the initial hurdles are overcome, members may decide to drop out. Progress and gains should be reviewed; re-entry at some later time should be encouraged. As the disabled child enters new developmental phases, with new age-specific tasks to be accomplished, such as entry into school or adolescence, parents may wish to re-enter the group, or to join another group of parents with parallel needs. Whichever choice is made, the parents will need continuing support in dealing with the tasks facing their family over time. This presumes an ongoing commitment on the part of the professionals involved in helping families to attain optimal development, both for themselves and their children.

CLINICAL EXAMPLE: COPING WITH THE DIAGNOSIS OF A HANDICAPPED CHILD

Mr. and Mrs. D., parents of a child with newly diagnosed cerebral palsy, were referred to the group by their pediatrician. Eric had been a "difficult" baby who was hospitalized twice for symptoms of failure to thrive. At eighteen months he had been diagnosed as being moderately afflicted with cerebral palsy, at which time the referral to the group was made. It took persuasion to get Mrs. D. to come to the group; her husband refused to attend because of work pressures. The family included another son David, four.

Mrs. D.'s attendance at the group was sporadic at first and she participated verbally only when asked to do so. Concern about her infrequent attendance, lack of participation, and evident distress resulted in concerted efforts on the part of the leaders and members to increase her participation in the group. Over time she was able to be more open, sharing her feelings of ambivalence and guilt over Eric's condition. Her husband's lack of involvement and his apparent rejection of Eric were serious problems for her. She was helped to understand that these behaviors were his way of coping with his own feelings of grief and guilt. As she worked through her own feelings, Mrs. D. was able to make renewed efforts to communicate with her husband. Several other fathers in the group talked about the ways in which their wives had helped them to deal with their feelings. From these discussions, Mrs. D. developed strategies which she role-played in the group setting. She was later able to use these, and eventually her husband responded to her efforts to have him join the group. In spite of his early resistance he soon became invested in the group. The couple's ability to communicate improved and both parents discussed the problems of caring for Eric. Previously, Mr. D. had refused to care for his son in his wife's absence. Now he talked about his fears of not being able to care for Eric adequately, but recognized the need to share the burden which he had left to Mrs. D. to manage alone.

The couple have been members of the group for more than a year. They both attend regularly and, while continuing to work on their own problems, they have assumed the role of experienced group members who reach out to support and encourage newer members in the group.

GROUP WORK WITH PARENTS OF DYING CHILDREN

Families in which a child has been diagnosed as having terminal illness are faced not only with the crises of diagnosis and death but also with the need to sustain their child as normally as possible throughout recurrent episodes of treatment and hospitalization. If other children are in the family, they also must be sustained in their developmental experiences. In addition, the parents as individuals and as a couple have needs that must be met throughout the illness and crisis of the child's eventual death.

Use of a group treatment model to support parents through this tragic experience has the advantage of providing contact with other parents who are coping with similar experiences. The group setting provides an atmosphere of empathy and understanding from people who are dealing with the same issues, a sense of "being in it together." Professionals functioning as group leaders bring to the situation not only their experience in providing psychosocial support but also their expertise regarding the issues to be faced. For example, the professional can provide information about the intrapsychic and behavioral phenomena which the parents may be experiencing, thus normalizing the experience and diminishing the sense of unreality or loss of control which they feel. In addition, the professional brings knowledge of and access to needed resources, thus functioning in an advocacy role. The members bring to the group much of their own experience in dealing with salient issues, and also form a supportive network which operates outside of the meetings and extends beyond the life of the group itself.

Ambulatory Health Clinics

The framework within which the group exists greatly influences its structure and progress. If the group is constituted as part of an ambulatory health clinic, it is likely that daytime meetings will include only one parent. Special attention should be given to this; meetings scheduled for evening hours when both parents can attend would be highly preferable so that the parents can deal together with issues. It has been noted that there is a differential rate of dealing with this type of family crisis by the two parents: men express their need to stay in control while women are more openly expressive of emotional responses to the crisis. Maintaining control, however, is expensive to the individual and is frequently viewed by the other spouse as withdrawal and rejection (Kennell, 1970; Helmroth and Steinitz, 1978; Lascari, 1978).

Ongoing Therapy   When the group is part of ongoing therapy in a special hospital unit, other problems with participation may develop. If the treatment unit is a referral center, only one parent (usually the mother) will be in attendance. There will be many occasions when a parent may be reluctant to leave the bedside of the critically ill child for any reason, thus making attendance at meetings irregular.

Group Participation by Health-Care Professionals

Leadership and staff participation in the group require careful consideration. A not uncommon reaction of parents to the stress they are experiencing is anger and hostility directed at the treatment staff. Should staff members from the unit directly responsible for the care of their child be actively involved in the group, this may inhibit the participants' willingness to be candid in the group sessions. If leadership for the group is provided by persons from outside the unit, leaders will need to establish good working relationships with unit staff before the group's inception. Ongoing work on communication between the group leaders and the unit staff will be of utmost importance.

When the group is organized to meet the needs of parents whose children are treated in different hospital units by various physicians, the communication between leaders, referring physicians, and nursing staff become even more critical (Heller and Schneider, 1978).

Assessing the Need for Psychiatric Referral It must be kept in mind that such a group is not a psychotherapy endeavor. Individual parents may very well present pre-existing psychiatric problems; marital difficulties of some couples may antedate the current crisis. The group leaders will need to be astute in assessing the need for immediate or future psychiatric referral in these circumstances. Should individual or marital problems intrude too heavily into the group task, a decision about having these persons continue in the group may be necessary, so that the overriding goals of the group can be facilitated.

Goals for this type of group should be based on principles of crisis intervention theory (Aguilera et al., 1970; Hoff, 1978) and on a knowledge of the task facing the grieving family (Lindemann, 1944; Kennell et al., 1970). The former include: the parents' perception of this crisis event; exploration of their situational supports; review of the coping mechanisms which they are currently using, as compared with those used in past crises; and exploration of the barriers which are hindering effective coping.

Understanding Grieving

Grieving entails both behavioral and interpersonal experiences which may be confusing and frightening. The group participants will benefit from information about such common reactions as irritability, anorexia, insomnia, difficulty with concentration, guilt about their child's illness, and anger at the treatment staff. The group leaders should know the probable course of the illness and the treatment protocol in order to correct misinformation and answer questions which parents raise. The leaders' awareness of behavior and expected reactions to treatment, based on the developmental level of the child, are critical, since the parents must help the child deal with the illness on a day-to-day basis. If there are other children in the family, the parents also must deal with behavioral reactions in these children as well.

Reactions of relatives to the crisis can be problematic for the parents (Lascari, 1978). If the parents are forewarned of this possibility, they are better prepared to avoid conflict between the advice of relatives and health-care professionals for management of the child's illness.

Structuring a Group

So many positive gains can be achieved by parents through exposure to others who are coping successfully that an open-ended group structure seems advisable for this population. Parents should be invited to attend by professionals and by members of the group. An initial refusal should not be accepted as final; rather, efforts should be made to meet the parents informally, at which time the purpose and goals of group participation can be explained. Group membership may include all parents of children being treated in a small unit. In a larger unit several groups may be necessary to keep manageable numbers in each group. Groups might develop logically around age of the child, since problems facing the child and parents will be different for different ages and developmental stages (Lascari, 1978; Tietz et al., 1977; Katz et al., 1980).

Time and place for the group meetings should be consistent. Proximity to the unit reduces the time parents must absent themselves from their child's bedside. A comfortably furnished room, allowing for quiet and privacy as well as informality, is desirable. The amount of time devoted to the group can vary depending on the size of the group and the leaders' time constraints. Given the nature of the issues to be dealt with, meetings of forty-five minutes to an hour, two or three times a week would seem to have great advantages over a weekly two-hour session.

Session Formats   Format for the sessions should include opportunity for questions regarding treatment as well as time for crisis intervention and anticipatory grieving. The issue of confidentiality must be confronted, particularly since parents need to ventilate feelings of frustration and anger toward the treatment team. Availability of the group leaders to parents outside of the sessions is advisable. It is unlikely that a group such as this can meet all the needs of these parents; individual contacts with other support staff such as social workers, nurse consultants, and clergy should be facilitated and encouraged.

Particular concern must be devoted to the parents after their child has died. Referral for grief counseling and follow-up is appropriate in all but exceptional cases. The family whose child is treated in a medical center far from home is particularly vulnerable, since the death of the child and the return home means the loss of an intensive support network developed during hospitalization. This is an area which requires the development of a methodology for adequate referral and follow-up services (Tietz, 1977).

Finally, a word about the professionals involved in leading such a group. The emotional toll on these persons can be enormous, and there is a need to develop support systems which meet their emotional and professional needs if they are to avoid rapid burnout (Kopel and Mock, 1978).

CLINICAL EXAMPLE: HELPING THE FAMILY OF A CHILD WITH TERMINAL CANCER

The B. family were referred to a university cancer center three thousand miles from home for a bone marrow transplant for their nine-year-old son, Greg. Mr. B. was the donor and therefore planned to be at the center approximately five weeks; Mrs. B. planned to stay the required four months while Greg was undergoing treatment. Two older children, Ken, fourteen, and Alice, thirteen, remained at their home in Georgia with their maternal grandmother. The B.'s had an advantage over other families seeking treatment at the center. Mrs. B.'s maternal aunt and her family lived thirty miles from the center. Greg had previously received two courses of chemotherapy, so the family had already been subjected to a great deal of stress, both emotional and financial, prior to their arrival at the center.

The B.'s were reluctant to join the parents' counseling group, but did so after several informal sessions with parents already participating. Because Greg's course of therapy was stormy, Mr. B. did not return home as planned; instead, he was present throughout the hospitalization. The parents initially took turns attending the sessions so that one of them could stay with Greg at all times. As Greg's condition became more serious, his siblings and grandmother also traveled to the center and this relieved the parents' vigil.

The B.'s were openly expressive in the group of their anger at the staff. They had many concerns about Greg's treatment, but were also concerned because of Greg's exceedingly demanding behavior. If Mrs. B. returned, at her husband's insistence, to their apartment for a night's sleep, Greg would telephone in the middle of the night and insist she remain at the center.

In the group sessions the parents were encouraged to talk about their frustrations and concerns. They were also encouraged to talk about experiences during Greg's previous hospitalizations. Emphasis was placed on their coping behaviors, and they were supported in their efforts to enhance coping measures during this experience. With other parents, they discussed the need to set limits on some of Greg's demands, and developed the strength to ask other people to relieve them in staying at Greg's bedside while they met some of their own needs. The B.'s were allowed to maintain hope in the face of a very poor prognosis for their son.

During the two months of Greg's hospitalization the B.'s went through recurrent stages in their experience in the group. Initially, they needed to trust the group members and the treatment team. As this was accomplished, they could share their fears and concerns, and accept help in dealing with them. With many setbacks in Greg's treatment, anger at the staff interfered with the parents' ability to use the group for help. Every time, however, their trust in the staff was more quickly renewed. In time they came to rely on the group and began to extend help to other parents.

At the end of two months of intensive treatment, Greg died in his sleep. Mr. and Mrs. B. were appropriately grief-stricken and were able to express their feeling that everything possible had been done for their son. The group leaders met alone with the family before their departure from the center. This was done to terminate the relationship and to review with the parents some reactions they might expect over the coming months. Mr. and Mrs. B. were encouraged to talk freely with each other about their feelings and to seek the help of a counselor when they returned home. Telephone follow-up was arranged at three-month intervals. In addition, an autopsy report was forwarded to their family physician; an appointment made to review this report provided opportunity for additional contact with the B. family during their grieving process.

SUMMARY

In this chapter marital therapy was viewed from a behavioral and psychological perspective which considered the work of Masters and Johnson, among others. Nuclear and network family therapy were contrasted in the context of problem-focused intervention. The necessity for giving priority to the needs expressed by the families was advised. Specific family problems responsive to group treatment included child abuse and wife beating, manifestations of which are frequently encountered by nurses working in clinical and community settings. The child within the child abuser and the infantilization of the battered wife were discussed in empirical as well as psychodynamic terms. Need for careful assessment was urged in preparing these individuals for group involvement.

The grief and recurrent crises in families with a handicapped child were perceived as especially suitable for group treatment. Self-help groups, as well as support groups with professional leadership, facilitate the long-term adjustment of such families. Intervention immediately after the birth of a handicapped child is essential. Parents can be greatly helped by being put in touch with others who have faced the same stressful events. Clinical examples of group intervention were provided for family problems described in the chapter.

REFERENCES

General

Ackerman, N.W. *The Psychodynamics of Family Life*. New York: Basic Books, 1958.

Attneave, C.L. "Therapy in Tribal Settings and Urban Network Intervention." *Family Process* 8, 1969, pages 192-210.

Barbach, L.G. "Group Treatment of Preorgasmic Women." *Journal of Sex and Marital Therapy* 1, 1974, pages 139-145.

Benningfield, A.B. "Multiple Family Therapy Systems." *Journal of Marriage and Family Counseling* 4, 1978, pages 25-34.

Blinder, M.G., and M. Kirschenbaum. "The Technique of Married Group Couple Therapy." *Archives of General Psychiatry* 17, 1967, pages 44-52.

Bowen, M. "The Family as a Unit of Study and Treatment." *American Journal of Orthopsychiatry* 31, 1961, pages 40-60.

Bowers, J.E. "Planning the Therapeutic Process with the Family." In *Family-Focused Care*, J.R. Miller and E.H. Janosik, Eds. New York: McGraw-Hill, 1980, pages 321-331.

Brownell, K.D.; C.L. Heckerman; R.J. Westlake; et al. "The Effect of Couples' Training and Partner Cooperativeness in the Behavioral Treatment of Obesity." *Behavior Research and Therapy* 16, 1978, pages 323-333.

Calvo, G. *Marriage Encounter*. St. Paul, MN: Marriage Encounter, 1975.

Caplan, G. "Organization of Support Systems for Civilian Populations. In *Support Systems and Mutual Help: Multidisciplinary Explorations*, G. Caplan and M. Killilea, Eds. New York: Grune and Stratton, 1976, pages 273-315.

Doherty, W.J.; P. McCave; and R.G. Ryder. "Marriage Encounter: A Critical Appraisal." *Journal of Marriage and Family Counseling* 4, 1978, pages 99-106.

Fogel, C.I. "Sexual Dysfunction: Etiology and Therapy." In *Human Sexuality in Health and Illness*, N.F. Woods, Ed. 2nd ed. St. Louis: C.V. Mosby, 1979, pages 132-189.

Frager, S. "Multiple Family Therapy: A Literature Review." *Family Therapy* 5, 1978, pages 105-120.

Gurman, A.S., and R.M. Knudson.   "Behavioral Marriage Therapy: I. A Psychodynamic-Systems Analysis and Critique." *Family Process* 17, 1978, pages 121–138.

Jackson, D.D., and J.H. Weakland. "Conjoint Family Therapy: Some Considerations on Theory, Technique and Results." *Psychiatry* 24, 1961, pages 30–45.

Jacobson, N.W., and G. Margolin. *Marital Therapy*. New York: Brunner/Mazel, 1979.

Jones, S.L. *Family Therapy: A Comparison of Approaches.* Bowie, MD.: Robert J. Brady, 1980.

Kaplan, H.S. *The New Sex Therapy.* New York: Brunner/Mazel, 1974.

Killilea, M. "Mutual Help Organizations: Interpretations in the Literature." In *Support Systems and Mutual Help: Multidisciplinary Explorations*, G. Caplan and M. Killilea, Eds. New York: Grune and Stratton, 1976, pages 37–93.

Langner, D.G., and D.M. Kaplan. *The Treatment of Families in Crisis.* New York: Grune and Stratton, 1968.

McCuan-Rathbone, E., and R. Pierce. "Intergenerational Treatment Approach: An Alternative Model of Working with Abusive/Neglectful and Delinquent Prone Families." *Family Therapy* 5, 1978, pages 121–141.

Maddock, J.W. "Sexual Health: An Enrichment and Treatment Program." In *Treating Relationships*, D.H.L. Olson, Ed. Lake Mills, IA.: Graphic, 1976, pages 355–382.

Messersmith, C.E. "Sex Therapy and the Marital System." In *Treating Relationships*, D.H.L. Olson, Ed. Lake Mills, IA.: Graphic, 1976, pages 339–353.

Papanek, H. "Group Therapy with Married Couples." In *Comprehensive Group Psychotherapy*, H.I. Kaplan and B.J. Sadock, Eds. Baltimore: Williams and Wilkins, 1971, pages 691–723.

Rueveni, U. *Networking Families in Crisis.* New York: Human Sciences Press, 1979.

Speck, R.V., and C.L. Attneave. "Social Network Intervention." In *Changing Families: A Family Therapy Reader*, J. Haley, Ed. New York: Grune and Stratton, 1971, pages 312–322.

Sussman, M.B., and L. Burchinal. "Extended Kin Networks in the United States." In *Readings in the Family and Society*, W.J. Goode, Ed. Englewood Cliffs, N.J.: Prentice-Hall, 1964, pages 170–175.

Zilbergeld, B. "Group Treatment of Sexual Dysfunction in Men Without Partners." *Journal of Sex and Marital Therapy* 1, 1975, pages 204–214.

Group Work with Child-Abusing Parents

Egan, K.J. *Stress Management and Child Management Training with Child Abusing Parents.* Unpublished Ph.D. dissertation, University of Washington, 1980.

Frew, M.J., and E.R. Alden. "Role of the Pediatric Nurse Clinician in Early Identification of Potential Child Abuse." *Military Medicine* Vol. 143, No. 5, 1978, pages 325–327.

Gil, D.G. *Violence Against Children: Physical Child Abuse in the United States.* Cambridge, MA.: Harvard University Press, 1970.

Helfer, R.E. *Child Abuse and Neglect: The Diagnostic Process and Treatment Programs.* U.S. Department of Health, Education and Welfare, Publication No. (OHDS)77-30069, 1977.

Justice, B., and R. Justice. "Evaluating the Outcome of Group Therapy for Abusing Parents." *Corrective and Social Psychiatry and Journal of Behavioral Technology and Therapy* Vol. 24, No. 1, 1978, pages 45-59.

Kempe, C.H., and R.E. Helfer, Eds. *Helping the Battered Child and His Family.* Philadelphia: J.B. Lippincott, 1972.

Krindler, S. "Psychiatric Treatment for the Abusing Parent and the Abused Child." *Canadian Psychiatric Association Journal* 21, 1976, pages 275-279.

Martin, H., Ed. *The Abused Child: A Multi-disciplinary Approach to Developmental Issues and Treatment.* Cambridge, MA.: Ballinger, 1976.

McCuan-Rathbone, E., and R. Pierce. "Intergenerational Treatment Approach: An Alternative Model of Working With Abusive/Neglectful and Delinquent Prone Families." *Family Therapy* Vol. 5, No. 2, 1978, pages 121-141.

Savino, A.B., and R.W. Sanders. "Working with Abusive Parents: Group Therapy and Home Visit." *American Journal of Nursing* Vol. 73, No. 3, 1973, pages 482-484.

Sideleau, B.F. "The Abusive Family." In *Comprehensive Psychiatric Nursing,* J. Haber, A.M. Leach, S.M. Schudy, and B.F. Sideleau, Eds. New York: McGraw-Hill, 1978.

Steele, B.F., and C.B. Pollock. "A Psychiatric Study of Parents Who Abuse Infants and Small Children." In *The Battered Child,* R.E. Helfer and C.H. Kempe, Eds. 2nd ed. Chicago: The University of Chicago Press, 1974.

Groups for Battered Wives

Elbow, M. "Theoretical Considerations of Violent Marriages." *Social Casework* Vol. 58, No. 9, 1977, pages 515-526.

Geller, J.A., and J.C. Walsh. "A Treatment Model for the Abused Spouse." *Victimology* Vol. 2, No. 3-4, 1977-78, pages 627-632.

Gelles, R.J. "Violence and Pregnancy: A Note on the Extent of the Problem and Needed Services." *The Family Coordinator* 24, 1975, pages 81-86.

Lynch, C.G., and T.L. Norris. "Services for Battered Women: Looking for a Perspective." *Victimology* Vol. 2, No. 3-4, 1977-78, pages 553-562.

Petro, J.S.; P.L. Quann; and W.P. Graham. "Wife Abuse: The Diagnosis and Its Implications." *Journal of the American Medical Association* Vol. 240, No. 3, 1978, pages 240-241.

Rounsaville, B.J. "Battered Wives: Barriers to Identification and Treatment." *American Journal of Orthopsychiatry* Vol. 48, No. 3, 1978, pages 487-494.

Ryan, W. *Blaming the Victim.* New York: Vintage Books, 1971.

Spiegel, J. "Emotional Reactions to Catastrophe." In *Stress Situations,* S. Liebman, Philadelphia: J.B. Lippincott, 1955.

Symonds, A. "Violence Against Women: The Myth of Masochism." *American Journal of Psychotherapy* Vol. 33, No. 2, 1979, pages 161-173.

Group Work with Parents of Handicapped Children

Johnson, S.H. *High-Risk Parenting: Nursing Assessment and Strategies for the Family at Risk.* Philadelphia: J.B. Lippincott, 1979.

Mercer, R.T. *Nursing Care for Parents at Risk.* Thorofare, N.J.: Charles B. Slack, 1977.

Waechter, E.H. "Developmental Consequences of Congenital Abnormalities." *Nursing Forum* Vol. 14, No. 2, 1975, pages 108–129.

Group Work with Parents of Dying Children

Aguilera, D.C.; J.M. Messick; and M.S. Farrell. *Crisis Intervention: Theory and Methodology.* St. Louis: C.V. Mosby, 1970.

Heller, D.B., and C.D. Schneider. "Interpersonal Methods for Coping with Stress: Helping Families of Dying Children." *Omega* Vol. 8, No. 4, 1977–78, pages 319–331.

Helmroth, T.A., and E.M. Steinitz. "Death of an Infant: Parental Grieving and the Failure of Social Support." *The Journal of Family Practice* Vol. 6, No. 4, 1978, pages 785–790.

Hoff, L.A. *People in Crisis: Understanding and Helping.* Reading, MA.: Addison-Wesley, 1978.

Jackson, P.L. "The Child's Developing Concept of Death: Implications for Nursing Care of the Terminally Ill Child." *Nursing Forum* Vol. 15, No. 2, 1975, pages 204–215.

Katz, E.R.; J. Kellerman; and S.E. Siegel. "Behavioral Distress in Children with Cancer Undergoing Medical Procedures: Developmental Considerations." *Journal of Consulting and Clinical Psychology* Vol. 48, No. 3, 1980, pages 356–365.

Kennell, J.H.; H. Slyter; and M.H. Klaus. "The Mourning Response of Parents to the Death of a Newborn Infant." *New England Journal of Medicine* Vol. 283, No. 7, 1970, pages 344–349.

Kopel, K., and L.A. Mock. "The Use of Group Sessions for the Emotional Support of Families of Terminal Patients." *Death Education* 1, 1978, pages 409–422.

Lascari, A.D. "The Dying Child and His Family." *The Journal of Family Practice* Vol. 6, No. 6, 1978, pages 1279–1286.

Lindemann, E. "Symptomatology and Management of Acute Grief." *American Journal of Psychiatry* 101, 1944, pages 101–148.

Tietz, W. "Family Sequelae After a Child's Death Due to Cancer." *American Journal of Psychotherapy* Vol. 31, No. 3, 1977, pages 417–425.

12

Group Work with Children and Adolescents

Lynn West Griffith

Anyone who has worked with children or adolescents realizes that the power of peer influence is compounded in group settings. Upon reaching school age, children are increasingly eager for inclusion into peer groups, both formal and informal. For teenagers facing the identity crisis of adolescence, rejection by the group is perceived as calamitous. When desired status is conferred by the group, feelings of self-worth are enhanced and the search for identity seems less hopeless. During childhood and adolescence, group pressures and the quality of peer group experiences attenuate the primacy of family influences for virtually all youngsters.

SUITABILITY OF GROUPS FOR YOUNG PEOPLE

An intense wish to be accepted by the group and to separate from parents lends importance and cohesiveness to adolescent groups. The desire to be like others of one's own age adds to the burdens of a teenager who is noticeably different. Young people with physical, mental, or emotional disabilities are often ostracized by members of available groups. Unless alternative experiences can be arranged, social isolation becomes an additional handicap for exceptional youngsters.

Peer group interaction is necessary for optimal growth and development, and groups organized for young people are an excellent medium for promoting healthy development and for treating developmental or other problems. For instance, a group organized for handicapped children may have both growth-promoting objectives and problem-solving objectives. Growth-promoting objectives fulfill a handicapped child's need for social acceptance by introducing the child to genuine peers whose understanding exceeds that of normal children. In the company of children with similar handicaps, the young group member may share experiences and discern commonalities, thereby feeling less alone.

In an early report, Slavson (1958) observed therapeutic benefits in adult parenting groups, some of which are equally applicable to groups for children and teenagers. It is interesting that the observations of Slavson presaged in some respects the curative factors formulated by Yalom (1975). The list of benefits includes the following:

- *Buttressing of Positive Trends:* As group participants buttress each other's strengths and progress and counteract hostile or destructive behaviors, a sense of hopefulness and optimism arises. Common problem solving operates to reduce defeatism.
- *Universalization:* Group participants are relieved to discover that others have similar problems.
- *Mutuality:* Common attention to the same problem induces a spirit of sharing and helping. Feelings of relaxation and acceptance follow reinforced member satisfaction and strengthen motivation to continue.
- *Identification with a Wholesome Parental Figure:* Group structure often resembles a family and can be used to foster positive family interactions. The parent-leader models a caring father or mother figure, providing opportunity for a healthy parent-child experience. The leader also encourages effective sibling relationships between members, which may not have been present in their original primary groups.
- *Acquisition of Knowledge:* Either through formal teaching or informal discussion, the leader imparts factual information, clarifies ideas, and corrects significant misinformation or misconceptions.

- *Widening the Field of Operations:* As comfort increases within the group, members begin to take risks, make friends, engage in new activities. Group members learn by following the example of others, by attempting and by practicing new skills. Trying out communication-interaction skills in the safe environs of the group enables members to transfer those skills into daily life.

CONCEPTUAL MODELS FOR CHILDREN'S GROUPS

When one contemplates leading a group for children or teenagers there is need for a broad conceptual model which explains characteristic dynamics of groups for young members. No one model can encompass all phenomena observable in the wide range of children's groups which exist at the present, nor is it profitable to adopt one model to the exclusion of all others. For a relatively new practitioner, however, it is helpful to utilize the model which accounts for typical phenomena in groups for young people. Adopting a suitable model simplifies the analysis of complex group interactions, aids in goal setting, in. planning sessions, and in recording observations.

The group models discussed earlier in this book have some value and some limitations in explaining dynamics present in groups for children or teenagers. In particular, the linear-progressive and life cycle models must be modified according to the developmental levels and capabilities of the young members in the group.

Linear-Progressive Model

This model of group development compares the growth of a group to the progress of an immature individual toward competent adulthood. The model is based on the premise that groups, like children, move from childlike dependency to productivity and interdependence. What must be remembered is that a group composed of young children may not progress through sequential stages, as outlined in the linear-progressive model, and that group goals and leader expectations must be modified accordingly. A nursery group of preschool children may progress no further than engaging in parallel play. Sharing or cooperation among members may be an unrealistic goal for such a group. In contrast to preschoolers, children between six and twelve years old are usually able to work together harmoniously to achieve the group task. Even at late stages of group development, however, these children will likely turn to the leader for direction and authority. Adolescent group members, on the other hand, are less inclined to tolerate close or continued direction from the leader. There may be a tendency among them to experiment with various roles in the group, and to prefer independence over dependence on the leader. Homogeneity in the ages of young members elected for groups allows leaders to set goals which challenge but do not overwhelm the abilities of members, whatever their developmental level. Kraft (1971) and Gazda (1978) confirmed the desirability of grouping children by age. Gazda recommended three chronological divisions: from five to nine years, from nine to thirteen years, and from thirteen years to young adulthood. It is essential that a group contain members whose ages are appropriate to the group objectives; homogeneity in other respects also contributes to the cohesiveness and effectiveness of the group.

Life Cycle Model

The life cycle model adds to the linear-progressive model a final stage in the form of separation or dissolution of the group. Unlike the linear-progressive model, which assumes a high level of productivity until the end of the group, the life cycle model takes into account the necessity for dealing with the demise of the group.

As a rule the experience of young people with death and loss is quite limited. It is therefore crucial for the leader to be responsive to feelings prevalent among young members facing imminent dissolution of a group which has become meaningful. Groups for children and teenagers tend to be time-limited. Often the groups are ad hoc, organized to serve the needs of members at a particular point in time. Once the group goals have been met, or the needs are no longer compelling, the group tends to disband. Members may simply leave the group one by one, or reorganize into new groups with different aspirations. In some affiliative groups such as scout troops, rites of passage are used to help members separate pridefully from lower level groups in order to move into higher ranks. If children or adolescents have found satisfaction and security in belonging to a group, they may react to threatened loss with expressions of anxiety, irritability, withdrawal, or disruptive actions. Sometimes premature concern about termination interferes with progress toward group goals, and this must be addressed. Even when an ongoing group must disband for a summer recess, regrets and fears may be manifested. Occasionally an interim reunion may be arranged as a way of reassuring members of the continued viability of the group. Encouraging discussion of feelings of regret, suggesting alternative ways of meeting needs, verbally reviewing the accomplishments of the group, or compiling an actual "book of memories" are among the strategies which mitigate grief among young group members.

Pendular or Recurrent Life Cycle Model

This model embodies the concept that impediments to the progress of a group toward its planned denouement are inevitable (Gibbard, Hartman, and Mann, 1974). Mills (1964) postulated that a group does not move forward in linear progressive fashion but must constantly attempt to maintain equilibrium against opposing forces which distract it from its legitimate task.

In groups for young people, reconciliation of opposing forces — trust versus mistrust, dependence versus independence, individual goals versus group goals — must be faced repeatedly. Thus the pendular or recurrent life cycle model is particularly applicable to groups organized for children and teenagers. Among such members, patterns of reconciliation and accommodation are rarely established once and for all. Regression to behaviors representing egocentric needs may result from situational factors outside the group, from interpersonal factors inside the group, or from intrapersonal insecurities. Leaders must exercise patience, tolerance, and flexibility when regressive behaviors are displayed by one or two members, or by the group as a whole. The latter is a more trying situation for the leader, since whole group regression denies the leader the constructive help of mature, group-oriented members. In many groups organized for young people the pendular swing from goal attainment to egocentric concerns contributes to a dynamic tension which challenges members and leaders alike.

CATEGORIES OF GROUPS

Developmental tasks are often addressed in groups for young people, and the degree of attention paid to developmental issues may be used to illustrate three categories of group work according to their relative scope and depth (Gazda, 1978) (Table 12-1). For *guidance* groups, resolution of developmental tasks is the goal with the highest priority. *Counseling* groups undertake to resolve remedial goals as well as developmental tasks. In *psychotherapy* groups, remediation or rehabilitation is stressed, with developmental issues given less priority.

In clinical practice the distinction among the three catagories is sometimes diffuse, but the classification is helpful to consider during the activities which precede and accompany group sessions. Membership selection and preparation, goal-setting, and leadership style may be held to a more consistent line if the three categories are kept in mind. There are similarities between the preventive, growth-engendering remedial processes of Gazda and the levels of prevention formulated

Table 12–1   CATEGORIES OF GROUPS ACCORDING TO SCOPE AND
DEPTH

Guidance Groups	Counseling Groups	Psychotherapeutic Groups
↓	↓	↓
Growth Engendering and Preventive	Growth Engendering and Remedial	Remedial and Growth Engendering
↓	↓	↓
(Primary Level of Prevention)	(Secondary Level of Prevention)	(Tertiary Level of Prevention)

by Leavell and Clark (1958) and Caplan (1961). Primary prevention, which focuses on health promotion and specific measures,
parallels group guidance. Secondary prevention, which deals with
early diagnosis and treatment, may be equated with group counseling. Tertiary prevention, which offers rehabilitation, is the goal of
group psychotherapy.

Group Guidance

The term *group guidance* simply means providing guidance in a group
setting. Gazda (1978) viewed guidance as an extension of educational
and vocational services, having as its goal the prevention of developmental problems. It is the most circumscribed of the three categories
of group work enumerated by Gazda.

Any group process in which young people build coping skills, clarify
values, or acquire information helpful in decision making constitutes
group guidance. Strategies used in group guidance may be elaborate
presentations involving sophisticated instructional aids, or they may
be simple, informal exercises or discussions. Young children learn
readily by means of puppetry, role-playing, or simulations, and these
methods are often employed in guidance groups. In junior and senior
high schools, significant amounts of time may be devoted to units on
personality development. School nurse-teachers of health education
classes use group guidance to help prepare young people for approaching developmental crises, and for possible physical and emotional
stresses. Life skills in activities such as dating, money management,
homemaking, and child care are no longer considered by educators
the natural results of growing up, but the results of affective, cognitive, and psychomotor learning, much of which can be accomplished
in groups.

Community Groups Special interest groups organized around central activities meet under the leadership of nurses, teachers, and community volunteers. Examples of community groups include, among others, scout troops, Campfire Girls, 4-H Clubs, and Big Brothers. Such groups, organized for recreation or the pursuit of specific goals, are growth-engendering and contain elements of group guidance.

Latency Groups *Latency clubs* is the term given to groups for children which support the critical tasks of the period from six to twelve years of age. This age period is one of steady growth and relative balance between physical, social, and psychological areas of development. It is generally a satisfying time, representing a plateau occupied with learning and growing. Through initiative and industry, the school-aged child strives to win a place at school, at home, and among peers. Latency clubs help children to become less self-centered and to derive satisfaction from cooperating with others. When peer interaction in latency groups is organized constructively, improved interpersonal communication and self-esteem follow. As a rule, leadership is active rather than laissez-faire, particularly during the early stages of the group.

Identity Groups Identity groups for adolescents resemble the latency groups of younger children in that both help in the successful resolution of age-appropriate developmental tasks. Adolescence is a time of rapid physical growth and great psychosocial uncertainty. A sense of identity emerges from association with peer groups and from recognition by others. During adolescence there is growing awareness of a unique identity. Among others, Erikson (1963) affirmed that for an adolescent to attain a positive ego identity, peer group affiliations must be established. Any group for adolescents, regardless of its primary objectives, must endeavor to foster positive identity formation. The leader of an adolescent group enters a relationship with group members which allows them to experiment with various roles and permits group autonomy to a safe and reasonable extent.

Adolescents are not too young to begin developing consciousness of the life cycle. In working with older patients, Butler (1973) studied the personal awareness of wholeness, rhythm, and pattern which evolves over a lifetime. This lengthy process of discovery begins in adolescence, as young people start to perceive similarities and differences among individuals, to learn the expectations of society, and to acquire adaptive means for achieving satisfaction. Learning what constitutes normal development, understanding what changes to expect, and recognizing the cyclic nature of existence are implicit tasks in many groups for adolescents.

Parenting Groups Examples of guidance groups are the parenting classes for teenagers which are sponsored by schools, churches, and community agencies. At all socioeconomic levels youngsters enter adulthood with little firsthand knowledge of small children. For some young people there may have been no parental models from whom to learn wholesome parenting behaviors. Some parenting groups include consideration of family planning, child rearing, and other concerns which perplex young parents or future parents. A volunteer leader or a professional from the same culture and background as the group participants may be most readily accepted. Co-leadership shared with a person of another ethnic or cultural background may help bridge distrust of strangers without causing undue anxiety. Parenting groups in the community are valuable for single parents and others with actual or potential child-rearing problems. Mental health agencies consider group support important in averting child neglect and abuse, and in maintaining family stability.

Sex Education Groups Sex education classes provide guidance at various levels, ranging from simple discussions of "growing up" to premarital groups for young adults. Groups of fifteen to twenty persons, led by health-care professionals who are comfortable in this role, are best suited for discussion of topics related to sex and marriage. Fifteen is a large enough number to monitor excessive disclosure, whereas groups of more than twenty may inhibit the timid from interacting. Here the responsiveness of the leader to emotionally-charged content must be carefully controlled so as not to close off the discussion.

In writing about sex guidance for the handicapped, Johnson (1975) offered guidelines which are appropriate for all leaders of sex guidance groups. The following recommendations were made.

- Select language which increases the cognitive level of discussion, clarifies meanings, avoids emotionality, and meets the needs of the participants.
- Avoid generalizing or presupposing the characteristics or feelings of others.

- Avoid setting oneself up as the norm or ideal.
- Recognize the hazards both of overteaching and underteaching.
- Avoid overconfidence in the extent of one's own knowledge, especially knowledge of physical or psychological causes for sexual inadequacies disclosed during group sessions.

GROUP COUNSELING

Group counseling is designed to foster growth in individuals, improve psychosocial skills, and overcome problems which have the potential of being chronic or exacerbated if left unattended. The goal of group counseling is to induce children and teenagers to modify attitudes and behaviors, to clarify values, to emulate healthy role models, and to utilize support systems. Best conducted in small groups of six to ten, group counseling is not suitable for all troubled children, but is indicated for those with certain specific or temporary problems. Through group counseling, individuals are often able to overcome difficulties with less emotional trauma than they would experience without group intervention (Gazda, 1978).

Organizing a Group

In organizing a counseling group, careful assessment interviews are necessary so that the leader may judge the suitability or readiness of the youngsters for the group experience. Age is an important factor, in both chronological and developmental terms, as are the child's presenting problem, verbal ability, self-perception, and previous group participation. Members who come into a group which has already entered a working phase must be oriented to group procedures. Delegating this task to older members often eases the entry of the newcomer. The use of succinct anecdotal records helps document group and individual progress. In groups for young people, reliance on the pendular or recurrent life cycle model greatly aids in understanding complex group interactions. In addition to managerial functions the leader of counseling groups must be a willing listener. Acceptance of negative as well as positive expressions of feeling stimulates group discussion. At the same time the leader of groups for young members must be a regulatory agent, alternately seeking a central or a peripheral position in the group, as conditions indicate. With children and adolescents, written group contracts which list group objectives, state the functions of the leaders and the responsibilities of members, set time frames, and define mutual expectations can become a reference point which guides group development and leads to satisfactory accomplishments by the group.

Group Work with Disabled Children

Group work with children suffering chronic illness has contributed to the adjustment of the children and their families (Noland, 1971). Hendry and Geddes (1978) described one community program for children with spina bifida and their parents. Soon after the birth of the defective child the parents are asked to attend newborn nursery sessions where they can meet and talk with other parents who are facing or have faced the same crisis. Continuity of service is provided through preschool activities which allow parents to meet one another and give the children a chance to interact with similar children. In this manner the entire family is helped to move together toward independence and self-help. The spina bifida group program was described as a vehicle for assisting the children and for counseling parents whose worries may not lessen as the children grow older.

An interesting variation of group counseling was described by Bolton (1976). This program was designed to meet the needs of young deaf adults whose social immaturity was compared with that of preadolescent hearing youngsters. Structured group situations were arranged which offered practice in paying attention, in discussing controversial subjects, and in respecting divergent points of view. Because of inherent communication difficulties, the groups for the deaf were limited to six to eight members. It was thought that sharing common problems and searching for consensus in a group setting was the dominant growth-producing feature of the program.

Group Counseling for Developmental Disabilities

Children and adolescents with developmental disabilities such as cerebral palsy, epilepsy, or mental retardation can derive substantial benefit from group counseling. Group work with developmentally disabled children is usually directed toward skill-building, socialization, and suitable educational and vocational goals. The trend toward blending developmentally disabled with normally developed children has enabled many developmentally disabled persons to live in the community. Siantz (1977) proposed an active role for nurses in coordinating health-maintenance services for these clients after they return to their own or to group homes. In addition to traditional services — such as periodic health assessment and appropriate referrals and care — the developmentally disabled can benefit from supportive group counseling. The key concept in group, as in individual, work with the developmentally disabled is the normalization of as many aspects of life as possible. Normalization refers to the right to live in the least restrictive environment. In group programs for adolescents who are developmentally disabled, members should be included in goal-setting and planning activities in order to heighten their interest and initiative.

Sex Education Sex education for developmentally disabled youngsters is a common concern of both parents and professionals, and is a matter which lends itself to group counseling. There is general agreement on the need to help these youngsters deal with sexuality, to learn to interact with members of the opposite sex, and perhaps to date or marry. In approaching these matters, emphasis should be placed not on the disability but on the human potential for finding sexual gratification in lasting rather than in promiscuous relationships (Gordon, 1976). Toward this end group meetings might include formal but simple teaching, audiovisual aids, and opportunities for questions. A matter-of-fact approach is indicated, employing terminology which meets the participants' level of understanding. Discussion of hugging, kissing, genital exposure, masturbation, and sexual intercourse should be frank and unevasive. Johnson (1975) noted that society is not yet tolerant either of mentally retarded persons or of sexual expression, and is even less tolerant of sexual expression by those who are mentally retarded. It may be assumed that most mentally retarded persons can learn to confine sexual expressiveness to appropriate times and places. Health professionals have an obligation to enlighten the general population concerning those who are intellectually or socially handicapped. Group counseling sessions are effective in assisting developmentally disabled youngsters to fulfill their sexual needs as normally as possible and in reassuring concerned parents who are reluctant to confront this aspect of normalization.

Groups for Siblings

An area which merits attention is sibling involvement in therapeutic intervention for disabled youngsters. Siblings play a major role in the climate of the family which must cope with a disabled child. Siblings as well as parents must adjust to a new baby's disability and to the reality of an altered family life. Parents who are struggling with their own pain and disappointment must also extend understanding toward normal siblings. In planning treatment strategies, professionals are advised to seek the involvement of older siblings in addition to parents. Siblings need help to reduce the negative effects of sibling rivalry and to understand the rationale of the therapeutic regimen. In an account of a program for the retarded, Wyatt (1976) reported on the results of training siblings to participate in behavior modification programs for their retarded brothers and sisters. The influence of the siblings on the behavior of the retarded children was observed to be greater than that of the parents.

Group Behavior Modification

In this group the one-to-one principles of behavior modification and a *token system* are used to eradicate problem behaviors. Since problem behaviors occur in a social milieu, the group method is appropriate and effective. In group behavior modification, leader and members react to behaviors, and provide the rewards and punishments which *modify, reinforce,* or *extinguish* behaviors. The group leader, who should be familiar with techniques of behavior modification and theories of group process, regulates interaction so that members adopt appropriate behaviors which may then be transferred from the group to interactions with family and community (Weathers and Liberman, 1978).

The potential of members to tolerate behavior modification in a group setting must be carefully evaluated. Controlled environments such as those found in residential or institutional facilities may be required for group behavior modification of some disabled or delinquent youngsters. The basic mechanism in both individual and group behavior modification was described by Marholin (1978), who stated that a child must learn that certain behaviors, if performed at the right time and place, will lead to positive consequences (*reinforcement*), and that other behaviors will either not result in positive consequences or will lead to negative consequences (*extinguishment*). Positive reinforcers might include candy, games, praise, or tokens, such as points or stars, to be redeemed by the individual member or by the group. Negative reinforcers include ignoring, censure, demerits, or other penalties levied for displaying undesirable behaviors.

Rewards In group behavior modification, rewards may be earned for the whole group, for teams and individuals within the group, or for individual members. Peer pressure to earn reinforcers strengthens incentives to cooperate. In very successful groups the children experience sufficient satisfaction from mastery and bestowed approval that they no longer need tangible rewards. Even when a group or team effort is being made, the leader may attempt to individualize each child's reward system. A successful method of individualizing and recording each member's progress was described by Marholin (1978). Each group member received a list of target behaviors for the day which could be checked as desired responses were noted.

Designing a Modification Program   Designing a group modification program includes: 1) assessing each member's baseline level of functioning; 2) analyzing target behaviors; 3) formulating behavioral objectives; and 4) planning interventions which foster peer pressure to achieve the target behaviors. In initial group sessions, reward systems are consistently applied and the leader evaluates the interaction. Over time the rewards may need to be adjusted as the group advances to higher levels of functioning, with more effort expected for fewer rewards. Marholin indicated that even very young children can function in behavior modification groups and become motivated to earn rewards. Groups can be designed to reinforce the expression of positive feelings, meaningful action and conversation, tolerance of others, and acceptance of decisions by the leader of the group.

Crisis Groups for Adolescents

Crisis groups generally use an approach similar to that of individual crisis work, with four stages of crisis resolution evident in the group: 1) assessing the nature of the problem and the resources available; 2) planning therapeutic intervention; 3) intervening to facilitate an intellectual understanding of the crisis, mobilize coping strengths, and utilize available resources; and 4) resolving the crisis and providing anticipatory guidance (Morley, Messick, and Aguilera, 1967).

In crisis groups for teenagers, members work to solve individual crises through group interaction. As in all crisis work the hope is that members will either return to a precrisis level of functioning or learn new coping skills which will then be available in the future. Crisis groups are usually small and open-ended, with members leaving and newcomers joining throughout the life of the group. In contrast to other groups, the time that a member may attend a crisis group is limited to about six sessions, since crisis is considered to be a time-limited phenomenon. Moreover, the limit of six sessions is thought to accelerate progress toward crisis resolution. Aguilera and Messick (1974) acknowledged that the overall success of crisis group work was mixed. Group intervention appeared to help some members. For other persons the crisis of each member was threatening; misunderstanding by some members of the predicament of other members led at times to maladaptive suggestions. Crisis groups are effective for some, but the potential of each person in crisis to benefit from group rather than individual work must be evaluated. Sometimes the nature of a crisis being faced is a factor which must be considered. Occasionally a maturational crisis of adolescence is better treated through individual or family intervention. Situational crises such as illness or death are often amenable to group work, as grieving families search for solace and meaning with the help of others who are also bereaved.

Group Work with Pregnant Teenagers

Statistics on teenage pregnancy show an alarming increase, especially among fourteen- and fifteen-year-old schoolgirls. The teenager who is pregnant faces the developmental crisis of motherhood superimposed upon the physical and psychological stresses of adolescence. Johnson (1979) wrote that the nine-month pregnancy period is insufficient to prepare a teenager for motherhood, and is hardly long enough for personal or social readjustment. The physiological and psychological immaturity of the pregnant teenager, her high risk of perinatal difficulties, and her family's distress amount to a formidable burden. After learning that she is pregnant, the unmarried teenager may be rejected by her boyfriend and her family, leading her to choose an abortion. Elective abortion is a decision which should not be made precipitiously, without determining the girls' investment in the decision, as well as the investment of the putative father. A family's shock and dismay may result in the girl's isolation or in her passive submission to the decisions of others, neither of which leads to a healthy resolution of the crisis. Maintaining open communication between the girl and her parents encourages rational planning and mutual support. An experimental school program described by Howard (1968) remains a model of an effective group program for pregnant teenagers. The girls in the program lived at home, attended public school, and at the same time participated in weekly group meetings, the goals of which were to foster responsible attitudes toward sexual behavior, parenting, and family relationships. The content of the sessions included information on pregnancy, adoption, foster care, abortion, and contraception, and was presented in terms of the quality of life for the girls and their families. Role-playing, audiovisual aids, case profiles, and member leadership of discussions characterized the group sessions. When the girls returned to school after giving birth, the group leaders made follow-up calls and arranged necessary modifications of the school program. During the period that the girls were participants of the program, their parents and guardians met regularly to discuss the social and sexual needs of adolescents, as well as how to provide supportive measures for the girls during their pregnancies and after childbirth. Prenatal and postnatal care was provided to the girls through referrals to appropriate health and social agencies in the community.

Teenage Fathers When a school girl becomes pregnant the feelings of the young father, who may feel very guilty and confused, are often overlooked. When included in the counseling program the putative father may prove an important source of support for the girl. Professionals should advise the couple of the risks inherent in a hasty marriage, but remain open-minded and accepting of whatever decision is made.

In group programs for pregnant teenagers, members receive the support of a peer group while extending help to others in the same predicament. Discussion of the physical changes of pregnancy leads to sharing of feelings and fears, and to new perceptions of themselves in relation to others. Ideally, group programs permit the girls to live at home when possible and to continue attending their neighborhood schools. Comprehensive health and psychosocial services are required after delivery. Group counseling sessions should be available for a year or more, with the girls encouraged to attend and to pursue their education with the assistance of child-care services.

GROUP PSYCHOTHERAPY

In the context of this chapter, group psychotherapy is defined as the regressive-reconstructive treatment of neuroses and other severe emotional disturbances by group therapists trained in personality theory and psychopathology (Gazda, 1978). Group psychotherapy is indicated for children and adolescents with severe emotional disturbances, chronic personality problems, drug addiction, severe delinquency, and other serious maladaptive disorders. In group psychotherapy, qualified therapists use psychoanalytic and group theories to help members achieve insight into their feelings and behaviors. It is the responsibility of the leader to regulate group interaction while eliciting emotional and intellectual understanding of feelings and behaviors. The recommended number of members of psychotherapeutic groups for children and adolescents depends on the needs and the ages of the members. A group of preschool children might contain only four members; an adolescent group might contain twice that number or slightly more. Group psychotherapy for children or adolescents often follows or is concurrent with individual or family work, and the leader must cooperate with other professionals without violating group rules about confidentiality.

Leadership Criteria

The leader of psychotherapeutic groups is a health professional with extensive training and experience in nursing, psychology, psychiatry, or social work. Among nurses, leadership is restricted to persons with graduate education on the master's or doctoral level, and should not be attempted without adequate preparation. Child psychiatry is a subspeciality within the fields of psychiatry and psychiatric nursing. Many nurses are involved in group work within the categories of guidance and counseling, but psychotherapy which has insight and personality reconstruction as a goal should be left to nurses and other health professionals with the requisite qualifications.

The qualifications required for group leadership relate directly to the purpose of the group. In guidance groups, positive attitudes toward the members and adherence to group goals constitute the chief prerequisite for leaders. Leaders may range from persons with college preparation in teaching or the helping professions to community volunteers without formal preparation.

The Joint Commission on the Mental Health of Children (1973) stipulated that minimum requirements for leaders of children's groups be a baccalaureate degree in psychology, human behavior, or early childhood education, and that such persons provide counseling under the supervision of more highly educated professionals. Assuming responsibility for leadership of a counseling group implies relating with the other professionals who provide supervision or consultation to the group.

NURSES AS LEADERS OF GROUPS FOR CHILDREN AND ADOLESCENTS

Nurses are eminently suited by their study of psychosocial needs, communication techniques, and crisis theory to lead guidance and counseling groups for young people. Carkhuff (1969) endorsed the importance of empathy, respect, and concreteness among counselors, along with genuineness, self-disclosure, confrontation, and immediacy.

Experiences in groups may have constructive consequences, destructive consequences, or no consequences at all. Gazda (1978) cited several instances in which the authoritarianism, impatience, excessive confrontation, and self-disclosure of leaders inhibited and even reversed the progress of groups for young people. Periodic evaluation of leader effectiveness through self-awareness, peer observation, supervision, and consultation is necessary to assure effectiveness as a group leader. The leader tries to create an atmosphere of safety, receptivity, and enthusiasm for the group's purposes so that the members can begin to develop trust. In groups for young people, initial uneasiness may be expressed as bravado or as silly behavior. If members are encouraged to participate in determining group rules and tasks, anxiety and distrust yield to a sense of belonging and to feelings of self-worth.

The leader encourages communication and directs attention to the sharing of meaning, at times interpreting for the group or seeking out ideas and reactions from members. Problem behaviors such as acting out, interrupting, or refusing to participate should be examined for causation. The inclination of many young people to proceed at their own pace presents a challenge for group leaders which should be handled with sensitivity and without recrimination.

CLINICAL EXAMPLE: GROUP WORK WITH EPILEPTIC TEENAGERS

A weekly group for epileptic teenagers between the ages of thirteen and eighteen was proposed, planned, and implemented by Mike, a social worker, and Doris, a nurse with a baccalaureate degree. The group leaders worked in an urban pediatric hospital, which was the sponsoring agency.

The original group goals were to encourage the teenagers to share their understanding of epilepsy and to talk about misgivings related to their illness. It was thought that the group would help members develop healthier self-concepts and more accurate perceptions of themselves in relation to others. The leaders also hoped that the group experience would assuage feelings of being misunderstood and excluded from school or community activities.

Richardson and Friedman (1974) asserted that many families with epileptic teenagers reported behavior problems, school difficulties, and depressive episodes in the youngsters. The time needed to accept the diagnosis of epilepsy varies, depending on the young person's own strengths, family support, and peer group status. Mike and Doris were unable to predict an optimum length of membership in their group, so the group was not time-limited. As most members reached the age of eighteen, they appeared to become ready to move into other peer groups and ceased to attend. No one was asked to terminate upon reaching eighteen, since it was thought that well-adjusted older members were valuable role models.

The group began with eleven members who were out-patients; it was coeducational, and most members were referred by a neurologist after diagnosis. The group met weekly from 5:00 to 7:00 P.M., with a summer recess. Membership varied between eight and ten members. Initially, whenever a member dropped out, a new member joined. As time passed the group grew more cohesive; it became more difficult to incorporate newcomers into the original group. When this became evident, a "junior" group was formed, and membership of the original group stabilized.

During the meetings, games, drawing, and painting were used to evoke discussion of the implications of epilepsy for adolescent sufferers. By means of artwork, fears about seizures, auras, and brain waves were given expression. Audiovisual aids such as films were used, and guest speakers from the community were invited to attend. A speaker from the local epilepsy association described adult programs and job opportunities for young members. At another session a geneticist advised the group on heredity — which was a matter of great concern to the members.

Although epilepsy itself seemed to be a concern among the members, normal adolescent interests, especially in the psychosocial realm, dominated discussions. Though planned as a counseling group, it gradually undertook guidance functions as well.

Coleadership of the group by a social worker and a nurse proved extremely effective. Their knowledge of the helping relationship, of leadership responsibility, and of group theory were essential to the success of the group. As a nurse, Doris's special contribution was her understanding of the physiological implications of epilepsy. The fact that the leaders represented both sexes enhanced the feeling of family in the group, and gave the members an example of open, adult interaction between a man and a woman.

The leaders committed four to six hours each week outside of group meetings to evaluating the previous session, writing anecdotal notes, getting in touch with absent members, and planning future meetings. Extensive documentation demonstrated the constructive effects of the group experience for the members and confirmed institutional support for the group. At the close of the meetings feedback from members was solicited about what seemed helpful during the session. Although the group members were the direct recipients of service, Mike and Doris realized that support at home was increased by parental understanding of epilepsy and of the group goals. Therefore parents of members were invited twice yearly to discuss their perceptions of the impact of the group experience and to make suggestions for the program. This was done with the concurrence of the members. Between meetings the leaders were available by phone during working hours, although members were instructed to call their physicians for any medical problems. When a member was hospitalized the leaders visited him or her in order to preserve this person's contact with the group. Since a common problem for the members was gaining acceptance at school, the leaders visited teachers and classes to explain the nature of epileptic seizures and constructive ways of helping epileptic teenagers.

Among the variables which contributed to the ongoing vitality of the group, the following factors were identified:

1. Coleadership by caring persons who fostered corrective recapitulation of the primary group experience.
2. Acceptance by the leaders that the group assumed characteristics of guidance and of counseling.
3. Formalized involvement of parents so that confidentiality of members was not violated.
4. Stabilization of membership when the group became too cohesive to accept newcomers readily.
5. Separation of group functions from the functions of other involved professionals such as physicians.
6. Extensive documentation to validate the value of the group to the suprasystem.
7. Liaison work by the leaders to preserve links with the group when members were ill or absent.

SUMMARY

In selecting a conceptual model for groups composed of children or adolescents, the recurrent life cycle model is most applicable. This model can be used to account for opposing forces, regressive and progressive, which contribute to tensions discernible in groups organized for young members. Regardless of more specific goals, developmental issues are often addressed in such groups. Three categories of groups were described, based on the relative scope and depth of the group task. Guidance groups were equated with primary prevention, counseling groups with secondary prevention, and group psychotherapy with tertiary prevention. Each of the three categories was described and several examples of each were given. Behavior modification and crisis intervention were presented as appropriate group treatment for selected members. Qualifications for leadership of the three categories of groups were cited according to recommendations of the 1973 Joint Commission on the Mental Health of Children. The unique qualities brought to group work by nurse leaders were discussed, along with appropriate limitations based on education and experience. Managerial responsibilities were emphasized for leaders of groups for young members. A climate of safety must be preserved in the group, as well as a climate of acceptance. Leaders were advised to move readily between a central position in the group and a peripheral position, as indicated by the leaders' perception of group needs.

REFERENCES

Aguilera, D.C.; J.M. Messick. *Crisis Intervention: Theory and Methodology.* St. Louis: C.V. Mosby, 1974.

Bolton, B., Ed. *The Psychology of Deafness for Rehabilitation Counselors.* Baltimore: University Park Press, 1976.

Butler, R.N., and M.I. Lewis. *Aging and Mental Health.* St. Louis: C.V. Mosby, 1973.

Caplan, G. *An Approach to Community Mental Health.* New York: Grune and Stratton, 1961.

Carkhuff, R.R. "Helping and Human Relations." *Selection and Training* Vol. 1. New York: Holt Rinehart & Winston, 1969.

Erikson, E.H. *Childhood and Society.* New York: W.W. Norton, 1963.

Gazda, G.M. *Group Counseling: A Developmental Approach.* 2nd ed. Boston: Allyn and Bacon, 1978.

Gibbard, G.S.; J.J. Hartman; and R.D. Mann, Eds. *Analysis of Groups.* San Francisco: Jossey-Bass, 1974.

Gordon, S. "Sex Education Programs: Guidelines and Materials." *The Exceptional Parent* Vol. 6, No. 1, 1976, pages 27–29.

Hendry, J., and N. Geddes. "Living with a Congenital Anomaly: How Nurses Can Help Parents of Children with Spina Bifida to Develop Lasting Patterns of Creative Caring." *Canadian Nurse* 74, 1978, pages 29–33.

Howard, M. *The Webster School Experiment: A District of Columbia Program for Pregnant Girls.* Children's Bureau, U.S. Dept. of Health, Education, and Welfare, 1968.

Johnson, S.H. *High Risk Parenting: Nursing Assessments and Strategies for the Family at Risk.* Philadelphia: J.B. Lippincott, 1979.

Johnson, W.R. *Sex Education and Counseling of Special Groups.* Springfield, IL.: Charles C Thomas, 1975.

Joint Commission on the Mental Health of Children. *The Mental Health of Children: Services, Research and Manpower.* New York: Harper & Row, 1973.

Kraft, I.A. "Child and Adolescent Group Psychotherapy." In *Comprehensive Group Psychotherapy*, H.I. Kaplan and B.J. Sadock, Eds. Baltimore: Williams and Wilkins, 1971.

Leavell, H.R., and E.G. Clark. *Preventive Medicine for the Doctor in His Community.* New York: McGraw-Hill, 1958.

Marholin, D., Ed. *Child Behavior Therapy.* New York: Gardner Press, 1978.

Mills, T.M. *Group Transformation: An Analysis of a Learning Group.* Englewood Cliffs, N.J.: Prentice-Hall, 1964.

Morley, W.E.; J.M. Messick; and D.C. Aguilera. "Crisis: Paradigms of Intervention." *Journal of Psychiatric Nursing* 5, 1967, pages 538–540.

Noland, Robert L., Ed. *Counseling Parents of the Ill and the Handicapped.* Springfield, IL.: Charles C Thomas, 1971.

Richardson, D.W., and S.B. Friedman. "Psychosocial Problems of the Adolescent Patient with Epilepsy." *Clinical Pediatrics* Vol. 13, No. 2, 1974, pages 121–126.

Siantz, M., Ed. *The Nurse and the Developmentally Disabled Adolescent.* Baltimore: University Park Press, 1977.

Slavson, S.R. *Child-Centered Group Guidance of Parents.* New York: International Universities Press, 1958.

Weathers, L., and R.P. Liberman. "Modification of Family Behavior." In *Child Behavior Therapy*, D. Marholin, Ed. New York: Gardner Press, 1978.

Wyatt, G. "Parents and Siblings as Co-Therapists." In *Professional Approaches with Parents of Handicapped Children*, E. Webster, Ed. Springfield, IL.: Charles C Thomas, 1976.

Yalom, I.D. *Theory and Practice of Group Psychotherapy*. New York: Basic Books, 1975.

13

Group Work with the Elderly

Ellen H. Janosik

Jean R. Miller

There is an erroneous impression among some health workers that group work is inappropriate for the elderly because they have little capacity for change or because the quality of life cannot be sustained during the sunset years. It can be argued, however, that the need for identity and self-esteem persists throughout the life cycle and does not diminish with advancing age. The alternative to ego integrity is despair (Erikson, 1963), and preservation of identity and self-esteem are crucial to the attainment of ego integrity, the final critical life task.

THE PROBLEM OF DISENGAGEMENT

In the later years of life there is demonstrable evidence of disengagement. During the fifth decade psychological *disengagement* appears; this precedes the psychological and social disengagement of the sixth and seventh decades of life. Furthermore, as disengagement proceeds, the sense of well-being declines. In a six-year study of several hundred subjects between the ages of fifty and eighty, a positive correlation was found between social interaction and psychological well-being. Correlations were higher among persons over seventy than among those between fifty and seventy years of age. Regret for bygone activities is not temporary but tends to increase with age. Despite disengagement, individuals seldom abandon social values acquired over a lifetime, and the reflected appraisal of others remains a source of identity and self-esteem (Havighurst, Neugarten, and Tobin, 1973).

It is true that one-to-one relations have great importance for the elderly, but these can be supplemented with group programs which are often more effective in opposing regressive or dependent tendencies. It may be stated categorically that present services for the elderly are less than adequate, and that group work with this population is effective in the restoration and maintenance of health.

Legislation has been enacted recently to safeguard the rights of handicapped persons who were denied access to opportunities and facilities available to others. For years society provided educational, vocational, and recreational programs in direct proportion to the ability of the recipients to make a contribution to society. Like the handicapped, the elderly were often considered incapable of contributing, despite a lifetime spent upholding social values. Accordingly, the needs of the elderly were rarely given priority and were often overlooked. With the number of senior citizens mounting yearly, and with awareness of their impact on political institutions and health-care facilities, state and federal programs for the elderly have become more available.

Coping with Loss and Isolation

In organizing groups for the elderly a prevailing goal is to give older persons the chance to establish new interpersonal relationships — not to replace those of early years but to alleviate feelings of isolation. The interpersonal transactions available in groups help older people define or redefine selfhood, and demonstrate how others like themselves are adjusting to the cyclic changes of aging.

The losses which inevitably touch the elderly mean that advancing age may erode the meaningfulness, confidence, and autonomy which previously guided adulthood. Elderly persons not only suffer the loss of loved ones but also the loss of roles and functions by which they measured their own value, and physical losses in the form of declining strength and vigor. They endure social losses which reduce the frequency and duration of meaningful interactions with others. Many of them must also cope with cognitive losses which narrow their view of the world and add to their feelings of depletion. In contemporary society the experience of the elderly is usually one of subtraction rather than augmentation.

Because of multiple losses encountered by the elderly, they may be reluctant to live in the present and to deal with the here-and-now. Unless a group is formed for the purpose of encouraging reminiscing, the usual course recommended for group leaders is to stress the importance of daily life and of immediate issues. The importance of the past is never negated, but group interaction among the elderly is often facilitated by attention to current issues (Burnside, 1980).

Curative Factors Groups established for the elderly can generate change within realistic limits. Among the twelve curative factors described by Yalom (1975), seven were identified as especially important in groups for the elderly (Burnside, 1980). The helpful curative factors included group cohesiveness, universality, interpersonal learning, input and output, catharsis, identification, and instillation of hope. The list of omitted curative factors included guidance, insight, corrective family re-enactment, and existential factors. Significantly, the curative factors deemed of lesser importance in groups for the elderly were those likely to be productive of substantive personality change rather than of improving or maintaining the status quo.

CLASSIFICATION OF GROUPS FOR THE ELDERLY

Types of Groups

Groups for the elderly may be organized for a particular purpose or they may be emergent informal groups resulting from propinquity or common interests. Health-care professionals are usually involved with more formal groups in a variety of community and institutional settings. Group work is carried out in institutions or homes for the elderly to prepare residents for discharge, improve disruptive behavior, raise staff morale and effectiveness, orient new residents, and increase social competence. In out-patient departments of health facilities, group work is used to offer psychosocial support and help solve problems in living. Social agencies operating in the community offer a wide range of group programs for the elderly which combine social activities with informational and supportive services (Goldfarb, 1971). Formal groups organized for specific purposes include: support groups, reality orientation groups, remotivation groups, reminiscing groups, and insight groups (Burnside, 1980).

Purpose

Decreased social interaction of the elderly has been attributed to difficulties about health, money, and transportation. One compelling reason for refusing social involvement are fears of elderly persons that they will be humiliated by being asked to perform tasks of which they may be incapable (Miller, 1971). Anticipation of failure haunts many elderly persons. This means that the purpose of any group program must be carefully delineated and its scope understood by prospective members. Unless the purpose of the group is clearly described during the selection process, there may be a tendency among prospective members not to join the group or to limit the activities in which they are willing to participate.

Participation

Many elderly persons are alert, able-bodied, and capable of making informed decisions about whether to make a commitment to a group. Such programs as Golden Age Clubs draw upon this segment of the elderly population. Others among the elderly may be reluctant to participate in groups either from fear of anticipated failure or from lack of energy. Unwillingness to take part in group activities may be attributed to one or more of the following concerns: inability to reciprocate or share responsibility because of family, money, or health problems; fear of requests for performance of which the member is thought to be capable but is not confident of fulfilling; errors or mistakes in performance which will reveal weaknesses to other group members (Miller, 1971).

When the fears of the prospective member are realistic, they should be regarded as valid and the decision not to participate should be accepted. Embarrassment which a failed member experiences is difficult for other group members to deal with and limits social roles in the group. Group members perceive the failed member as someone who must not be allowed to fail again. Protective maneuvers from the group have the effect of subverting the group from its stated purpose. It is essential to place elderly members in group situations which demand only interactions within their social repertoire. When their fears of failure are unrealistic, persuasive measures may be used. If the purpose of the group is one which a prospective member has the potential to meet, fears of anticipated failure are unwarranted. In such instances, reassurance regarding the group goals and behaviors expected of members may effectively counter resistance to joining.

Once the members have joined the group, regular attendance should be recognized and rewarded. Failure to attend should be investigated not only to discover the cause but to stress the importance to the group of a member's presence. Coercive measures regarding membership or attendance should not be invoked. An exception to this rule applies to orientation or discharge groups organized to acquaint newcomers with a residential facility or to plan for the adjustment of returning home.

Leaders who are organizing a group may have to persuade and reassure reluctant candidates who are thought to be appropriate members. In other cases, leaders may have to limit the number of willing group members. When the number of persons wishing to join precludes accomplishment of the group task, it is advisable to organize other groups similar or different in purpose to give interested persons the opportunity for a group experience. In residential facilities for the elderly, group membership may be considered a privilege, and residents who are not invited to join may become resentful. Resentment may be expressed covertly by disclaiming any interest in the group, or by making disparaging remarks about the leaders or members. Others who are more direct may ask to be admitted to the group or to be placed on a waiting list if the group is full. Burnside (1980) urged that requests for admission be honored whenever possible, since the action denotes healthy assertiveness and a desire to be responsible for oneself.

Structural Properties

When groups for the elderly are held in the community, geographic location is a paramount consideration. Availability of public transportation or services of volunteers to escort disabled members may mean the difference between failed and successful group programs. In residential facilities, logistics are less of a problem, but other considerations intrude. If personnel are needed to bring members to the meeting room, they should be inconvenienced as little as possible. Since the goodwill of the staff is crucial to the group, meeting times and places should be arranged with their full involvement and consent. The following measures are helpful in assuring the success of groups offered in residential facilities for the elderly:

- Organize the group to fit into the time frame of the institutional program and the everyday routine of members and their visitors.
- Arrange for staff to remind members of meetings and to escort them to the meeting room if necessary. A "buddy" system is effective in bringing forgetful or apprehensive members to meetings, and reduces the demands on the staff.

- Limit the length of meetings so that members are physically comfortable. Frequent micturation or inability to sit in one position for a long time may cause members to be absent. Recess periods during which members can move about or leave the room if needed, help them attend to physical needs without embarrassment.

Early Issues Early issues to consider are whether a group shall be ongoing or time-limited, closed or open to new members. Intrinsic factors such as group goals, membership composition, and leader preferences are included in those considerations. Extrinsic factors such as time, space, and institutional preferences must also be considered. One argument for ongoing groups for the elderly is that the issue of group termination need not be faced. On the other hand, ongoing groups must deal with arrivals and departures of members, some of whom will leave because of illness or death.

Closed Groups Time-limited groups are likely to be closed to the admission of newcomers. Closed groups tend to be more cohesive, and setting a time limit for a group helps motivate members to deal with the task. Termination is a stressful event for elderly members, but may be dealt with therapeutically if time and attention are given to grieving. Feelings of loss as a group ends are attenuated by pride in the accomplishments of a successful group. Time-limited groups may be less anxiety-provoking for members who are fearful of a prolonged commitment or of their own performance failure.

Group Size Group size varies according to the purpose of the group, the number of members who are suitable and available, and pragmatic considerations of time and space. The most influential variable affecting group size is the nature or type of group which is contemplated. Table 13-1 presents a range of recommended sizes for particular groups.

Selection of Members

Group work has been attempted among elderly persons with varying physical and psychosocial needs by leaders representing the major health-care disciplines of medicine, nursing, psychology, and social work. Because of its diversity, group work can do many things for the elderly, but not the same things for all people (Goldfarb, 1971). In selecting members for gerontological groups, advanced age alone is insufficient to insure a positive group experience. Burnside (1980)

Table 13-1 TYPE OF GROUP AND NUMBER OF MEMBERS

Type	Number of Members
Support Groups	12 Members (Murray, Huelskoetter, and O'Driscoll, 1980) 6 Members, if regressed (Burnside, 1980)
Reality Orientation	8-10 Members (Murray, Huelskoetter, and O'Driscoll, 1980) 4 Members, if confused (Burnside, 1980)
Remotivation Groups	15 Members (Burnside, 1980)
Reminiscing Groups	8 Members (Ebersole, 1980)
Insight Groups	7-9 Members (Fried, 1971)

advised that personality considerations are important in organizing any group, regardless of the ages of members. Personality is an abstraction which is sometimes difficult to assess. Leaders engaged in member selection may choose to examine specific personality traits or to divide personality assessment into affective, cognitive, and other components.

Maintaining Affective Balance In selecting members it is wise to maintain a balance in the affective realm so that the group is not dominated by any prevailing mood. Members who are consistently anxious or consistently depressed should be offset by members whose affect is not symmetrical. If all group members exhibit a retarded or depressed affect, the group may be immobilized by inertia and hopelessness. Whenever several depressed members are in the group it is essential that their interactional styles not be the same. Similarity of affect and of interactional style are mutually reinforcing and may inhibit group development or individual growth. This means that effects of a very anxious member should be counteracted by the presence of members who are more serene. Heterogeneity of affect and of interactional style are recommended in group work with the elderly (Burnside, 1980).

Maintaining Homogeneity Homogeneity is advised in the cognitive realm, since members with limited cognitive ability may be unacceptable to those who consider themselves more capable. Competent members may be threatened and upset by being placed in groups with very regressed persons. Declining capability in the cognitive realm is common among the elderly and their self-esteem may be lowered by prolonged contact with others whose mental powers are seriously impaired. Cognitive ability should not be associated with educational level. Members with good cognitive skills and little formal education are often able to help well-educated members whose adeptness at intellectualization is used to avoid problem-solving.

The Noah's Ark Principle Psychomotor ability or disability among group members may be mixed. When all members must use wheelchairs, there is great physical distance between members. Wheelchair members and ambulatory members can benefit from the same group experience, particularly if the Noah's Ark principle is adopted. If only one group member must be in a wheelchair, that person may be able to swing into a sofa or comfortable seat, thus easing feelings of differentness which might otherwise isolate the wheelchair member.

Other Factors Unless there is a reason for limiting group membership solely to men or women, both sexes should be represented. Because elderly women outnumber men this recommendation may pose a problem. Persons with a physical disability should not be arbitrarily excluded from a group, but the prospective member must be able to get to meetings, to stay for the allotted time, and to be able to communicate effectively. Blatant psychiatric disability in the form of psychosis intimidates other members who are not psychotic. Residual psychiatric disability is not sufficient to exclude members who are able to stay in touch with reality. Organic brain damage evidenced by symptoms of senility often frightens elderly persons who are lucid and comprehending, for they see their own future in the rambling incoherence of senile members.

Group Dynamics

The developmental stages and levels which characterize most groups can be identified in groups for the elderly. (Extensive discussion of group development is found in Chapter 5.) There is as much difference in the behaviors of older people as there is among younger ones, with the proviso that elderly persons tend to remain the same sort of people they were at a younger age. Individuals who were anxious in their more productive years continue to be anxious, only more so. Persons who were spontaneous and enthusiastic in midlife usually carry these qualities into old age. Nevertheless, there are intensifications of problematic behaviors which occur among the elderly and should be kept in mind by group leaders (Bellak, 1975).

Callousness Because of repeated encounters with loss, some elderly persons appear to become detached or indifferent toward death, illness, or the misfortunes of others. Instead of commiserating, some of them seem to exhibit feelings of triumph because they have survived less fortunate family and friends. This is a defensive behavior which makes them seem indifferent, but is actually protective in nature.

Compartmentalization The elderly use focal awareness and selective inattention (Sullivan, 1953) to deal with issues which seem manageable and ignore issues which seem unmanageable. Because of physical or mental deficits, the elderly tend to put each task or responsibility into a separate compartment. In this way the elderly are able to handle one thing at a time and avoid being overwhelmed by events.

Somatic Preoccupation Sleeping, eating, and excretory problems are among the somatic preoccupations of the elderly. This is attributable to anxiety about mysterious changes occurring in the body of the aging person.

Verbosity Loquaciousness from the elderly represents an overture to others and is motivated by a desire for attention or interest. When there is little or no response from others, or when the response is withdrawn abruptly, the insecurity of elderly persons is intensified.

Denial When reality is frightening, elderly people may resort to excuses or blaming. Confabulation or the concealing of amnesia by inventing details is a form of denial used by old people who are frightened by their memory lapses and confusion.

Regression Some elderly persons combat regressive tendencies in themselves by becoming fiercely independent while others become clinging and demanding.

Selfishness Inconsiderate behavior displayed by the elderly may be a sign of dependency or insecurity. The elderly person who insists on having the same chair for every meeting may be exerting control over a life which seems out of control. Insignificant things take on overriding importance to the elderly, who attach such significance to possessions and territory that their behavior at times seems asocial.

Repetitiousness Like verbosity, this may indicate a wish for attention or for reassurance that one is still competent and accurate. Giving reassurance and trying to ascertain the purpose of repetition are appropriate responses from the group leader.

INTERVENTION PRINCIPLES

In determining appropriate interventions for group work with the elderly it is helpful to keep in mind the theoretical formulations of Erikson (1963) and the struggles inherent in the critical task of ego integrity versus despair. This concept offers an approach which helps the members accept the implications of aging but balances acceptance against efforts to make daily life satisfying and enjoyable.

As in all groups, the leader must attend to socioemotional functions which maintain the group and instrumental functions which enable members to accomplish the group task, whatever that may be. The behaviors of the leader have been divided into active and passive functions. Among the passive behaviors are attentive listening and being a target for the ventilation of members' emotions (catharsis). Among the active behaviors are directing, comforting, explaining, desensitizing, analyzing, negotiating, managing, deciding, and commenting (Goldfarb, 1971).

Members of groups for the elderly seem to benefit from active leadership which is not authoritarian but may at times be directive. Often elderly persons must give up control of their lives to others, and the group experience should avoid replicating this. Nevertheless, members are inclined to look to the leaders for information and guidance. This should not be withheld, especially in the initial stages of group life. If the group indicates that it wishes to be more autonomous, or if group members show leadership traits, the group deserves praise and encouragement. The group leader should intervene to oppose passivity of elderly group members.

Leaders who undertake this kind of group work must equip themselves with the following knowledge and abilities.

- Knowledge of the physiological, psychological, and social implications of aging, normal and abnormal.
- Knowledge of theories of group process and development.
- Knowledge of communication techniques and skills.
- Ability to tolerate dependency without fostering it.
- Ability to understand the interactional foibles of the elderly.
- Ability to accept incremental rather than drastic change.

Encouraging Participation

Serving light refreshments during group meetings is one method of increasing the interest and involvement of members. Delegating responsibilities of preparation and serving promotes self-esteem and altruism within the group. Spatial distance between members should be monitored so that no member is physically isolated. Touch can be used gently by the leader to reassure anxious members or to restrain monopolistic ones. Social and sensory deprivation accompany old age, and touching is often a source of comfort among the elderly. It would be appropriate, for example, for leaders to institute hand-shaking at the beginning of a session, or to ask members sitting in a circle to clasp each other's hands for a few seconds before the meeting ends.

There are many ways of evaluating the outcome of a group experience, some of which are simple but fairly satisfactory. Any observable improvement in level of social functioning is indicative of success. Reports of improved functioning from persons outside the group also indicate that the group experience is having a beneficial effect. Pre- and post-group questionnaires concerning group outcomes may be administered to members. Some leaders employ a checklist of behaviors or interactions exhibited by each member to validate random observations.

An objective evaluation of group results was reported by Wolk and Goldfarb (1966), who studied the effects of group therapy with elderly patients in a state hospital. Subjects were clinically and psychologically tested before and after group treatment using a mental status examination, double simultaneous stimulation (face-hand test), and the chromatic/achromatic house-tree-person tests. After a year of weekly group treatment consisting of one-and-a-half-hour sessions, retesting showed improvement in interpersonal relationships, and in depression and anxiety levels, which agreed with clinical observation of improvement.

SPECIFIC PURPOSE GROUPS

Support Groups

Support groups for the elderly have multiple purposes, chief of which are the promotion of self-esteem and the development of problem-solving skills needed to accommodate the changes of aging. More specifically, supportive health education groups provide information and encouragement for a population which is often at risk. Church sponsored groups give solace and spiritual support to the elderly while providing opportunities for congenial socialization. Participation in support groups is usually voluntary; duration may be time-limited or ongoing, depending on the group goals. Murray, Huelskoetter, and O'Driscoll (1980) cited the common themes present in support groups as depression, social isolation, and sensory losses. Leader interventions dealt with topics of memory, vision, hearing, interpersonal relationships, health, housing, death and dying. Emphasis was on problem solving and anticipatory planning; role-playing and other exercises were used to encourage active participation of the members.

Another study of supportive group work among the elderly (Nickoley, 1978) identified the following major themes: loss; need to be viewed as individuals; loneliness; awareness of "slowing down"; attitudes toward aging; management of the aging process; use of community, material, and personal resources. The same study suggested that group leaders utilize the following interventions.

- Focus on the present.
- Provide an atmosphere of acceptance.
- Emphasize strengths rather than limitations.
- Solicit group assistance in managing individual anxiety.
- Use minimal interpretative intervention.
- Encourage active rather than passive learning.
- Provide cognitive information.
- Foster preventive health measures.

Reality Orientation Groups

The term orientation is derived from the fact that the sun rises in the east and that its movements are a reference point for the human and animal world. The purpose of reality orientation is to maintain contact with the environment and reduce confusion experienced by the elderly regarding time, place, and personal identity. Reality orientation groups are held daily for a half hour with the same leader.

The number of members depends on the degree of disorientation: if they are severely confused, four members are the maximum number; otherwise eight to ten members may constitute the group. It is desirable that the group leader be familiar with the total health-care plan and needs of every member.

Usually, reality orientation groups are held in institutional settings, where the content covered in the small group sessions can be reinforced throughout the day by other staff members. Clocks with large numbers are on view and time is noted. Calendars with holidays marked are prominently displayed. Basic information is given repeatedly and recall is asked for by the leader. Sessions are relatively brief so that members are neither bored nor overwhelmed. Since reality orientation may be humiliating for those who are not altogether confused, it is important that leaders present the simple content in an adult manner. Members should be treated with dignity and respect, and given whatever time they need to complete an act or to recall facts. Careful explanations are required for all group proceedings, with the leader imparting person, time, and place information with infinite patience and concern.

Remotivation Groups

Remotivation groups may be offered in combination with reality orientation groups, or they may be offered to persons who are withdrawn rather than disoriented. The goal of such groups is to stimulate thinking and task performance related to everyday life. Persons suitable for remotivation programs should be fairly well-oriented to reality, possess adequate speech and hearing faculties, and not be preoccupied with hallucinatory stimuli. A competent leader should be able to handle a remotivation group with up to fifteen members. Although the time frame may vary, remotivation groups are time limited. The group may meet one hour a week for twelve weeks or three hours a week for four weeks (Robinson n.d., cited in Burnside, 1980).

Five specific steps contribute to the achievements of a remotivation group, as presented by Murray, Huelskoetter, and O'Driscoll (1980).

1. Create an atmosphere of acceptance by spending the first five minutes of the session greeting and welcoming each member by name.
2. Build a pathway to the world by spending fifteen minutes discussing whatever topic was selected by the group at the previous meeting.
3. Expand the pathway to the world by exploring the topic through the use of pictures, poems, audio tapes, and so on.

4. Relate the topic to the lives, experiences, and interests of members.
5. Create a climate of appreciation for the contributions of members while selecting a topic and arousing anticipation for the next session.

The format for remotivation groups is quite structured, and there is a didactic aspect to part of the proceedings. Visual aids are used to help members adhere to the selected topic. Leader interventions are employed to sustain attention and to avoid discussion of individual or family problems not relevant to the topic.

Reminiscing Groups

The purpose of reminiscing groups is to allow members the opportunity of a life review by sharing their thoughts and past experiences with the group. Reminiscing is considered an adaptive process for the elderly and a method of preserving identity and self-esteem at a time when physical abilities are diminished and social roles are narrowed. The reminiscing group need not adhere to a strict format but should follow the will of the members. The group may be time-limited or ongoing, structured or free-flowing. Topics may be selected in advance and visual aids may be introduced if necessary to stimulate discussion. As members begin to feel comfortable, reminiscing may move from superficial content to deep affective issues. The leader is responsible for preserving a democratic milieu, but may at times intervene to protect the group from disclosures which are too startling or too intimate. Troubled members who display obsessive preoccupation with remorse and guilt should be referred for individual counseling.

Intergenerational Groups An interesting variation of reminiscing groups is one which transcends generations. Elderly people who have survived personal vicissitudes and cataclysmic social events such as war and economic depression, have much to tell young people. Many elderly persons have already told their treasured memories to the people they encounter every day and welcome the chance to share memories with a new, receptive audience.

Compatibility is an important factor in reminiscing groups and it may be prudent to let prospective members know who else will be in the group. Residential care for the elderly sometimes means that hostilities develop between people. While disagreement among members during group sessions is unavoidable, it is disadvantageous to include in the same group persons who are already resentful and antagonistic toward one another (Ebersole, 1980). Having prospective members suggest others they would like to have in the group is a positive method of ensuring compatibility. In addition, this strategy adds to feelings of being autonomous and influential.

Insight Groups

Insight groups are reparative groups which seek to induce some personality change; therefore, they are thought to have limited effectiveness with elderly members (Wolff, 1967). If the major goal of the insight group is to increase social effectiveness, reduce psychological distress, and improve self-esteem, then there is a place for insight work with the elderly. Like most other people, the elderly are capable of transferences, which can be explored in a group setting and which sometimes increase self-awareness. Leading an insight group requires advanced education in group and psychodynamic theory, and should not be attempted by a beginner. While advocating group psychotherapy with the elderly, Altholz (1980) described it as a difficult modality, partly because sharing intimate problems with a group is difficult for older people who grew up in a more reticent time.

Leader interventions in insight groups consist of exploration, interpretation, and working through. A prominent curative factor is the corrective re-enactment of the primary group experience (Yalom, 1975). Elderly people who have difficulty in their current relationships with others can learn that early experiences with significant others contribute to some present-day problems. Some elderly persons are capable of introspection and of making the abstract connections which lead to self-awareness, insight, and changed behavior. In insight groups the regressive wishes of elderly members must be combated. An active leader who dilutes transference phenomena by clarifying and explaining will be able to circumvent regression and dependency among group members.

If possible, insight groups should contain members of both sexes, all of whom are capable of speaking, hearing, and comprehending the exploration of past conflicts. Psychotherapy group members may have similar problems, but should present differing affective styles. The groups are usually long term, extending over a period of several years. When careful selection occurs, an insight group enables elderly members to examine past and present relationships analytically in order to resolve residual conflicts and face the rest of life less defensively.

Social isolation is often a defense used by the elderly to avoid further experiences of loss (Barnett, 1978). To interact with others and to form attachments means remaining open and vulnerable, and for some elderly persons isolation is preferred to vulnerability. The medium of group interaction effectively reduces the effects of social and psychological isolation which are the lot of many elderly persons. Regardless of its specific purpose, every group for the elderly has the potential of improving the quality of life. Talking to other people about facts or feelings, eating together, or working together are social events which promote self-esteem and reduce feelings of loneliness. The ultimate result is to share the joy and memories of a long life, and to move in the direction of ego integration.

CLINICAL EXAMPLE: DEATH CONFRONTED IN A SUPPORT GROUP

A group of elderly residents in a church home met every Wednesday under the leadership of the nurse assigned to their care. Usually the meetings were attended by all ten residents on the fourth floor, but Millie, a faithful member, was absent on a particular day. When the leader was questioned about Millie, he told the group that Millie was too upset to come to the meeting because Perry, her loved canary, had died the night before. The reactions of the members varied. Helen, a pert little woman, in a bright dress, shook her head sadly saying, "He was such a little bird — ate hardly anything and never did any harm." Jim, a big, slow-moving man, shrugged helplessly and remarked, "Well, when you gotta go, you gotta go. Me, I never had no pets." Lulu sat silently for a while, then rose suddenly and shut the door. Max, who had been rocking back and forth in his chair, asked loudly, "What are we going to do about it? That's what I want to know, what're we going to do about it?"

This question seemed to release a great deal of group tension. Several members looked at one another and repeated Max's remark. "What are we going to do about it?"

Evelyn's sad eyes circled the group as if appraising their financial capabilities. "Well, we could take up a collection and buy Millie another canary — or even a pair of love birds. Then she wouldn't miss Perry so much."

The mention of love birds drew an exclamation of disgust from Jim. "Better buy her a parrot instead," he suggested. "She could teach it to talk. Maybe it would swear at her and she could pretend it was her husband." Jim laughed loudly, but no one joined in.

After several minutes of heated discussion about what each of them could afford to contribute, what kind of bird to buy, and who would shop for it, the members turned to the leader for approval and confirmation of their plans.

During the discussion the group leader had been thinking about the individual responses of the members. Helen obviously identified with the helpless, insignificant bird who died. Jim reacted stoically and indicated that when you loved anybody, even a canary, you were likely to suffer pain. He avoided pain by not having pets. Lulu symbolically shut death out of the room. Her act in shutting the door indicated her fears for the group members. And Max, who was always agitated, sought action from the group. Practical Evelyn offered a practical solution to the group.

Because he realized that immediate restitution is not the most therapeutic response to loss, the leader temporized. "Your idea of getting Millie another canary is a good one, and it's nice to see that you care so much. But maybe for today Millie just needs to think about Perry and cry for a little while. She has asked me for a shoebox and she is planning to bury him in the garden this afternoon. Maybe she needs some help with that. You might ask her."

This information turned the attention of the group from the shopping trip to sharing in the funeral rites for Perry. It was agreed that two members would visit Millie after the meeting to hear how Perry died and to help bury him in the garden, if Millie agreed. Evelyn said she had a nice box with satin lining that would hold Perry and she would offer it to Millie. The final comment of the meeting was made by Jim, who said it was a shame Perry died, but at least it wasn't a group member, and Millie had better show up next week because he sure missed her. The leader suggested that Jim should tell Millie that he missed her, and he agreed.

SUMMARY

Group work is appropriate for elderly persons whose lives are characterized by loss of loved ones and loss of valued roles. The critical task of the elderly is that of reaching ego integration rather than despair, and groups which offer opportunities for meaningful social interaction can contribute to the resolution of this age-appropriate task. Types of groups for the elderly are support groups, reality orientation groups, remotivation groups, reminiscing groups, and insight groups. Issues of participation, member selection, and the structural properties of groups were discussed. Certain behaviors typical of elderly persons which pose problems in groups were described. These included callousness, compartmentalization, somatic preoccupation, verbosity, denial, regression, selfishness, and repetitiousness. The underlying motivation for these behaviors was discussed and some intervention principles cited.

Outcome evaluation of groups was outlined in a general way; several subjective procedures were suggested and one sophisticated outcome study was described. Each of the previously mentioned special purpose groups was presented briefly; distinctions among the five types of groups were contrasted and compared.

REFERENCES

Altholz, J.A.S. "Group Psychotherapy with the Elderly." In *Working with Elderly Group Processes and Techniques*. I.M. Burnside, Ed. North Scituate, MA.: Duxbury Press, 1980.

Barnett, J. "On the Dynamics of Interpersonal Isolation." *Journal of the American Academy of Psychoanalysis* 6, 1978, pages 59–70.

Bellak, L. *The Best Years of Your Life*. New York: Atheneum Press, 1975.

Burnside, I.M. *Working with Elderly Group Processes and Techniques*. North Scituate, MA.: Duxbury Press, 1980.

Butler, R. "The Life Review: An Interpretation of Reminiscence in the Aged." *Psychiatry* 26, 1963, pages 65–76.

Ebersole, P.P. "Establishing Reminiscing Groups." In *Working with Elderly Group Processes and Techniques*, I.M. Burnside, Ed. North Scituate, MA.: Duxbury Press, 1980.

Erikson, E.H. *Childhood and Society*. New York: W.W. Norton, 1963.

Fried, E. "Basic Concepts in Group Psychotherapy." In *Comprehensive Group Psychotherapy*, H.I. Kaplan and B.J. Sadock, Eds. Baltimore: Williams and Wilkins, 1971.

Goldfarb, A.I. "Group Therapy with the Old and Aged." In *Comprehensive Group Psychotherapy*, H.I. Kaplan and B.J. Sadock, Eds. Baltimore: Williams and Wilkins, 1971.

Havighurst, R.J.; B.L. Neugarten; and S.S. Tobin. "Disengagement and Patterns of Aging." In *Middle Age and Aging*, B.L. Neugarten, Ed. Chicago: University of Chicago Press, 1973.

Miller, S.J. "Social Dilemma of the Aging Leisure Participant." In *Comprehensive Group Psychotherapy*, H.I. Kaplan and B.J. Sadock, Eds. Baltimore: Williams and Wilkins, 1971.

Murray, R.; M. Huelskoetter; and M.S. O'Driscoll. *The Nursing Process in Later Maturity*. Englewood Cliffs, N.J.: Prentice-Hall, 1980.

Nickoley, S.E. *Promoting Functional Level of Health and Perception of Control in Elderly Women in the Community Through Supportive Group Interaction*. Unpublished Master's thesis, University of Rochester, 1978.

Robinson, A.M. *Remotivation Techniques: A Manual for Use in Nursing Homes*. Philadelphia: American Psychiatric Association, and Smith, Kine and French Laboratories, Remotivation Project, n.d.

Sullivan, H.S. *The Interpersonal Theory of Psychiatry*. New York: W.W. Norton, 1953.

Wolff, K. "Comparison of Group and Individual Psychotherapy with Geriatric Patients." *Disorders of the Nervous System* 28, 1967, page 384.

Wolk, R.L., and A.I. Goldfarb. "Response to Group Psychotherapy of Aged Recent Admissions Compared with Long-Term Mental Hospital Patients." *American Journal of Psychiatry* 10, 1966, page 123.

Yalom, I.D. *Theory and Practice of Group Psychotherapy*. New York: Basic Books, 1975.

14

Groups for the Chronically Ill

Madeline H. Schmitt

The dramatic growth of both professionally led and self-help groups for chronically ill patients is attributed to a variety of causes. Prominent among them is recognition that the present health-care system does not offer adequate emotional support, adjustment, and adaptation to chronic illness; instead it focuses on the treatment of the disease *per se.* The increasing autonomy of nurses and social workers has contributed to the ability of these professionals to respond to expressive needs. The greater public awareness of chronic illness problems coupled with increased consumer involvement in health-care issues has encouraged self-help approaches to these needs. Self-help groups in chronic illness, unlike the self-help approaches to addictive disorders, have often been organized with the active assistance of health-care professionals, and may operate as components of a local voluntary health agency. For example, stroke groups may be sponsored by the local heart association, and various cancer self-help groups for ostomy patients, laryngectomy patients, or for terminally ill patients may be sponsored by a local voluntary cancer organization.

The kinds of groups that can be organized are numerous. Theoretically, any chronic illness requiring persons to make significant changes in life-style, to acquire new personal care skills, or which results in social isolation by virtue of some stigmatizing aspect can provide the basis for organizing a group experience.

HISTORY OF GROUPS FOR CHRONICALLY ILL PATIENTS

Some of the earliest group therapeutic efforts in the United States were organized on behalf of patients with chronic physical illness. Histories of the development of group psychotherapy identify Dr. Joseph Pratt, a Boston internist, as the American founder of the group psychotherapy movement (Anthony, 1971; Mullan and Rosenbaum, 1962). In the early 1900s Pratt organized tuberculosis classes consisting of about twenty-five patients, which he conducted weekly. He lectured about the importance of various aspects of treatment and had patients follow their progress by keeping records of such items as their temperature, diet, and rest periods. In addition, the class was viewed as a time during which patients could experience supportive social relations with each other. Pratt's talks were apparently not only educational but inspirational, leading Mullan and Rosenbaum to label him as the "father of the repressive-inspirational movement in group psychotherapy" (p. 6). Written treatments of Pratt's contributions to the group movement tend to emphasize his rudimentary concepts of psychological dynamics operant in the groups, his growth in understanding these over his lifetime, and the relationship of his ideas to the contributions of others who were establishing group psychotherapy as a treatment for mental illness. Group therapeutic efforts on behalf of chronically physically ill patients did not become popular immediately and the work of Pratt initially was of greatest interest to psychiatrists.

The application of group techniques to problems other than mental illness has emerged since the 1940s. Two trends have been significant. Among professionals, psychiatric social workers began to use group skills outside mental health settings (Marram, 1973). During the 1970s, persons other than mental health workers began to explore the usefulness of group approaches to a variety of patient problems including those of the chronically ill.

Another trend of the 1940s, aided by the formation of Alcoholics Anonymous, was the self-help approach to shared problems. Such groups did not rely on professional motivation and leadership, but formed a peer group to meet common needs, to overcome common handicaps, and to bring about social and personal change (Tracy and Gussow, 1976). In recent years, these groups have expanded to include persons who share a common chronic illness.

A FRAMEWORK FOR CONCEPTUALIZING GROUPS
FOR THE NURSING CARE OF THE CHRONICALLY ILL

Current Frameworks

Marram (1973) and Loomis (1979) have provided typologies for relating other types of groups to psychotherapeutic groups. It is of interest to compare these typologies with the one provided by Janosik in Chapter 3 of this book. The basis of Janosik's typology is the degree of personality change sought in the group context. Leadership behaviors are identified as critical variables in creating a group context that fosters or limits personality change. A continuum of five types of groups expresses variation from regressive-reconstructive groups, where maximum personality change is sought, to repressive-inspirational groups where minimum personality change is sought.

Marram's distinctions of group psychotherapy, therapeutic groups, self-help groups, plus growth and self-actualization groups also indicate that one implicit dimension is the degree of personality change sought. Thus, group psychotherapy encompasses regressive-reconstructive and reparative types of groups which focus on the alleviation of emotional disturbance. Therapeutic groups, in which treatment of emotional distress is secondary include those that Janosik terms adaptational and supportive. In distinguishing self-help groups from psychotherapy and therapeutic groups, Marram moves from personality change to concern with who the leaders are. Noting that leaders of self-help groups are typically not professionals, Marram adds that the goals of such groups emphasize repression of impulses and improved socialization. In Marram's final category — namely growth and self-actualization groups — the goals include education and self-enhancement of psychologically normal individuals. Thus, except for the distinction as to type of leader (professional versus nonprofessional) and the addition of growth and self-actualization groups, the typologies of Janosik and Marram are basically similar.

Loomis (1979) is another nurse-writer who developed a typology of groups. Omitting reference to self-help, Loomis includes most of the group types discussed by Marram and Janosik, sometimes using different labels. A noteworthy addition is the "task accomplishment" group, which is not usually referred to in literature dealing with group therapy formats. In some respects the task group is the antithesis to groups whose goals focus on the individual. Task groups typically involve the suppression of individual needs in order to accomplish a goal related to the common good. The categorization by Loomis of task groups seems to incorporate them in an adaptational or therapeutic frame of reference because they are organized more for the purpose of teaching people basic skills of working together than for accomplishing a greater good.

Typologies can be useful in theory building if they assist in the isolation of critical, rather than superficial, dimension. Typologies have practical value if the isolated dimensions help diagnose problems systematically and formulate alternative solutions. Finally, particular typologies may lend legitimacy to the isolated dimensions, while suggesting that other neglected dimensions possess lesser value. The typologies discussed here have strengths and weaknesses relating to theory building, practicality, and questions of legitimacy. When taken together the various typologies draw attention to the poles of a continuum, representing personality repair and personality enhancement, but do little to visualize the middle of the continuum, which involves supportive and adaptational processes arising from normal life crises, physical illness, and social maladjustment. Nonpsychiatric nurses and other health workers are often called upon to conduct groups in this middle range, and clarification of salient dimensions in these groups would benefit theory building and facilitate a consistent approach to problems and solutions in these middle range groups.

None of these typologies directs attention to the functions of groups *qua* groups nor to relationships between group functions and personality systems. In other words these typologies give no hint as to why group intervention as opposed to one-to-one intervention is either desirable or preferable in achieving stated goals of personality change, support or enhancement.

Two requirements, then, for an adequate framework within which to visualize the use of groups for chronically ill patients are the analysis of the impact of chronic illness on the personality system, and a typology of groups suggesting basic aspects of group life which can be systematically activated to help individuals cope with the impact of chronic illness.

Life Cycle View of the Impact of Chronic Illness

One way to conceptualize the impact of chronic illness is to adopt a life cycle perspective. Since the meaning of illness differs for individuals at different life stages, people can be expected to react differently to the experience of illness at these different stages. Their reactions reflect the impact of illness on their role responsibilities, psychological status, and interpersonal relations.

For the general population in the United States the incidence of chronic illnesses such as heart diseases, cancers, and disabling musculo-skeletal disorders rises dramatically with early middle age. In addition, people at this stage of life are coping with a number of midlife issues: decline and death of their own parents, independence of their children, leveling off in their achievements at work, and changing relationships with spouses. A chronic illness which induces serious disability or a foreshortened life span is likely to complicate and lend urgency to the solution of normal developmental issues. One good indicator of the ability to cope successfully with mid-life issues is the degree of success a person has had in dealing with prior life cycle problems. Those who have made only marginal adjustments previously are most vulnerable to "mid-life crisis" (Farrell, Rosenberg, and Schmitt, 1976). Chronic illness may either be a concomitant of crisis and contain psychosomatic dimensions or it may contribute to the stresses already evident in inadequate response to mid-life issues. On the other hand, individuals who have successfully coped with prior life issues may find new sources of strength and meaning in their confrontation with chronic illness, which, though lending a different character to the resolution of the normal life issues, nevertheless results in successful adaptation.

Disabling or life-threatening chronic illness appearing at any earlier stage of the life cycle is likely to result in the need to adjust to permanent alterations in the normal, expected life course (Neugarten, 1973). Such alterations include changes in employment capabilities, social life, intimate relationships, daily routine, and plans for the future.

In addition to having implications for the resolution of current life cycle issues, the physical impact of chronic illness in the form of increases in dependency and reductions in autonomy may contribute to a revival of past conflicts. For example, at an age when an individual may reasonably expect to achieve independence financially, occupationally, and socially, the necessity of being cared for by others may be a profound blow.

Psychological Impact of Chronic Illness

Psychologically, the impact of chronic illness on physiological and social functioning is one of identity or ego threat. This threat is expressed as anxiety or fears of one kind or another. The response to this threat, in an effort to contain the anxiety or control the fears, may take the form of defense mechanisms whose aim is the protection of ego integrity and identity. Such phenomena as repression, suppression, denial, displacement, isolation, regression, withdrawal, projection, identification and sublimation may characterize the person's psychological reaction to the presence of a chronic illness (Schwartz and Schwartz, 1972).

Often, the reactions of those close to the individual exacerbate the psychological impact of the illness. Rejection because of altered physical appearance or fears of contagion, anger at the inability of the person to meet responsibilities, or refusal to accept increased responsibility on the part of significant others may add to the ill person's sense of worthlessness, powerlessness, and isolation.

The nature of the illness itself is often an important variable in predicting the kinds of problems blocking resolution of life cycle issues, the psychological reactions manifested, and the interpersonal responses encountered. For example, problems associated with and reactions to cancer often differ substantially from those associated with stroke, diabetes, hypertension, or chronic renal failure and dialysis.

Although there may be considerable variation in individual reactions to a particular chronic illness based on a unique life history, people at the same stage of the life cycle confronting chronic illness problems are likely to have similar problems in the areas of role responsibilities, and in the reactions of others toward them in interpersonal situations. Furthermore, they are likely to have similar ranges of defensive patterns and similar needs for information and instruction in techniques for managing their illness. All of these factors suggest the desirability of organizing groups according to life cycle stage and type of chronic illness as a means of capitalizing on the therapeutic properties of groups.

The Functional Model of Groups: A Comprehensive Typology

Parsons, Bales, and Shils (1951) developed a model of social systems originating from studies of large social systems (societies) and of small groups. The model identified four interrelated demands of social systems, large or small. Parsons noted that every social system must, over time, focus attention on these four demands in order to maintain equilibrium. Though the usefulness of the model has been questioned in studying whole societies, it has been a productive model for thirty years in empirical research and theory building about small group processes.

The four interrelated demands are shown in Table 14-1. When groups are focusing on the latency or "L" box, they are dealing with the intrapsychic tension in their members. When the members are involved in productive work the focus is on the attainment of group goals, represented by the "G" box. The "I" or integration box emphasizes the building of interpersonal ties resulting in group solidarity, while

Table 14–1   DIAGRAM OF THE PARSONS-BALES VIEW OF THE
SOCIAL SYSTEM

Adaptation "A"	Goal-Attainment "G"
Latency-Tension "L"	Integration "I"

Expressive Demands:
Latency-Tension Management
Integration

Instrumental Demands:
Adaptation
Goal Attainment

the adaptation or "A" box deals with the acquisition and utilization of resources such as skills and knowledge required for goal attainment. Theoretical ideas about the interrelationship of these demands, particularly the expressive demands characterized by the "L" and "I" boxes and the instrumental demands characterized by the "A" and "G" boxes, have led to empirical studies of these relationships extending over three decades. The studies start with Bales' observations of the cyclical pattern of attention to the instrumental or task demands followed by attention to the expressive or socio-emotional demands in small *ad hoc* task groups, and distinctions between two types of leaders responsive to these key demands of group life. Recent ideas about the interrelationship of these demands involve complex models of group development and changes in leadership function over time consistent with the developmental cycle (see earlier chapters of this book; also, Tuckman, 1965; Farrell, 1976; and Tuckman and Jensen, 1977).

Newer models emphasize the links between individual and group growth. In a reworking of the Parsons, Bales, and Shils model, growth dimensions of the four demands were outlined as these relate to the group and the individual in it (Mills, 1967). In terms of tension management, the individual shows capacity for deeper emotional experience coupled with ability to convey this experience to others in a positive fashion. As group members increase in this capacity, the group as a whole acquires a culture and structure which encourages emotional growth among new members. When individuals learn to accept themselves and others, including acceptance of altered aspects of the self without loss of identity, the group as a whole develops greater power to accept and integrate a variety of individual responses.

Finally, as a person learns how to achieve goals, modify goals, and accept new goals, the overall ability of the group to identify and address objectives relevant to the membership increases. In addition, there is a clear link between individual growth in each of the four demand areas and growth in group capabilities, for the capacities of individual members influence the collective capacity of the group (Mills, 1967). The total group structure and process also may determine the extent to which individual capabilities are utilized or thwarted in the modification and expansion of the resources of the group as a whole.

ORGANIZING GROUPS FOR CHRONICALLY ILL CLIENTS

Groups may devote more attention to one demand than another. Task-oriented groups emphasize goal attainment while therapy groups emphasize tension-reduction and personality integration. Through their involvement with various demands of group life, members can participate in experiences that improve their individual functioning in these dimensions. Involvement in task groups results in improvement of work-oriented skills; involvement in therapy groups results in improved emotional functioning. An example of a goal attainment group in the area of chronic illness would be a committee of patients and health providers organized to make community facilities accessible to the physically handicapped. An example of latency-tension management group might be a therapy group for persons at high risk for heart disease because of personality factors. Most needs of chronically ill patients, however, are likely to fall in the areas of adaptation and integration. The need for reducing social isolation and resolving communication problems in the family arising around the illness, are problems of integration. A group specifically organized to deal with these issues can provide the context for working out these problems. These groups are often called "support" groups. The need to acquire new knowledge and new coping skills as well as to apply old solutions to new problems in order to manage aspects of daily living are adaptational problems. While these issues might be dealt with on a one-to-one basis, addressing them in groups may well be more efficient. Traditionally, these constitute a type of "class" for patients conducted for diabetic teaching, cardiac teaching, and so forth. On the other hand, problems of integration can uniquely benefit from group approaches. The "curative factors" of Yalom (1975) heavily emphasize the integrative demands of group life.

Therapy groups that concentrate only on emotional problems of chronic illness convey an implication of personality disturbance into the experience that is unwarranted, while ignoring other dimensions such as the social isolation imposed on ill persons by others, and the need for new knowledge and skills in order to cope. On the other hand, "classes" that are conducted for the purpose of conveying information and teaching skills, such as giving insulin injections or using home dialysis equipment, may ignore the emotional consequences of adjusting to the presence of a chronic illness.

Setting

Practically, the utilization of group approaches for chronic illness problems requires an adequate population base from which to draw participants. Several settings lend themselves to large enough populations to organize particular kinds of groups. Hospitals have provided the context for short-term groups for selected inpatients. These have often taken the form of instructional classes, such as those for newly diagnosed diabetics. One nurse may have the responsibility for conducting a series of classes for all newly diagnosed diabetics. Specialized wards such as oncology wards or dialysis units may also provide a context for the organization of an ongoing group. Utilization of groups in inpatient settings is limited by such things as scheduled tests (although using evening hours opens the possibility for inclusion of family members who may work during the day), the physical ability of the patient to participate, and the length of hospitalization.

Few outpatient settings lend themselves naturally to the use of group approaches. The staggered appointments characteristic of most private medical practices, outpatient clinics, or health maintenance organizations work against building a group approach into the medical appointment structure. Exceptions are when patients come at the same time for a period of treatment such as institutionally based outpatient dialysis units, cancer treatment centers, or rehabilitation centers. One spouse of a patient described an informal support group that began in a waiting room of a radiation treatment center. The fact that patients diagnosed at the same time were scheduled for radiation treatments on the same days for several weeks created the potential for building a supportive group experience (Gardner, 1980).

A group may be organized on a community-wide basis. A voluntary agency may be more willing to provide initial sponsorship than an institution. This may be the way a newly recognized need for a particular kind of group is integrated into the community. If the group is successful in drawing a large number of participants, it may divide into subgroups which are geographically dispersed and closer to the membership of the subgroup. Successful self-help organizations have experienced this pattern of growth. The creation and success of an initial group may also reveal a need for a more integrated service to health professionals, and individual institutions may then choose to create such groups for their clients. An example might be the success of a local *Make Today Count* group for terminally ill patients leaving large hospitals with cancer treatment facilities to establish institution-ally-based groups for these patients.

Currently, the use of group modalities to respond to the non-medical needs of chronically ill patients is often seen as an embellishment which can be cut from the budget during hard times. Outcome re-search documenting the contributions of group approaches is still seriously lacking.

Focus and Frameworks of Chronic Illness Groups

The focus or overall goals of a group for chronically ill patients can encompass any of the four demands (adaptation, latency-tension management, goal attainment, and integration) of the functional model, depending on the predominate needs of the patients. These needs are likely to vary by type and stage of illness as well as by indi-vidual developmental status. Depending on the overall goals of the group a variety of conceptual-theoretical frameworks are available in the literature which emphasize one or the other of the demand areas. These frameworks guide the organization, implementation, interpre-tation, and evaluation of the group experience.

Coping Skills Following diagnosis, most chronically ill patients have a need for information about the disease process and treatment, including medication regimens, nutritional modifications, recreatio-nal and daily living activities, communication skills, and relaxation-meditation techniques. Many of these adaptational needs may be met more efficiently in groups. A variety of resources including the crea-tion or use of audiovisual aids such as movies, the use of demonstra-tions, and the presentations of experts are feasible when the recipients are a group rather than individuals. Discussion can be focused on problem-solving among group members as they encounter obstacles to implementing changes. Methods used successfully by some group members can be shared with the others. Professionals may even find that ideas generated in this fashion have potential for systematic evalu-ation and research as means to improving patient care.

Frameworks for patient groups which identify teaching-learning processes for either informational purposes or the acquisition of coping skills as a major focus are not well applied in nursing. Most teaching done in groups reflects traditional approaches to education. The content often reflects some prejudgment by the nurse as to what people need to know or superficial assessment of "what people would like to hear about." Little use is made of the unique abilities of the group to foster learning. Some current approaches of nurses to teaching chronically ill patients individually emphasize behavioral theory and techniques (see, for example, Steckel, 1980). These have been applied to health-related groups (Rose, 1977) and offer potential for working with chronically ill patients in groups, particularly for patients whose illnesses require major modifications in usual behavior. A systematic behavioral approach to learning, the positive reinforcement built into a well-functioning interpersonal support system, and aspects of modeling could all be meaningfully utilized in a group approach.

Emotional Reactions A second potential focus is aimed at dealing with powerful emotional reactions to the onset of a chronic illness. Because particular illnesses have shared negative cultural meaning, generate similar integrative and adaptational problems at different stages of the illness, and have similar consequences for individual development, it is possible for these common and shared emotional reactions (which may be avoided and defended against, thereby becoming negative factors in overall coping) to become the focus of group work. This focus often predominates in "therapy" approaches to group work with the chronically ill.

Because of the history of the development of group work as a form of psychotherapy, the greatest variety of models available are in the area of tension management or emotional relations. Many of the models share an attempt to conceptualize the avoidance of anxiety and resistance to confrontation and working through of emotional relations among members of the group. These conceptualizations rely on an understanding of individual defense mechanisms used to contain anxiety and the creation of group defensive strategies in shared efforts to contain anxiety as characteristic of group situations where there are powerful emotional issues.

Bion (Rioch, 1970) described these group defenses as dependency, fight-flight, and pairing; or what he called "basic assumption" modes of interaction. In dependency, anxiety and the pressures to work are reduced by members' reliance on an all-powerful, all-knowing leader who is expected to share member problems and protect members from the emotions whose expression is feared. Such unrealistic dependency must be distinguished from real needs for information and other resources to which a professional leader may have access in facilitating coping with chronic illness. Anger is an emotion which characterizes the "fight" defensive reaction. Rather than taking responsibility for action group members may attribute their difficulties to the leader or figures outside the group such as doctors, institutions, or even God. It is important to remember that these models focus on irrational emotions and that the anger expressed at the leader or figures outside the group is not justified by objective events. Rational anger resulting from mismanagement of an illness, poor professional-patient relations, a lack of needed services, job discrimination, and so forth requires the mobilization of group effort directed at social change, not therapy. Flight is expressed as a defense against work demands and anxiety when the group disintegrates into subgroups to avoid talking about anxiety-provoking issues. The transformation of the interaction into that of a social group may be another means of avoidance. Again, these phenomena as *defensive* reactions must be distinguished from sub-grouping that may be appropriate to accomplishing tasks or a social group climate that assists the group in integrative demands. The final defense, pairing, is one of fulfilling the hoped for wishes of the group by delegating an idealized pair of members who will work for the group and whose imagined success provides the group with a vicarious sense of gratification. This pairing is not to be confused with the importance of role models whose coping with chronic illnesses are causes for optimism and hope among other members.

Whitaker (1976) and Lieberman (1973) developed the concept of *group focal conflict*, observing that therapy groups often create shared themes that capture the group attention and emotion for a time, only to change and reappear in a different way. These themes have two aspects — shared wishes and shared fears. The conflict itself tends to be hidden, but the interaction and content reflect the group's wishes, fears, and more or less adequate solution to the conflict. Whitaker described two types of solutions: enabling solutions that alleviate fear while allowing exploration and expression of the wish, and restrictive solutions that alleviate fear but prevent the exploration or expression of the wish associated with it. Whitaker suggests that restrictive solutions characterize early group interaction. Barring a group membership that is so homogeneous in defensive avoidance mechanisms that enabling solutions are prohibited, a skillful group leader can move the group in the direction of safe exploration of the wish after several beginning sessions. Themes mentioned in the literature as appearing in groups of chronically ill patients include fears of rejection, isolation and loneliness, dependency, loss, and death.

Social Isolation A third focus is especially appropriate in responding to the social isolation which characterizes some of our major chronic illnesses. A group may be the vehicle by which individuals whose self-esteem has been affected by physical stigma or a "dread" diagnosis find acceptance of their "new" selves, empathy from others who are experiencing similar problems, a reduction in the sense that they are unique or alone in their problem, and a sense of real meaning or purpose in being able to be of assistance to other members who may need help. Such groups are especially effective if supportiveness among members includes the family, either by directly incorporating family members in the group or by providing a context in which isolation from family can be worked on in a problem-solving fashion. Such groups encourage reintegration of the individual into the family unit or offer an alternative support system in the absence of family support. This process is reinforced if contacts among members extend beyond meetings to other activities such as telephone contacts and mutual aid. Whether this kind of group is called a "support" group or "resocialization" group or something else, its central goal is the need of the members to be integrated into a meaningful interpersonal environment.

Changing the System The fourth focus of the group may involve a common desire to change the way people with a particular chronic illness are managed by the health-care institution or the larger society. Lack of needed health services, job discrimination, architectural barriers, legal problems, or special education needs may provide the impetus for a task group whose major goal is the solution of this larger problem. Groups are more efficient and effective than individuals in such situations because several people can divide up the work in ways that recognize the special interests and skills of the membership.

Bales and Strodtbeck (1951) originally proposed a series of three stages that small groups pass through in moving toward a goal: orientation, evaluation and decision making, and reintegration. Tuckman (1965) expanded on the sequence by proposing four stages of group life: *orientation*, which involves identifying the relevant dimensions of the task and the manner in which the group will go about achieving it; *emotional response to the task demands*, which involves individual resistance of the group members to doing their part; *open exchange of relevant interpretations*, which involves the actual work of exchanging information relevant to accomplishing the work; and *emergence of solutions*, which involves constructive attempts at task solution. More recently a final stage of *termination* was added (Tuckman and Jensen, 1977).

Leadership

The expertise of the leaders of any chronic-illness group should reflect the demands emphasized. Groups organized for the purpose of conveying information and teaching adaptive skills should include a leader who has clinical expertise in the adaptive problems of patients who have particular chronic illnesses, as well as background in teaching-learning frameworks. Groups that focus on integrative demands need leaders with skills in community building. Groups in which a major focus is on an attempt to alter the care system or the response of the larger society to the illness should involve leaders with skills in social change; and, groups that focus on emotional demands should utilize leaders with experience in individual psychodynamics and group defensive cultures. The different areas of emphasis and expertise require somewhat different styles of leadership: teacher, facilitator, activist, and therapist, respectively. These styles bear some resemblance to the categories of leadership behaviors identified by Lieberman, Yalom, and Miles (1973) in their study of encounter-group leadership. Four styles were identified, each characterized by different types of leadership behaviors which included: meaning attribution, caring, executive function, and emotional stimulation.

A broader scope of problems can be systematically dealt with by using a coleadership model, designed to include leaders with skills in two different and complimentary demand areas. Thus, a psychiatric nurse-clinician and a social worker might create a group emphasizing emotional and integrative demands. A nurse-clinician specialist and social worker might create a group emphasizing information, skill, and integrative demands.

All leaders should be sensitive to the limits of their expertise and should be aware of the entire scope of problems which confront patients during the course of a particular chronic illness. Leaders should also be aware that they are susceptible to the same stereotypes, fears, and defenses expressed by their patients in confronting the chronic illness experience. Such leader susceptibilities can hinder the leader's ability to fully utilize the potentials of the group experience.

Membership

Reports of groups organized for chronically ill patients emphasize their "openness" in a number of ways: they often include family members; they include patients of all ages (adults); they include individuals at all stages of the chronic illness; and they permit members to come and go at will. In many instances, members are not screened for pre-existing psychological problems. Although such an open membership may be necessary initially while leaders identify demands by type and stage of illness, life issues, and so forth, such an open membership is probably too diverse to permit leaders to develop a group experience that successfully deals with any one of the demand areas. Patient and family member concerns may be sufficiently different, making it difficult to find a common basis for discussion. The life issues being dealt with by a majority of the members may be sufficiently different so as to isolate one or two members who are much younger or older. Individual, divergent concerns at various stages of illness — such as trying to maintain a normal life during chronic illness and preparing for one's impending death — may also create problems for groups because of the dissimilarity of these concerns. The leader's time will be spent inappropriately in trying to develop and maintain a minimum group cohesiveness, which will be able to be built only on very generally shared concerns.

When members are allowed to come and go freely with no minimal attendance expectations any attempts to build cohesiveness and cumulative experience in the group will be impossible. If individuals with pre-existing psychological problems are admitted rather than excluded by screening, the group will be unable to deal with chronic illness needs in addition to pre-existing psychological problems. Thus, the group may be diverted from addressing the shared needs of the total membership by attempting to deal with the severe and unignorable needs of a particular individual.

Group Size, Meeting Length, and Duration of the Group Experience

Didactic portions of a group meeting, or groups that emphasize primarily informational and skill demands, can be somewhat larger than those that focus on discussion of emotional matters or on problem solving around integrative and adaptive concerns of individual members. The course of some chronic illnesses is punctuated with crisis. If a group is too large, it is impossible to respond to individual members during times of crisis. Though the leader may want to keep the group small, a fairly large roster of eligible individuals may be kept since varying states of illness may prevent the attendance of individual members. The roster should be kept large enough so that six to eight members attend with some regularity.

Meeting length should be manageable for members whose physical tolerance may be limited. Attention should be given to the overall comfort level of the meeting room. Dank, unattractive, or cold rooms are not conducive to the physical or psychological comfort of chronically ill individuals. These types of meeting places may characterize community-based programs that rely on donated or low-cost space. Chairs should be as comfortable as possible. The group should be supportive of those members who must move about periodically to relieve physical discomfort. Meetings should end at the agreed upon time so that people whose physical condition does not allow them to linger are not embarrassed by leaving while the group is still in session. Family members caring for seriously ill persons may feel guilty about staying away longer than they planned to. Usually, sessions should be limited to about one and one half hours. If part of the session is didactic, ample time should be left for discussion of individual concerns.

Group duration should be determined by the time required to meet the chosen goals. Goals that cannot be accomplished within available group duration should not be attempted. For example, development of a support group is likely to demand a long-term commitment. Informational needs may be met in a short-term group. Groups in which there is a likelihood of rapid turnover, such as in an acute-care inpatient facility, should choose goals that can be accomplished within a single or a few meetings when membership might be expected to be stable. Attention should also be given to the frequency with which meetings are held. Some goals such as building a supportive community cannot be accomplished when groups meet infrequently. Groups expected to be of short duration usually accomplish more by increasing the frequency of meetings.

Groups may continue over a long time and maintain their focus through controlled changes in membership. As some members die or are rehabilitated and find they no longer need the group, new members can be added at specified times.

THE ROLE OF SELF-HELP GROUPS IN CHRONIC ILLNESS

Health related self-help groups are not a new phenomenon. Thomas Mann, in *The Magic Mountain*, writes of a Half-Lung Club formed among tuberculosis patients who were together in a Swiss sanatorium and had undergone a therapeutic pneumothorax. Since the 1940s, considerable attention has been given to the rapid growth of health-related self-help groups, which typically arise around chronic illness. Self-help groups may be divided into two types: "type 1" groups "provide direct services to patients (and relatives) in the form of education, coping skills, peer encouragement, and other supporting activities" (Tracy and Gussow, 1976, p. 381). "Type 2" groups focus "on promoting biomedical research, fund raising, public education, and legislative and lobbying activities" (p. 382). Some groups encompass both types, but a division seems to occur on the basis of whether rehabilitation efforts are likely to be successful. Where there is no such hope, groups tend to emphasize more the need for biomedical research into basic causes.

The typology that was developed earlier in this chapter is useful in revealing areas of concern shared by self-help groups and groups led by professionals. Self-help groups of the "type 1" variety fit the adaptive and integrative concerns; while "type 2" groups can be characterized as goal-directed. Some resources of self-help groups distinguish them from professionally-led groups, however. In self-help groups leadership is assumed by "older" or "senior" members whose adaptation to the particular illness serves as a particularly positive role model. Observing and listening to persons who have successfully coped not only gives hope but also may show behaviors and attitudes, which, if adopted, will provide ways to cope with the situation being faced. Second, self-help group members rely heavily on each other for support and mutual aid through holding frequent meetings and engaging in a lot of informal contact between meetings. A key dimension of many self-help groups for chronic illness is a visiting program in which "senior" members talk with newly diagnosed persons to initiate the supportive pattern of interaction. The interaction is also thought to benefit the "senior" member. The importance of utilizing "senior" members even in professionally led social-support groups have been noted (Caplan et al., 1976). Continuing motivation, rather than information, may be more important in maintaining long-term changes in life style necessary to adapt to a chronic illness. The supportive aspects of ongoing self-help groups, because they are long term, provide a vehicle for inspiring motivation considerably beyond the potential of most time-limited professionally led groups to build meaningful and enduring support networks.

Self-help groups, just because they are so labeled, cannot guarantee the quality of the group experience offered. Self-help groups must follow similar principles of clarity of focus, qualities of leadership, organization of the membership into groups whose concerns are similar enough to generate helpful peer interaction, and policies concerning frequency of meetings, group size, meeting length and so forth. Many of the older self-help groups have a clear structure encompassing these issues. Outsiders, including health professionals, may experience the structure as oppressive, inflexible, and limiting. While there are elements of this, such a structure endures beyond the involvement of any particular individual or set of individuals who may benefit from the group during a particular period of crisis or rehabilitation and who then move back into the broader community. The familiar, ongoing self-help structure provides available social reinforcement when people require extra resources in order to manage difficult times in their illness.

Another characteristic of self-help groups, particularly "type 2" groups, which helps to explain the suspicion of many health professionals towards them, is their goal of changing the health-care system to improve its responsiveness to the broader needs of chronic-illness patients. These social-movement qualities tend to alienate health-care professionals precisely because the emphasis is on shortcomings of the current system of care. It is possible for a self-help group to get caught in dynamics which unrealistically blame health-care professionals for allowing the disease to occur in the first place, for failing to cure, or for otherwise generally failing to relieve patients and their families from facing the implications of the illness. Such dynamics may be fed by one or two particularly angry, hostile individuals who gain leadership in the self-help group. The problem is enhanced when there is avoidance of the group by the health-care professionals in the community. Such dynamics can have disastrous consequences if the emotion leads patients and their families to reject services that *are* available. Most self-help groups organized around chronic illness desire the expertise of professional advisors and speakers. It is important in building cooperative, complementary relationships for professionals to respond to requests for assistance from self-help groups. Some institutions are able to demonstrate supportive relationships by providing a meeting place, advisory staff, and aid with programs (Tracy and Gussow, 1976).

VARIED APPROACHES TO GROUPS FOR CANCER PATIENTS

Adaptational and Tension-Management Needs

Krumn, Vanatta, and Sanders (1979) cited the needs of cancer patients for information and management strategies for minimizing side effects of chemotherapy. The group for patients undergoing chemotherapy in a hospital outpatient department and their family members was conducted by nursing staff with consultation from a psychiatric mental-health nursing specialist and a health educator. Classes presented information about chemotherapy, controlling side effects, preventing infection, and maintaining nutrition, rest, and exercise. Appropriate visual aids were developed; patients engaged in problem-solving discussions. Acceptance of the group experience was evaluated by a questionnaire, in which patients indicated that they appreciated the thoroughness with which information was presented directly by health professionals and opportunities to talk with other patients. No evaluation was used to determine whether the sessions actually helped reduce side effects.

Reflecting the predominance of therapy approaches to the needs of chronically ill patients, a number of articles on group work with cancer patients emphasize the resolution of emotional problems associated with the disease. Though these problems encompass a variety of themes, the overall emphasis seems to be on death and dying.

Corder and Anders (1974) reported on an outpatient group held on oncology clinic day. Any patient or family member visiting the clinic was invited to the weekly one hour sessions. A chaplain led the group, while a medical oncologist, a psychiatric nurse-clinician, and an oncology clinic nurse attended. The open-ended group met for fifteen months. Attendance ranged from one to fifteen with an average size group of five. No framework was used to structure the group. The general goal was to enable patients to "ventilate" their thoughts and concerns. Many concerns were raised: adjusting future expectations, living in the present, quality of medical care, and group members' deaths. Group members' deaths were considered to have a "powerful" impact.

Wellisch, Mosher and Van Scoy (1978) described an open-ended group for family members (and, later, patients) which met one evening per week for two hours in the waiting room of the offices of a private oncology practice. The purpose was described as assisting families in coping with "difficult and unique psychosocial problems." These problems were "inevitable intrapsychic conflicts." Another goal was to work toward an "appropriate death, psychologically." The leader was a clinical psychologist, working in a team with a nurse-oncologist and the office staff. Attendance ranged from four to sixteen with six members as the average. The framework used was multiple-family therapy and crisis theory. Attendance was also associated with crisis periods in the illness. Those families with previous serious psychological disturbance among the members had the greatest difficulties in adjustment. One theme among family members was guilt at leaving the patient while attending the group session. The professionals were surprised to find that including patients in the discussion resulted in better attendance; reduced fear, awe, and avoidance of the patient; and, did not seem to cause additional stress for the patient.

Whitman, Gustafson, and Coleman (1979), described the establishment of an open-ended inpatient oncology unit discussion group for patients and their families. The group was co-led by a nurse and a psychiatrist. Regularly one or more of the patients might be confronting life-threatening stages of the disease or treatment, which made some meetings "incredibly sad." The leaders saw their role as one of recognizing the group's defenses for avoiding confrontation with feelings about suicide and death. Discussions dealing with such topics as causes of cancer, treatments of cancer, quality of medical care, and available social support were viewed as "safe subjects" and were preferred by patients to dealing with powerful emotional issues of death and dying.

Integrative Needs

Wood, Milligan, Christ, and Liff (1978) described a time-limited, closed group for patients all in the same stage of illness. Eight weekly evening sessions of one and one half hours were led by two professionals, a psychiatrist and a social worker, and focused on issues of "living and coping with cancer." The authors emphasized the strong feeling of support that developed between members and extended to mutual help outside of group time. Following the first eight weeks, the group became open-ended for five months. Attendance then fluctuated markedly and the supportive aspects of the group were seriously undermined. A re-evaluation of the experience led to the re-establishment of the closed, eight-week series. The group's purpose was to function as a support system for patients, many of whom would otherwise lack significant support. Many subjects or themes were raised, with the issue of death and dying being most denied and avoided. The coleaders of later group experiences, a nurse and a social worker, encouraged an attitude of living in the present and permitted some denial and avoidance of feelings about death.

Kelly and Ashby (1979) reported the use of a five session group for newly diagnosed patients and their families in initial stages of hospital outpatient treatment. The emphasis was on problems of daily living, with considerable attention paid to themes of loneliness, isolation, grief over physical and social losses, family communication problems and desire for specific information on aspects of the illness. Patients participated in short-term goal-setting around specific needs and in identifying content of future didactic sessions. Suggested topics included nutrition, community resources, and relaxation therapy. The authors noted that patients signed up for more than one five-session series, reflecting, perhaps, their desire for continued group involvement.

The most complete description of a group emphasizing integrative needs was that of Speigel and Yalom (1978). This open-ended group, which met for four years, was specifically for women with metastatic breast cancer and stressed care of the dying patient. The framework for the group was a combination of a group psychotherapy model, a self-help and community support model, and the psychodynamics of individual treatment of the dying patient. The group met weekly for ninety minutes, holding occasional special pre-sessions on self-hypnosis or relaxation techniques. This group of outpatients incorporated hospitalized members when possible. Attendance ranged from three to twelve members, with an average of six to seven present. Spiegel and Yalom identified seven members as an optimal group size. Over a period of four years, forty patients were involved in the group. The leaders maintained an active roster of ten members at any given time. Fifteen deaths occurred during this four year period. Separate sessions of four to six weeks duration were held periodically for family members.

The focus of the group was described as "living in the context of dying." Goals extended beyond facing up and expressing feelings about dying to maintaining meaningful family ties and careers. Psychologically the goal was to help people preserve a sense of purpose by avoiding denial or depressive preoccupation. Special exercises helped people maintain a sense of enduring identity despite the loss of valued attributes of themselves. Active and supportive group involvement with dying members helped reduce fears and fantasies and clarified for living members their own preferred values and actions in facing their own deaths. The intense support network created among patients had a positive effect on family members. Patients derived a sense of meaning, control, and expertise which could be shared with others. Acceleration in personal growth, rise in self-esteem, improvement in communication, and lessening of depression and loneliness were observed among members. The writers clearly attribute many of the observed positive outcomes to success in meeting integrative needs of members, noting that they resisted members' requests to "do psychotherapy."

Goal Attainment Needs

There are few descriptions of groups designed to help cancer patients achieve changes in treatment or rehabilitation processes or influence political-legal processes. Such goal-oriented activities tend to fall to self-help groups. The leader of one such group of cancer patients was Orville Kelly, founder of *Make Today Count*, Inc. Kelly was, until his death, active in fighting job discrimination against cancer patients and in obtaining veterans' benefits for cancer victims who, as military personnel, had been exposed to high amounts of radiation and suspected chemical carcinogens. His autobiography (Kelly, 1975) recounts his own massive exposure to radiation during nuclear testing in the Pacific.

THE FUTURE OF GROUP WORK WITH CHRONICALLY ILL PATIENTS

The potential of group work with chronically ill patients is still to be realized. Progress has been made in recognizing emotional concerns of patients and families faced with various chronic diseases. Models for working out emotional concerns in group settings are available, even if opportunities for such groups are limited in health-care settings. Assessing and planning for the informational needs and adaptational needs of the chronically ill requires a high level of expertise. The benefits derived from providing social support and integration into a larger community during the course of chronic illness are only beginning to receive attention. Close and continuous contact with patients on a day-to-day basis has given nurses the potential for making an enormous contribution in this respect. In the absence of systematic research in these areas, only the pragmatic experience and the empathetic response of patients, who through trial and error have found solutions to their own problems, can be offered to others undergoing the same adjustment problems. Herein lies the major strength of the group approach at the moment, and an explanation as to why self-help approaches are presently so popular.

As additional research is accomplished regarding patients' informational and adaptational needs in coping with specific chronic illnesses, this research can be applied in group settings where information may be efficiently and creatively conveyed. A major virtue of group approaches may be their ability to meet supportive, integrative needs, thereby enhancing the effects of other interventions which more directly affect members' disease adaptation (Caplan et al., 1976). The separate effects of information giving and group support at various stages of the disease may require special research designs since it has been difficult to limit supportive interaction in groups emphasizing information dissemination, as opposed to groups establishing supportive environments (Caplan et al., 1976).

A common theme in research and in group work with chronically ill patients has been an emphasis on living in the present, "making today count," gaining control through short-term goal setting, and preserving a sense of purpose by avoiding denial or depressive rumination. Further knowledge of the integrative and adaptive needs of patients is required so that chronic illness patients have maximum opportunity to overcome the serious obstacles that tend to separate and isolate them from the rest of society. The addition of group approaches at all stages of chronic illness may well be the most effective antidote in minimizing separation and isolation, maintaining a sense of purpose and worth, and facilitating utilization of specific strategies in coping with chronic illness.

SUMMARY

In this chapter, the roots of group work with chronically ill patients were traced to Joseph Pratt's efforts with tuberculosis patients. Early development of group work for psychiatric disturbances strongly influenced professional approaches to working with a wider variety of social and health problems, beginning in the 1940s. These approaches emphasize emotional disturbances characteristic of various problems, and certain typologies of group work indicate the ways in which personality change can be achieved in a group context.

The problems of chronically ill patients are diverse and their needs may be met through a variety of group approaches. A viable typology of groups was offered which identified various categories of individual need which could be met by acknowledging four different demands characteristic of all groups. Organization of groups for chronically ill patients was discussed in terms of the varying emphasis on the four types of demands: tension management, integration, adaptation, and goal attainment. Variation in leadership styles was related to these four emphases. General information concerning populations in need, settings conducive to group work, membership selection, group size, meeting length, and duration of the group experience was presented. The role of self-help groups is chronic illness was discussed. An example of group approaches to meeting the needs of chronically ill patients with cancer was presented through an examination of related literature. The importance of developing information on the adaptive and integrative needs of chronic illness patients to be applied meaningfully in group settings was noted. Clarification of various group approaches in meeting patients' needs was identified as a task for future research and evaluation. The unique and major contribution of group work may lie in the ability to meet supportive, integrative needs, while enhancing the results of other interventions more specifically affecting individuals' adaptation to chronic illness.

REFERENCES

Anthony, E.J. "The History of Group Psychotherapy." In *Comprehensive Group Psychotherapy*, H.I. Kaplan and B.J. Sadock, Eds. Baltimore: Williams and Wilkins, 1971, pages 47–117.

Bales, R.F., and F.L. Strodtbeck. "Phases in Group Problem-Solving." *Journal of Abnormal and Social Psychology* 46, 1951, pages 485–495.

Caplan, R.D.; E. Robinson; J.R. French; J.R. Caldwell; and M. Shinn. *Adhering to Medical Regimens: Pilot Experiments in Patient Education and Social Support*. Ann Arbor, MI.: Research Center for Group Dynamics, Institute for Social Research, University of Michigan, 1976.

Corder, M.P., and R.L. Anders. "Death and Dying-Oncology Discussion Group." *Journal of Psychiatric Nursing and Mental Health Services*, July/August 1974, pages 10–14.

Farrell, M.P. "Patterns in the Development of Self-Analytic Groups." *Journal of Applied Behavioral Science* 12, October/November/December 1976, pages 523–542.

———; S. Rosenberg; and M.H. Schmitt. *Identity, Alienation and the Life Cycle; The Effects of Age and Status on Male Identity Development*. American Sociological Association Annual Meeting, New York City, August 1976.

Gardner, M.E. "Notes from a Waiting Room." *American Journal of Nursing* 80, January 1980, pages 86–89.

Kelly, O. *Make Today Count*. New York: Delacorte Press, 1975.

Kelly, P.P., and G.C. Ashby. "Establishing a Group." *American Journal of Nursing* 79, May 1979, pages 914–915.

Krumm, S.; P. Vannatta; and J. Sanders. "Group Approaches for Cancer Patients: A Group for Teaching Chemotherapy." *American Journal of Nursing* 79, May 1979, page 916.

Lieberman, M.A.; I.D. Yalom; and M.B. Miles. *Encounter Groups: First Facts*. New York: Basic Books, 1973.

Loomis, M.E. *Group Process for Nurses*. St. Louis: C.V. Mosby, 1979.

Marram, G.D. *The Group Approach in Nursing Practice*. St. Louis: C.V. Mosby, 1973.

Mills, T.M. *The Sociology of Small Groups*. Englewood Cliffs, N.J.: Prentice-Hall, 1967.

Mullan, H., and M. Rosenbaum. *Group Psychotherapy*. Glencoe, IL. : Free Press, 1962.

290 Chapter 14 Groups for the Chronically Ill

Neugarten, B. *Middle Age and Aging.* Chicago: University of Chicago Press, 1973.

Parsons, T.; R.F. Bales; and E. Shils. *Working Papers in the Theory of Action.* Glencoe, IL.: Free Press, 1951.

Publer, D., and H. Skippy. "How Patients Help Each Other." *American Journal of Nursing* 75, August 1975, page 1345.

Rioch, M.J. "The Work of Alfred Bion on Groups." *Psychiatry* 33, 1970, pages 56–66.

Rose, S.D. *Group Therapy: A Behavioral Approach.* Englewood Cliffs, N.J.: Prentice-Hall, 1977.

Schwartz, L.H., and J.L. Schwartz. *The Psychodynamics of Patient Care.* Englewood Cliffs, N.J.: Prentice-Hall, 1972.

Spiegel, D., and I.D. Yalom. "A Support Group for Dying Patients." *International Journal of Group Psychotherapy* 28, April 1978, pages 233–245.

Steckel, S.B. "Contracting with Patient Selected Reinforcers." *American Journal of Nursing* 80, September 1980, pages 1596–1599.

Tracy, G.S., and Z. Gussow. "Self-Help Health Groups: A Grass-Roots Response to a Need for Services." *Journal of Applied Behavioral Science* 12, 1976, pages 381–396.

Tuckman, B.W. "Developmental Sequence in Small Groups." *Psychological Bulletin* 63, 1965, pages 384–399.

———, and M.C. Jensen. "Stages of Small Group Development Revisited." *Group and Organizational Studies* 2, December 1977, pages 419–429.

Wellisch, D.K.; M.B. Mosher; and C. Van Scoy. "Management of Family Emotional Stress: Family Group Therapy in a Private Oncology Practice." *International Journal of Group Psychotherapy* 28, April 1978, pages 225–231.

Whitaker, D.S. "A Group Centered Approach." *Group Process* 7, 1976, pages 37–57.

———, and M.A. Lieberman. *Psychotherapy Through the Group Process.* New York: Atherton Press, 1964.

Whitman, H.H.; J.P. Gustafson; and F.W. Coleman. "Group Approaches for Cancer Patients: Leaders and Members." *American Journal of Nursing* 79, May 1979, pages 911–913.

Wood, P.E.; M. Milligan; D. Christ; and D. Liff. "Group Counseling for Cancer Patients in a Community Hospital." *Psychosomatics* 19, September 1978, pages 555–557, 561.

Yalom, I.D. *The Theory and Practice of Group Psychotherapy.* New York: Basic Books, 1975.

15

Group Work with Substance Abusers

Ellen Hastings Janosik

In groups organized for alcohol and drug abusers the common problem is addiction, and dealing with substance abuse is the primary group task. Because of social disapproval, alcohol and drug abusers feel rejected and therefore require alternative support systems which provide acceptance as well as encouragement for change.

COMMON-PROBLEM GROUPS

The remarkable success of Alcoholics Anonymous in promoting sobriety among problem drinkers has helped to establish group programs as the treatment of choice not only for alcoholics but also for other individuals facing problems of substance abuse. In joining a common-problem group these individuals enter a milieu in which their problems

Portions of this chapter were supported by the Center for Naval Analysis, Office of Naval Research, Grant - N0014-76-001.

need not be hidden. When interacting with other problem drinkers the alcoholic need not feel inferior or different. The same may be said of most substance abusers joining common-problem groups. Within the group, hardcore drug addicts discover that their anti-establishment attitudes are comprehended and that they are not unique. Thus, support and socialization are important aspects of common-problem groups for substance abusers.

In addition to providing socialization, common-problem groups for alcohol and drug abusers permit members to see their maladaptive behaviors reflected in the actions of fellow members and to witness their self-destructiveness being replicated in the lives of others. The opportunity to observe the rehabilitation of successful members refutes beliefs that alcohol and drug abuse are insurmountable problems.

Leadership by Group Members

Although professionals often lead groups for alcohol and drug abusers, the idea of self-help has permeated programs dealing with addiction. This is attributable in part to the Alcoholics Anonymous approach which stresses leadership by group members for group members. Distrust of outside leadership and certain exclusive claims by Alcoholics Anonymous have provoked caustic reactions in some professional quarters. In recent years there have been shifts on the part of Alcoholics Anonymous and various professional organizations toward rapprochement and an end to rivalrous claims of superiority. At the same time Alcoholics Anonymous continues to emphasize self-help and eschew professional leadership (Fontana, Dowds, and Bethel, 1976).

Counterparts to the self-help of Alcoholics Anonymous are found in drug abuse programs in which reformed addicts function as role models and group leaders. This does not mean that common-problem groups for drug abusers are always led by previously addicted members. Many programs for alcoholics and drug addicts use interdisciplinary health teams while also employing reformed abusers as counselors and group leaders. In programs for drug abusers, where the concept of self-help prevails, professionals who are not former users may be unwelcome. When dealing with such programs the nurse may find that contributions are limited to making referrals and to validating the worth of the group to prospective members.

Norms

Norms which are gradually established in common-problem groups operate to make continued abuse reprehensible. This means that to be a valued member one must comply with group norms or risk being a deviant inside the group as well as outside. Because the problem of substance abuse is shared, group goals are similar for the members, although there may be differences of degree.

After joining the group, members learn that external status is inconsequential. Power and influence in the group are contingent on the progress one makes toward goals (Feeney and Dranger, 1976). Group norms repudiate the abuse and group emotion is harnessed to the task. The successful member receives praise and approval. The unsuccessful member may or may not be censured, but is given no reward for noncompliance except in the form of proffered assistance. Usually the group includes role models in the person of "good" or abstinent members whose achievements inspire the others. Intermittent drinking of "bad" members is met with regretfulness mingled with expressions of confidence that the struggle against the abuse will continue.

The prevailing opinion is that common-problem groups are efficacious for alcohol and drug abusers, regardless of whether the group is self-led or professionally led. When leading this type of group the nurse should realize that substance abuse may indicate considerable individual or family pathology. In some common-problem groups the focus is on altering behavior, while in others it is the focus on modifying individual or family dynamics. In all cases the extent to which underlying dynamics are addressed depends on the group contract, the capabilities of the members, and the qualifications of the leaders. Common-problem groups which deal only with behavior are repressive-inspirational; Alcoholics Anonymous is an example. A common-problem group consisting of housewives who abuse barbiturates might be termed regressive-reconstructive if the task is not merely to eradicate the symptom but to explore causation and bring about intrapsychic change in members. In the latter group, as in any regressive-reconstructive group, qualified professional leadership, adequate supervision, and careful selection of members are essential.

GROUP WORK WITH ALCOHOLICS

Alcoholics Anonymous

Founded in 1935 by two alcoholics, Alcoholics Anonymous is a worldwide organization boasting almost thirty thousand autonomous chapters with over one million members. Designating itself as a "fellowship," Alcoholics Anonymous has a policy of cooperating but not affiliating with other organizations. Committed to anonymity for its members, the program has no membership lists and requires no dues. The Alcoholics Anonymous fellowship considers itself a society of equals dedicated to the promulgation of certain principles rather than the promotion of any therapeutic modality.

The Alcoholics Anonymous program is concerned with sobriety rather than with drinking, and the causes of alcoholism are not explored. Single-minded pursuit of sobriety is a unifying theme, but is sometimes thought to inhibit the individuation and differentiation of members. The doctrine of Alcoholics Anonymous has the effect of bonding members to each other and to the program, but may not be equally effective for every alcoholic. Inherent in the program is the idea that sober persons require sober companions and that association with friends who are still drinking may subvert abstinent alcoholics. New members are urged to rely on the "Twelve Steps" of the program and on a higher power in order to stay sober. Meetings are held frequently and are considered healthy alternatives to tavern friendships.

Fostering Dependency   At Alcoholics Anonymous meetings the dependency needs of members are not only met but fostered. Anxiety is considered detrimental to the well-being of alcoholics and is held to minimal levels. In everyday life members are advised to avoid situations which cause excessive anxiety and to call upon fellow members for help whenever the urge to drink becomes overpowering. Meetings are safe, comfortable, and predictable. Members often eat together at meetings and engage in such rituals as reciting the Serenity Prayer in unison. Alcoholism is identified as an illness which the alcoholic cannot control without help. The member is advised to deal with the disability day by day while looking to the fellowship and a higher power for assistance.

Open meetings are held at which members testify to the help they have received through Alcoholics Anonymous. Friends and relatives of members as well as interested outsiders may attend the open meetings. Closed meetings are attended only by alcoholic members. At the closed meetings members discuss on a personal level their problems related to abstinence. In these closed sessions the Twelve Steps of the program are often cited. The Twelve Steps and the way they are presented form a major part of the recovery program. The First Step consists of admitting to a drinking problem which is out of control; the Second Step consists of calling upon a higher power for help. The final or Twelfth Step involves the recovering alcoholic in carrying the message to others. Each of the Steps is phrased not as a negative injunction or prohibition but as a litany of positive actions already taken.

Although the emotional climate of Alcoholics Anonymous is one of acceptance, departures from sobriety are considered serious, even though the erring member is forgiven and encouraged to begin again. Lapses from sobriety are called "slips" and are deemed ominous but not hopeless. It is considered necessary for members to admit to their episodes of alcohol ingestion. Despite the emotional supplies available in the form of peer support and divine help, the ultimate purpose of Alcoholics Anonymous is to increase personal responsibility and self-determination. The program emphasizes behavioral change primarily, discounts causality, and uses member-centered rather than group-centered problem solving.

Programs for Family Members   Al-Anon and Alateen are two family programs cooperating with Alcoholics Anonymous. The aim of both is to help marital partners and children of alcoholics improve the quality of their own lives regardless of the drinking habits of the alcoholic family member. Nurses and other health professionals who encounter children of alcoholics should identify them as high risks for delinquency, truancy, and depression (Janzen, 1978). These troubled children are often the victims of physical, sexual, and psychological abuse from drunken parents. Al-Anon and Alcoholics Anonymous members often serve as Alateen sponsors in an attempt to aid the children of alcoholics. All three programs use an approach which combines spiritual values with social support networks.

Although Alcoholics Anonymous is available to all drinkers admitting to a problem which is out of control, its accomplishments are greatest among alcoholics who retain vestiges of family and community stability. Of all self-help programs, Alcoholics Anonymous is the most prominent, and its impressive record may be attributed to its simple, idealistic format and constant, unchanging message.

Therapeutic Groups for Alcoholics

In contrast to Alcoholics Anonymous meetings, most therapeutic alcoholism groups led by nurses and other health professionals explore the reasons for problem drinking. Since the etiology of alcoholism is complex, exploration may include various aspects of the members' lives. The notion that alcoholics are psychologically fragile and that treatment must proceed delicately has been challenged by practicing clinicians who assert that the best group for alcoholics is one which provides a reality-based experience. At times dysfunctional individuals set standards for themselves which are excessive. In such cases the nurse must try to neutralize the effects of a punitive conscience or superego. The conscience of an alcoholic may be punitive at times, but these effects are quickly eroded by alcohol. Principles of reality therapy may be used to advantage in helping alcoholics view themselves and their lives realistically. Reality therapy proposes that persons become dysfunctional not because their personal standards are too high but because their performance is too low. Some individuals drink to eradicate feelings of inadequacy which can only be removed by learning to accept the world as it is rather than the world as they wish it to be (Glasser, 1966). Most of the difficulties in the interpersonal relationships of alcoholics can be traced to their distorted construction of reality. Many alcoholics are extremely self-oriented, and the inner values they live by do not conform to the values of society at large (Thompson, 1979).

In alcoholism groups the initial tendency of members is to engage in protective maneuvers which maintain self-esteem. If the group is cohesive and if members reach consensus regarding group expectations, protective defenses are lowered and the group is able to move toward self-awareness and change. A paradoxical factor is apparent in alcoholism groups. The paradox lies in the fact that although any problem drinker may be welcomed into the group, approval is withheld until the member shows some commitment to group goals (Feeney and Dranger, 1976).

Entering Treatment Comparatively few alcoholics enter treatment unless they are in a condition of medical, social, or economic crisis. At times persuasion from relatives may be the compelling force. Coercion from employers or from the courts constitutes another reason for seeking treatment (Heyman, 1978). This means that the entry of an alcoholic into treatment is often involuntary and precipitous. The new member of an alcoholism group is likely to be angry, fearful, and reluctant. Therefore the leader must extend warmth and support, particularly if the group is not mature enough to do so. In addition to welcoming and orienting new members, the leader of an alcoholism group should encourage anticipatory planning and problem solving. When a group member who has been drinking appears at a meeting the experienced leader will have already prepared for this contingency by working out in advance appropriate group responses. Some groups prefer that intoxicated members not be admitted, but more often the group interprets the attendance of an inebriated member as a plea for help and hesitates to expel the offending member. If a rule has been made that intoxicated members may remain but not participate in group discussion, the leader need not intervene except to uphold the decision already reached by the group. In subsequent sessions when the intoxicated member is again abstinent, the leader may allude to the incident in order to stimulate discussion of the lapses which are typical of most alcoholics. Certain members may engage in repeated episodes of drinking and regularly attend meetings while intoxicated. When prolonged, these behaviors can be disruptive to the group. Here again a problem-solving approach and a decision which involves the whole group should be sought. If the group decides that the drinking member is insufficiently motivated, termination may be recommended. In order to forestall later resentment of the leader's power, termination should be a consensual rather than a unilateral decision. Needless to say, a mechanism should be provided for the drinking member to rejoin this group or a similar group at a later time. Most alcoholism groups are long term and open-ended. Termination, voluntary or involuntary, should not be considered irrevocable.

Cohesion   The group leader who is not an alcoholic may be challenged by members who believe that only alcoholics can understand one another. Cohesion is established early in alcoholism groups because of the shared problem; and intimacy seems to be an immediate consequence. This early cohesion is rather superficial in nature and the intimacy is circumscribed. Among alcoholics there is a tendency to restrict interactions to alcohol-related matters, and to establish a fraternity of drinkers which is tribal rather than familial (Janosik, 1977). It has been suggested that the early cohesion characteristic of alcoholism groups is of dubious worth, since it is chiefly related to the members' collusive identification with drinking (Mullan and Sangiuliano, 1960). This premature closeness may be interpreted as resistance to change rather than potential for change. A nurse functioning as leader may reduce pseudocohesion by recognizing group members as distinct individuals rather than merely alcoholics. Because the health professional leading an alcoholism group is usually not an alcoholic, premature group cohesion sometimes excludes the leader.

Leadership   Flexible leadership is needed to provide acceptance and limits, both of which are required in alcoholism groups. The group leader must be equipped by temperament as well as training to fulfill these requirements. Scott (1976) classified leaders of alcoholism groups as A or B types, concluding that A types were more effective than B types in relieving the subjective distress of abstinent alcoholics, while B types were more effective in dealing with impulse control problems. A reasonable inference is that A-type leaders performed socioemotional functions, whereas B-type leaders performed task-oriented functions. The A-type leader was more therapeutic in responding to the pain and anxiety of sober alcoholics, but B-type leaders were more able to uncover anger in members. Encouraging the appropriate expression of anger during sober intervals seemed to lessen extreme outbursts of anger during drinking episodes. Some leaders are able to perform A-type functions and revert to B-type functions when necessary. This is not an easy accomplishment, particularly after a group becomes accustomed to one type of intervention from a leader. A practical solution is to organize the alcoholism group under dual leadership, with one leader offering supportive, or A-type interventions as the second leader tries to elicit appropriate verbalization of anger.

Fostering Dependency A psychoanalytic approach is not usually adopted for alcoholism groups, although causes and consequences of drinking may be addressed in the meetings. Battegay (1977) noted that analytic group therapy is not effective with alcoholics or other abusers because their egocentric demands are excessive and must be dealt with constructively. During the early phases of an alcoholism group the leader must respond actively to all members. The activity of the leader opposes regressive forces, particularly if the leader adopts a moderate approach. If the leader does not gratify the needs of the group to some extent, unrewarded members may leave the group. Having acknowledged and responded to the dependency needs of the members, the leader must then begin to direct them toward interdependence and eventually toward independence. The egocentricity of alcoholics causes them to become very dependent on the group — this is an inclination which is not discouraged but is successfully exploited by Alcoholics Anonymous. One cannot argue with the statement that dependence on a group is preferable to dependence on alcohol or other substances.

Alcoholism group leaders must avoid working harder than the alcoholic members, since members should be encouraged to search for their own solutions. Judicious interpretation and confrontation are advocated for alcoholism groups, particularly when members resist problem solving or a reality experience by resorting to monologues which prevent spontaneous interaction. In alcoholism groups confrontation is a nonjudgmental explication of the facts coupled with suggestions for alternative coping methods. Therapeutic confrontation in alcoholism groups should not be mistaken for accusation. In therapeutic confrontation the alcoholic is not simply told to stop drinking but is given to understand that entering treatment constitutes the beginning of a difficult but rewarding way of life (Gust, 1979).

Exchange Theory

It is not unusual for alcoholics to spend an entire group session recounting drinking adventures, their own and those of others. In some groups members compete for the position of "worst" drinker. If a member cannot aspire to this honor, friendship with a "worst" drinker may be claimed. These anecdotes seem to enhance the self-esteem of the alcoholic. When the alcoholism of any member is described as especially severe, any effort to stay sober is more impressive. Becoming a "special" member of the group also explains occasional lapses when these occur. One account of a prison alcoholism group described the undue attention given to legendary drinking companions whom the inmates had known. Although they were never members of the group, the exploits of "Red Eye," "Whistling Willie," "Mad Dog," and others whose nicknames described their drinking behaviors were related with mingled fear and admiration (Janosik, 1977).

Preoccupation with drunken adventures and misadventures allows members an opportunity to displace ambivalent feelings about drinking. A plausible explanation is that regaling one another with these stories is a form of resistance which allows members to ignore the serious nature of their own drinking. The leader who believes that reminiscing about the escapades of friends is a form of resistance might reinforce reality with interpretations derived from *exchange theory*. Exchange theory asserts that actions produce certain reactions, and that it is important to identify the quid pro quo exchange which accompanies human behavior. In using exchange theory the leader might begin by asking what rewards members find in discussing the drinking behaviors of persons not present in the group. If this draws no response, the leader might then ask the present whereabouts of the drinkers being discussed. It is customary for members to acknowledge that many of the legendary drinkers have already suffered accidents or serious illnesses. The climate of the group will change as the members begin to consider the multiple misfortunes which invariably pursue unregenerate alcoholics. There is no humor or whimsy to be found in recalling the consequences of uncontrolled drinking or the price paid by drinkers.

When a member vies for the position of "worst" drinker or admits repeated episodes of drunkenness, exchange theory may be used again. A nurse leading the group might observe that behaviors which are rewarding continue, and then ask group members to explain why Joe goes on drinking when he is in danger of losing his job and his family. Explanations from members might range from "Joe is getting back at his wife by getting drunk" to "Drinking lets Joe drop out of the rat race at work. He doesn't have to worry about getting ahead when he can blame his mistakes on drinking." Exchange theory requires the group to look for the hidden rewards the alcoholic finds in drinking and helps replace various avoidance tactics with meaningful exploration.

ISSUES IN ALCOHOLISM GROUPS

Abstinence

The primary objective in the Alcoholics Anonymous program is abstinence. In traditional groups for alcoholics an early decision must be made regarding this objective. Abstinence is extremely difficult for alcoholics to maintain without interruption, and the group leader may decide not to insist on total abstinence, nor to equate abstinence with success and drinking with failure. Although lapses should not be ignored, neither should they be used to excoriate the alcoholic. Many leaders of traditional alcoholism groups modify insistence on sobriety in order to prevent members from feeling alienated from the group because of occasional drinking. In the opinion of Brown and Yalom (1977) stressing total abstinence over other measures of group outcome tends to produce an uneasy, authoritarian relationship between leader and members.

Even if group leaders choose not to demand sobriety, patterns develop whereby the members take note of one another's drinking. This is less intimidating to the group than questions from the leader, since alcoholics are apt to be more open with one another and to be less threatened when interrogations are reciprocal. Permitting members to share this responsibility allows them to express concern for one another and increases group autonomy. Adhering to group decisions about members who come intoxicated to meetings is another reminder to members that the group can monitor its own processes.

When group issues are expanded beyond abstinence, leaders as well as members avoid discouragement. Alcoholism is a chronic disorder in which improvement is slow and unpredictable. If a broad perspective is adopted which includes treatment outcomes other than sobriety, signs of progress are discernible even when sporadic drinking intrudes. Giving up alcohol means a resurgence of anxiety, depression, and turmoil for the members. An alcoholic who is not drinking must exist without the substance which made life endurable. It is not surprising that periods of sobriety are broken and that the alcoholic must be persuaded to begin anew.

There is a tendency in some alcoholism groups for members to protect one another, which is another form of self-protection. Members who distrust their ability to control alcohol intake hesitate to confront drinking members lest they themselves be the target of confrontation at a later time. If this self-serving behavior persists, leaders might intervene to point out that growth involves risk-taking and that members must care enough about each other to deal with the drinking behavior of fellow members.

Leader Expectations

Leaders who require continual rewards for their work or who do not believe that alcoholics can be helped are not suited to work with alcoholism groups. Few persons are more susceptible to the expectations of others than an alcoholic (Gilmour, 1973; Hyde, 1971; Moody, 1971). Leader attitudes toward the success or failure of members help determine how the group fares. When a recovering member begins to drink and this behavior is equated with failure, there is little incentive for the alcoholic to try again. If the group is encouraged to find indications of progress in a member who has "slipped," the failure will be less stressful. Research has shown that the expectations of others significantly affect the performance of alcoholics involved in mutual interactions. In an investigation of the effect of counselor expectations on the recovery of alcoholics, Leake and King (1977) reported the following data.

- Alcoholic clients from whom counselors expected recovery actually confirmed the expectations by showing improvement.
- Alcoholic clients in the control group from whom counselors did not expect recovery did not show improvement.
- Alcoholic clients in the control group from whom improvement was not expected had significantly higher drop-out rates than clients for whom the leaders had greater expectations.

Equally interesting was the finding that alcoholics from whom counselors expected improvement were more highly valued by fellow members, even though the expectations of improvement were not divulged to group members. Since the members had no knowledge of the expectations communicated to leaders, the higher value attached to some members was subtly transmitted by the leaders. An implication of the data is that expectations of members regarding their potential for recovery is crucial. In alcoholism groups where leaders foster the idea that occasional insobriety obliterates all gains, needless pessimism intrudes. Leaders must convey the expectation that alcoholics are capable of growth, that progress is possible, and that potential for recovery persists in spite of occasional failure.

Dependency, Denial, and Anger

Individuals dealing with dependency conflicts may behave in any of several ways. Those who accept their dependency needs are not difficult to assess — they are compliant, clinging, and insatiable in their search for security. Those who are less tolerant of their dependency needs may present themselves as grandiose and challenging. These individuals fear dependency so much that they use reaction formation and become counterdependent.

The category of overt dependency includes persons whose hunger for reassurance causes them to substitute the leader for the comfort once found in alcohol. Since their expectations of the leader cannot be met, it is wise to present the group rather than the leader as the source of emotional supplies. The resources of the group exceed the resources of the leader; redirection to the group diffuses demands on the leader and offers recovering alcoholics the opportunity to stabilize their gains by turning to fellow members (Brown and Yalom, 1977).

Counterdependent members behave in ways which may disturb the leader. Some counterdependent members defy and question the leader. Others ally themselves with the leader, avoiding closeness with other members by trying to be cotherapists. The latter tactics are less threatening to the leader, but if continued they perpetuate the denial used by alcoholics reluctant to admit their problem.

Denial   Alcoholics engage in denial of their problem and in denial of responsibility for their actions. Denial may lead to projecting responsibility to others (*blaming*) or finding reasons for drinking (*rationalization*). Use of denial in the group allows alcoholics to avoid introspection and to hold interaction to superficial levels. In some alcoholism programs, characterological deficits are thought to be the basis of alcoholism, and personality change is attempted (Seelye, 1979). When alcoholism groups are inspirational or supportive, insight is not usually a goal and denial may be permitted until members are ready to discard this defense. On the other hand, Alcoholics Anonymous groups are inspirational and supportive, but insist that members must forego denial upon entering the program.

An implicit manifestation of dependency has been described by Brown and Yalom (1977). This was identified as fear of recovery which is revealed by the alcoholic's inability to trust or enjoy success. Because success means renouncing alcohol, attainment of sobriety may be accompanied by a sense of loss and a dread of subsequent failure. The recommended response for leaders is to reassure members that neither success nor failure means abandonment or expulsion from the group. This reassurance helps remove the fear of alcoholics that if they become successful they must then continue on their own, and terminate involvement with the group.

Anger Appropriate expression of anger is difficult for alcoholics, many of whom believe themselves inferior to other people. Remorse and contrition, which often follow drinking, help convince alcoholics that they do not have a right to express anger. These convictions may be aggravated by interactional patterns in the families of alcoholics. When sober, alcoholics tend to avoid situations which heighten their own anxiety or add to the discomfort of others. Their reluctance to express anger directly sometimes causes group interactions to become constricted. When the alcoholic is sober, politeness and conciliatory behavior are customary, but when drunk the same alcoholic may become very aggressive. Getting drunk permits the alcoholic simultaneously to express and deny anger, since any expression of anger made while intoxicated may be attributed to alcohol. An effective intervention by the leader is to solicit verbalization of anger by sober members in the group. Negative as well as positive feedback from members may be interpreted by the leader as a form of caring, while avoidance of sensitive topics may be interpreted as self-serving indifference. In absorbing and redirecting challenges or provocation issued by counterdependent members, leaders demonstrate by example that anger can be tolerated without defensiveness or retaliation.

Inconsistencies in the behavior of alcoholics place a burden on group leaders trying to assess the meaning of behavior. Alcoholics are distrustful of praise but yearn for it. Fear is evident among alcoholics, many of whom experience fear of success, fear of failure, fear of offending, and fear of competing. Helping the alcoholic sort out these tumultuous feelings and to separate fact from fantasy should be included in the agenda of the alcoholism group leader.

Selection in Alcoholism Groups

Some alcoholics can participate both in Alcoholics Anonymous and in traditional alcoholism groups without being confused by the contrasting approaches. Other alcoholics are steadfastly devoted to the principles of Alcoholics Anonymous and cannot deal with the complexity of traditional group therapy. A third group finds the philosophy of Alcoholics Anonymous to be simplistic and unhelpful. Fontana, Dowds, and Bethel (1976) formulated the hypothesis that incompatibility between Alcoholics Anonymous and traditional groups for alcoholics was attributable to the cognitive structures used by alcoholics to organize their life experiences. An earlier theorist (Pepper, 1942) had categorized four ways in which individuals confer meaning on life experiences, and Fontana, Dowds, and Bethel built on this work. These four categories of cognitive orientation were identified as characteristic ways of viewing the world, and a questionnaire was devised to classify the cognitive orientation of subjects to whom the instrument was administered. The four categories of cognitive orientation identified in the questionnaire are shown in Table 15-1.

Contextual/Organicistic vs. Formistic/Mechanistic Thinking

Contextual and organicistic modes of thinking are antithetical to formistic and mechanistic thinking in several ways. The latter modes of thinking are fairly objective, with relationships between objects or events either connected or classified. The former are subjective, with relationships altered by circumstances or participation. In administering the questionnaire, Fontana, Dowds, and Bethel (1976) attempted to show that formistic thinkers related positively to Alcoholics Anonymous and negatively to traditional group therapy. Their results substantially supported the first hypothesis and partially supported the second. Alcoholics low in contextual thinking seemed to benefit from Alcoholics Anonymous, and alcoholics high in contextual thinking were unlikely to commit themselves to principles of Alcoholics Anonymous. There was evidence that alcoholics who were mechanistic thinkers related argumentatively in traditional group therapy and disputed the interventions of leaders. Alcoholics who understood the world in terms of labels and categories found the Alcoholics Anonymous approach more congenial and group therapy less attractive than did alcoholics who were relatively unstructured in their thinking.

Another investigative team (Janosik, Trimborn, and Milanese, 1978) administered the same questionnaire to eighty-three alcoholics in group treatment. This study produced data consistent with those of

Table 15–1   WORLD HYPOTHESIS FORMULATION

Cognitive Orientation	Characteristic Features
Formism	1. Classification is the primary basis for organizing experience 2. Meaning is obtained by placing an object, event, or experience in a category which considers commonalities and ignores differences 3. Experience is not unified but is composed of separate elements
Mechanism	1. Events are given meaning through connections between events, their antecedents, and their consequences 2. Each component of experience is separate but interacts with other components in a cause-and-effect relationship 3. Experience is made meaningful by means of an operating system of distinct but related components
Organicism	1. Meaning is conferred by placing experience in a pattern of events 2. Experience is made meaningful by means of continual integration and reintegration. Partially integrated experience proceeds until ultimate synthesis is reached
Contextualism	1. The quality of subjectivity is superimposed on experience 2. The individual is part of the event 3. Events are unstable and shifting 4. The context in which the event occurs is as important as the event itself

Fontana et al. The subjects who were members of Alcoholics Anonymous tended not to think in organicistic terms. Afro-American alcoholics in the study were characterized by organicistic thinking; Irish-American alcoholics were likely to be formistic thinkers. Subjects with a high school education were more likely to be formistic thinkers than were subjects with a grade school education. Preference for formistic thinking among high school graduates indicates that Alcoholics Anonymous programs may be less effective for persons with a grade school education. This is consistent with the documented appeal of Alcoholics Anonymous to middle-class problem drinkers.

These studies call attention to selectivity in referring alcoholics to traditional therapy groups or to Alcoholics Anonymous. An organicistic- or contextually-oriented alcoholic might be more receptive to a traditional group approach, which explores inner dynamics and reasons for drinking. The finding that Afro-Americans may be organicistic thinkers argues for referrals of these alcoholics to traditional group programs rather than to Alcoholics Anonymous. Although the data of these investigations are tentative rather than conclusive, they represent efforts to predict which group approaches may prove effective and to place alcoholics in treatment programs compatible with their view of themselves and the world.

GROUP WORK WITH DRUG ABUSERS

In a broad sense, any substance taken for nonmedical reasons in amounts or ways which are not medically sanctioned constitutes drug abuse. This definition, then, includes most of us, for countless individuals adjust drug doses in idiosyncratic ways, often in defiance of accepted medical practice. Many drug abusers are contributing members of society whose lives are not adversely affected. In contemporary life drug abuse may be caused by a wish for a nonrational, extraordinary experience. A majority of abusers use drugs periodically to relax or relieve the tedium of everyday life. For these persons drug use is ritualistic rather than compulsive, and is a response to the ready availability of drugs and to social pressures to experiment (Weil, 1972).

User or Abuser?

A dichotomy of drug abuse was developed which separated casual drug users from compulsive drug abusers (Wurmser, 1972). In this dichotomy compulsive drug use was explained as a way of coping with inherent psychological problems which antedated or complicated drug dependence. Because compulsive drug use indicates psychological deficits, withdrawal from one form of addiction is likely to lead to other forms. The problem of compulsive drug use is not physical dependence per se but the conflicts which are the core of the problem. In a comparison of alcoholics and drug addicts, alcoholics did not differ significantly from their nonalcoholic control group in essential respects; heroin addicts had significantly more neurotic and characterological deficiences than their nonaddicted control group (Lachar, Gdowski, and Keegan, 1979).

Drug abuse has been linked to powerful social forces such as poverty, racism, or rootlessness. Peer influences and family interactional patterns have also been cited as causes of compulsive drug abuse. Identifying psychological deficits as the core of the problem does not necessarily reject other factors but does put them in perspective. Concentric rings of predisposing factors, as shown in the following figure, help explain the etiology of drug abuse. The complexity of factors which contribute to compulsive drug abuse has had the effect of expanding the scope of drug-abuse programs.

Compulsive drug abuse begins with psychological needs which are met by the drug. Alleviation of psychological distress gratifies the user and reinforces drug dependence. If one substance is unavailable or insufficient, others are tried and multiple addiction follows. The illusion of the compulsive abuser is that the outlines of reality are softened. In actuality, drug abuse introduces a new reality in which motivation is limited to activity necessary to obtain the supply. Unless

Figure 15-1 CONCENTRIC ETIOLOGY OF DRUG ABUSE

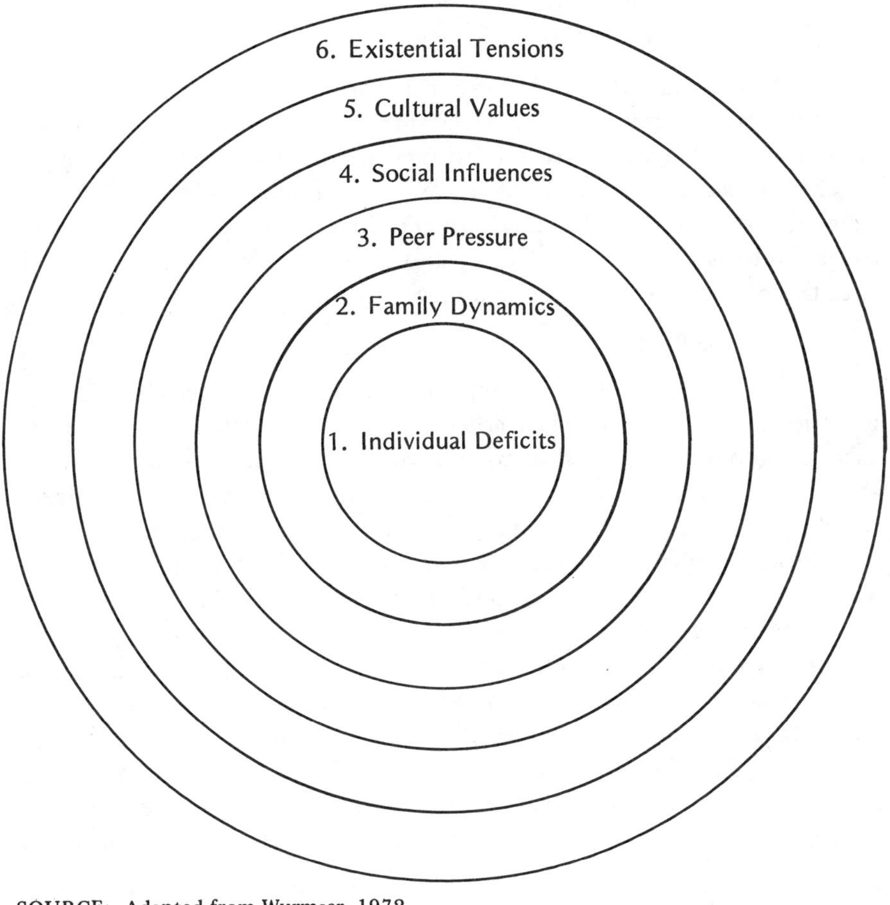

6. Existential Tensions
5. Cultural Values
4. Social Influences
3. Peer Pressure
2. Family Dynamics
1. Individual Deficits

SOURCE: Adapted from Wurmser, 1972.

interrupted by therapeutic intervention, drug abuse dominates the life of the addict.

Frequently Abused Drugs   Most drugs have some potential for misuse, but the following categories of drugs are most frequently abused. Representative drugs in each category are listed.*

Narcotics:	Natural Opiates — Morphine, Heroin, Codeine
	Synthetic Opiates — Demerol, Methadone
Depressants:	Sedatives — Equanil, Dalmane
	Barbiturates — Seconal, Nembutal, Phenobarbital
	Minor Tranquilizers — Librium, Valium, Alcohol
Stimulants:	Amphetamines
	Cocaine
Hallucinogens:	D-Lysergic Acid (LSD)
	Mescaline
	Phencyclidine
	Psylocybin

Marijuana   Many of these drugs are available on prescription, while others, such as heroin or cocaine, are unobtainable except by illicit means. Marijuana is a substance which is difficult to categorize, but in sufficient amounts it has hallucinogenic effects. Current legislation in some states has reduced first possession of marijuana from a felony to a misdemeanor, and research is in progress to evaluate the properties of this substance.

Abuser Profile

There is some evidence of similarities among persons abusing any specific category of drugs (Yowell and Brose, 1978). Barbiturate users in general feel unable to control their lives and have doubts about their ability to cope. These feelings are reduced by drugs which precipitate social isolation and disengagement. More often than not, barbiturate users are passive-dependent individuals. The opiate abuser is discontented and frustrated, but is less passive than the barbiturate addict because difficulties in obtaining illegal drugs preclude total passivity. Opiate abusers tend to be passive-aggressive individuals who want to feel euphoric and powerful. This existential dilemma is solved by opiate addiction. Amphetamine abusers are usually people who fear not being able to meet their own demands or those which others make upon them. Abusers of hallucinogenic drugs are often thrill-seekers who find ordinary life dull. It must be added

---

*Alcohol is a depressant; but because alcoholism is such a pervasive disorder, the problem has been discussed separately.

that identifying personality types which are prone to certain forms of drug abuse is less important than treating drug abusers as individuals who must begin to live in ways which make drug abuse unnecessary. Generalities have limited value since experiential states such as anxiety, depression, hostility, and boredom are as prevalent among nonabusers as abusers. At the same time recognizing dominant patterns of behavior among addicts may be helpful to neophyte leaders and counselors (Burkhalter, 1975).

The Drug Culture

A striking difference between abusers of legal drugs and abusers of illegal drugs is that the latter follow a life-style which removes them from conventional society. Compulsive abusers of prescription drugs break laws but try to preserve a semblance of respectability. Individuals who are addicted to illegal drugs soon enter a culture whose norms are antiestablishment. After renouncing conventional society, users of illegal drugs seek a sense of community in the drug culture and security is found in behaviors which support the addiction. Obtaining the drug from dealers, using paraphernalia for injections, and feeling the pleasurable effects of the drug are actions which eradicate feelings of loss. Abusers of illegal drugs ignore meaningful relationships and are unlikely to be overly concerned with concealment of drug dependence. Unwillingness to trust and poor impulse control are among the common behaviors of abusers of illegal drugs. Since illegal drugs are expensive, the abuser may resort to crime in order to support the habit.

"Culture" refers to qualities and attributes which characterize a particular way of life, and individuals adopt the values in the surrounding culture which are important to them (Anderson and Carter, 1978). For drug abusers, group therapy is a social encounter intended to replace the drug culture and help them re-enter the community. The group represents a step away from the drug culture and toward the restoration of earlier values and a return to conventional society.

Treating the Abuser

No one program can meet the needs of all drug abusers, and organizing a drug abuse group is an arduous process. Persons addicted to the same substance may have the capacity to interact effectively, but age, sex, length of addiction, social history, and motivation are variables which merit consideration. Compulsive drug use may be part of a schizophrenic process, and sound clinical judgment is needed to determine whether such an individual can tolerate sustained group interaction of high intensity. In preparing prospective members for a drug abuse group the nature of the contract must be explicitly stated and clearly understood. Among school children and adolescents, drug education groups are considered helpful in countering peer pressure to experiment. If the group is solely preventive, it is unwise to include addicts or former addicts as members, although they may be asked to contribute as visitors or speakers.

Compulsive drug abusers require treatment for extended periods of time in order to alter maladaptive behaviors which perpetuated abuse. Treatment of compulsive drug abuse is often carried out in a psychiatric facility. Detoxification or withdrawal precedes group treatment and occurs in a general hospital or detoxification unit. Some drug treatment programs exclude heroin addicts because of the severe problems surrounding this addiction. The antagonism of heroin addicts toward representatives of mainstream culture makes them extremely negativistic. Their provocative behavior is best handled in a heroin abuse program administered by staff members with special expertise.

Treating the Heroin Addict   The proliferation of heroin addictions after the Vietnam War did not change restrictive policies toward these addicts but led instead to comprehensive heroin abuse programs, many of which substituted methadone for heroin addiction. Methadone is a synthetic opiate which blocks the effects of heroin, reduces the addict's craving for heroin, but does not produce the same orgastic pleasure. The effects of methadone last for about twenty-four hours, and it is thought that an addict receiving methadone daily can function in society and perform productive work. Addicts participating in a methadone program are carefully screened and their potential for rehabilitation is evaluated. There is a four-to-six-week period in a residential facility or day treatment center during which the addict is withdrawn from heroin and stabilized on methadone. While enrolled in the program the addict receives medical treatment and is tested periodically for heroin or other forbidden drugs. A methadone program is usually multifaceted, offering individual, family, group, and vocational counseling to the addict. The purpose is to prepare the addict to return to the community by providing re-education along with daily amounts of methadone. Some addicts who enter the program gradually decrease their dependency on methadone and become drug free, but they are a minority. Other addicts simply substitute one addiction for another, and do not separate entirely from the deviant drug culture. Although methadone maintenance programs are not a panacea for heroin abuse, they are representative of comprehensive programs devised for the rehabilitation of compulsive abusers of illegal drugs. Methadone maintenance is a controversial treatment and discussion of its worth is not within the scope of this chapter. What is relevant are the techniques used in group programs for hardcore drug abusers. Group work with heroin abusers will be discussed at length, since these rigorous programs have implications for drug abuse groups in general.

ISSUES IN DRUG-ABUSE GROUPS

Motivation

The reasons which impel drug-dependent persons to enter treatment markedly influence behavior and attitudes brought to the group. Motives for entering treatment may be construed as pragmatic physiological, legal, or existential, although the reasons an addict gives for entering treatment may bear little resemblance to the facts. The motives which cause an addict to enter treatment include the following (Burkhalter, 1975).

- *Economic:* Hope of reducing the drug habit in order to curtail amounts of the drug needed to produce the desired effect.
- *Physiological:* Desire to undergo withdrawal or detoxification with minimal physical discomfort.
- *Legal:* Imposition by a judge or court of mandatory participation in drug abuse treatment.
- *Existential:* Determination to cease drug abuse and undergo rehabilitation.

Group Goals

The question of abstinence in drug-abuse groups is a difficult one for members and leaders. If total abstinence is demanded of addicts in order to continue to be eligible for treatment, the number of members remaining in the group is reduced. Conversely, if standards are lenient, members may not persevere. Problems are compounded when the abused substance or substances are illegal. Even when addicts are being maintained on methadone, they often have recourse to other substances such as cocaine or amphetamines. The operations of a methadone maintenance program are subject to legal surveillance, and in some localities personnel must report all infractions of drug laws by program members. Preparation of addicts entering the program should include detailed explanation of the legal obligations of staff members. Program policies must be legally correct, and rules must be enforced equally for all members. Since infractions are to be expected, anticipatory planning should consider staff and group responses to these contingencies. Even though a group leader may wish to emphasize incremental steps to rehabilitation, the illegality of most drug abuse makes total abstinence a more pressing goal than in alcoholism programs.

It is possible to continue a therapeutic relationship with recalcitrant drug abusers if there is some evidence of motivation or progress. An effective way of avoiding possible estrangement between a member and a group leader after an infraction is to classify group goals as immediate, intermediate, and ultimate (Burkhalter, 1975). Group goals may be presented to members as progressive or developmental. This insures that temporary return to drug abuse will partially but not totally erase progress.

Immediate Goals
1. Withdrawal or detoxification.
2. Medical treatment for physical complications.
3. Cessation of criminal activity.

Intermediate Goals
1. Full participation in the aftercare program.
2. Exploration of reasons for drug abuse.
3. Sustained efforts to maintain abstinence.
4. Improvement in social functioning.

Ultimate Goals
1. Successful maintenance of abstinence.
2. Development of insight and awareness.
3. Stabilization of family relationships.
4. Completion of vocational rehabilitation.

Discipline is strictly enforced in drug-abuse programs and staff members must be alert to the manipulative operations of members. Attendance is required at all scheduled meetings and punctuality is demanded. In residential facilities chores are assigned to addicts, with newcomers given the most menial jobs. When an addict has advanced sufficiently in the program, negotiations may be initiated with the staff and the other residents to modify assignments. Until negotiations are completed the assigned chores remain the responsibility of the addict. On these issues, as on all matters, communication is expected to be direct and forthright. Incongruence, obliqueness, or failure to negotiate are confronted, as are excuses and double messages.

Confrontation

Techniques of confrontation common in encounter groups are a form of strategy used in drug-abuse groups. In methadone maintenance programs, where freedom from all addiction is not a goal, confrontation in the group is less forceful, although rules for attendance, punctuality, and responsibility are upheld just as rigidly. Group therapy meetings convene several times a week and are a fundamental part of drug-abuse programs. The members are expected to participate aggressively in confronting one another. Those who fail to do so are reminded of their dereliction by leaders and fellow members (Gust, 1979). Physical aggression in the group is forbidden, but catharsis is permitted in the form of profanity, crying, and shouting. Authentic behavior is welcomed, but behavior which is considered false or manipulative is attacked by the group. Attention is directed to immediate problems of relating and coping rather than to antecedent events. The here-and-now interactions of the group are used to point out dysfunctional communication engaged in by members. Levels of intensity rise and fall during the sessions as group events take the form of exploratory questioning or accusatory probing (Lowinson and Zwerling, 1971).

Coleadership Strategy The group leader monitors interaction and must not be intimidated by emotional intensity. Because of the uninhibited nature of group interactions, coleadership may be advisable for drug-abuse groups. A nurse and an ex-addict often combine their skills in order to regulate the group. Sharing with members the rationale for certain interventions reduces the anger and bewilderment which group incidents may evoke. In order to moderate the impulsiveness of members, group leaders model reflective thinking and the careful interpretation of group events. During the meetings leaders identify maladaptiveness and suggest more appropriate responses. Group pressure is applied to extinguish communication which is distracting or extraneous. When one leader confronts a member directly, the second leader may offer a cognitive explanation or expand the interaction to include others in the group. Confrontation is deliberate and measured by the leaders who work cooperatively, with each assuming a stance complementary to the position of the coleader (Goldstein and Wolpe, 1971). Confrontation which takes place in drug abuse groups may appear harsh but is actually purposeful. Deception and circumstantiality are repeatedly challenged in a way which cuts through evasion. Clinicians working with compulsive drug abusers have learned that unmitigated acceptance is not therapeutic and that support for group members must be joined with firm limit-setting. Drug-abuse groups may seem conflict-ridden, but conflict is guided in order to effect change. The group leaders perform whatever regulatory functions are appropriate. At times a leader may intervene to control volatile group elements.

Summarizing Sessions At the conclusion of each session leaders try to create an atmosphere of hopefulness and universality so that the meeting ends on a positive note. Summarization and clarification of the proceedings may be used to achieve this purpose. Verbal summarization by the leaders may be augmented with a written summary of each session, prepared by the leaders and distributed at the following meeting. These written summaries may contain hypotheses about group transactions or acknowledge mystification felt by leaders about certain issues. Solicitude or praise may be extended to some members, particularly when leaders feel that closure has not been reached. Amounts of disclosure contained in the summaries can be titrated to group needs. An added benefit of written summaries is that unrealistic expectations of leader omnipotence are reduced. At the same time members are reassured that the leaders are in charge and that the group is a safe place to be. Group attitudes toward the leaders of drug-abuse groups are ambivalent, even when the leader is an ex-addict. Distrust and apprehension are expressed, along with many counterdependent behaviors. Summarization of the meetings, whether written or oral, helps to correct distorted impressions of what happened in the group meeting.

Rules and Norms

The intense reactions in drug-abuse groups may pose problems for members who fear that the group is unmanageable. Therefore the leaders must go to some lengths to build the group normative system. This is done by crediting the group with the ability to establish rules of behavior which then become group norms. Newcomers to the group are told by senior members what the rules are and why they must be respected. Drug-abuse groups are usually long-term and open-ended, with members entering and leaving the group as necessary. Reiteration and compliance hasten the incorporation of rules into the normative system of the group. Once established, group norms prevail even though group composition is altered (Mills, 1967). A strong normative system is needed to maintain order and to prevent attenuation of group cohesion as members enter and leave.

Manipulative Behaviors Deviations from group norms are easier to confront than are the avoidance behaviors used by some members. Because members of drug-abuse groups are skilled in duplicity, they are well able to defend themselves against confrontation tactics. Several manipulative ploys used by drug-dependent persons have been described by Burkhalter (1975). *Rounding* was described as verbal facility in eluding unpleasant topics by changing the subject or counterattacking the interrogator. *Imaging* was described as the ability of an addict to present onlookers with the image of a responsible, well-intentioned individual. Through imaging, skeptics and experienced professionals may become convinced that an addict is deserving, committed, and responsible. A third technique used by addicts to thwart rehabilitative efforts is known as *gaming*. This is the ability to falsify events and circumstances in order to deceive the "straight" world. It is difficult to say whether these propensities were present before addiction, but they undoubtedly were confirmed through experiences in the drug culture.

Among the topics discussed in groups are requests for information about drugs, especially if methadone is being used; complaints about work assignments in the treatment facility; misgivings about being accepted by respectable society; anxiety about sexual problems; and conflicts among members, or between staff and members. As a result of confrontation tactics, contentious and dissembling behaviors, plus the high turnover of members, the drug-abuse group demands the utmost in leadership skills.

Family Meetings

Family dynamics may exacerbate drug dependence or speed the progress of the recovering addict. For this reason family meetings are a component of a comprehensive drug-abuse program. These meetings are held under the leadership of a health professional who may be a nurse or social worker qualified in family assessment and intervention. Multifamily meetings may be held, or one family may be seen as a unit. It is recommended that the addict always be present so that family sessions are witnessed by everyone concerned rather than recounted secondhand. The meetings may be devoted to acquainting families with the drug program and securing their understanding of the changes which lie ahead. In family meetings the leader has an opportunity to observe interactional patterns and estimate resistance to change. If a nonaddicted spouse appears threatened by the prospect of living with a competent, rehabilitated partner, marital counseling may be suggested. As the addict recovers, marital interactions which were asymmetrical may become symmetrical. A struggle for dominance may ensue which hampers rehabilitative work but is amenable to intervention.

Multifamily meetings are especially helpful for addicts as they re-enter the community and become involved with work or study programs. Evening meetings allow recovering addicts and family members to continue some involvement with the treatment program. Spending time with other addicts who are trying to "make it" eases the transition of an addict into respectable society until durable ties with other support systems can be formed.

Community Meetings

Day treatment centers and residential facilities serving drug abusers employ daily community meetings to plan activities, orient new members, and review pertinent issues related to the program. Discussions may include progress reports from members or reactions to decisions taken by staff. Attendance at community meetings is compulsory for staff and clientele alike. There may be no formal leader, or leadership may be rotated among staff members. Proceedings of the community meetings are handled in a fairly democratic fashion, although order is maintained. Confrontation is not a prominent technique of the community meetings, and the issues addressed are often procedural or informational.

Role of the Nurse

In comprehensive programs for compulsive drug abusers the nurse is a central member. During withdrawal or detoxification, the assessments and interventions of nurses are crucial. When methadone maintenance is part of the program, dispensing the drug is the responsibility of professional nurses. Since the nurse is the dispenser of a highly valued substance and a caretaker during withdrawal or detoxification, acceptance of the nurse by the addict is accomplished rather quickly. Functioning in various capacities in the drug abuse program, the nurse is regarded as a person of some consequence. Moreover, popular acceptance of nurses as care providers and patient advocates helps the addict to develop trust. These appraisals heighten a nurse's effectiveness as a group leader and add weight to interventions in the group.

CLINICAL EXAMPLE: AVOIDANCE BEHAVIORS AND CONFLICT IN A DRUG-ABUSE GROUP

A number of heroin addicts in a residential facility for drug abusers were members of a therapy group which met three times a week. The group was heterogeneous in terms of age, sex, and race. All of the members had been withdrawn from heroin and were receiving methadone.

Monica was a nineteen-year-old prostitute who was five months pregnant. According to Monica, her boyfriend, who was the father of the baby, had recently been "busted" and was serving a prison term for armed robbery. Monica was taking methadone in gradually smaller doses and asserted that she intended to be drug free by the time her baby was born. Woodrow was an intelligent thirty-five-year-old black man who was being maintained on methadone and was not attempting to lower his intake. He had a grade school education and was enrolled in a work-study program through which he hoped to get a high school equivalency certificate. His progress toward the certificate was impeded by erratic attendance. Woodrow was afraid of not being able to function in the straight world but tried to conceal this by swaggering and boasting. Sheila was a twenty-one-year-old addict who spent weekends with her divorced mother, and relied on her mother for financial help. Ronnie was a twenty-two-year-old Vietnam war veteran who had become addicted to heroin while overseas. Like Sheila, he spent considerable time in his parents' home, but he resented their efforts to control his life. Ronnie's father was the custodian of a local church and both parents were devout and active in church affairs. They were deeply ashamed of their son's addiction and were afraid that friends and parishioners would learn that Ronnie was participating in a drug abuse program.

The therapy group was led by a psychiatric nurse and an ex-addict who was a staff member. Preparatory sessions held with group members had established specific contracts with each member regarding goals. The individual goals of the members were recorded in the group journal or diary which was available to all members. The individual goals of the above four members were recorded in the group diary as follows:

Monica: To be drug free two months before her expected delivery date.

Woodrow: To obtain a high school equivalency certificate and enter job training.

Sheila: To move into her own apartment and be less dependent on her mother.

Ronnie: To make some friends and to use his veteran's benefits to return to college.

Since Ronnie was the newest member to move into the residence, he had been given the chore of cleaning up the kitchen after dinner. After two weeks of this assignment Ronnie was extremely resentful and began complaining to the group. He compared his work in the kitchen to cleaning up after pigs, and stated angrily that everybody used the kitchen in the evening and thoroughly messed up his work. Because he was a veteran, Ronnie thought that he should have more privileges than other members. "I'm no welfare bum like the rest of you in this place," he said vehemently. "I shouldn't have to do any work — I pay my own way here" (*imaging* and *rationalization*).

Woodrow responded to Ronnie with this rejoinder. "You don't pay your own way here any more than I do. The Man pays for all of us — your money just comes out of a different pocket, that's all. What are you bad mouthing us for? You ain't so big, Ron — you're just about where I was a couple of months ago" (*rounding* and *denial*).

Monica jumped into the argument at this point and joined Woodrow in attacking Ronnie. "Yeah, you don't pay any more here than the rest of us, Ronnie. What a baby you are, complaining and still hanging on to your mommy and daddy — and they can't even stand having you around. At least Woodie and I know how to stand on our own two feet. Stop your damn whining, Ronnie. If my baby ever grows up to be anything like you, I'll drown it" (*gaming* and *reversal*).

Sheila then joined the battle on Ronnie's behalf and began yelling at Monica. "What do you know about it, Monica? You haven't got a home except for this place. Your mother threw you out on the streets when you were twelve. You're just jealous because Ronnie and I have folks and some place to go. Woodie and you are really weird and I bet your kid turns out to be weird, too. Maybe you *should* drown it, especially if it takes after you" (*rounding* and *displacement*).

As the arguing continued, the decibel level in the room became deafening. Before the dispute could escalate further the leaders insisted that everyone stop shouting and begin to examine what was happening. The interventions of the leaders were stated emphatically and their directions were clear. All four adversaries were asked to listen quietly and reflect as uninvolved members of the group discussed the incident. With the disputants transformed into onlookers, the following points were made by the members who had not been involved in the argument.

1. Ronnie had three demands, one of which was reasonable. His current assignment was to clean the kitchen and rules dictated that he spend two more weeks on that job. As a Vietnam veteran, he had no more privileges than anyone else. His complaint that people continued to use the kitchen after he cleaned it was valid and legitimate. Ronnie was advised to bring this up at the community meeting the next morning.

2. Woodrow's remark that Ronnie was just about where he had been a few months ago was interpreted as a hostile response to Ronnie's statement that veterans should have higher status. If Woodrow wanted to compare his progress with Ronnie's, that was permissible. But it had nothing to do with the real issue, which was Ronnie's complaint about cleaning the kitchen. Comparing himself favorably with Ronnie was Woodrow's way of denying his own doubts about the progress he was making.

3. Monica introduced another irrelevant issue by accusing Ronnie of hanging on to his parents. This was probably related to Monica's own conflicted feelings about becoming a mother and wanting to be mothered at the same time. In stressing her independence Monica was trying to reverse or undo the past, which still troubled her. Despite her facade of strength and determination, Monica distrusted her ability to accomplish her goals. Actually, she was frightened at the prospect of raising her child alone.

4. Sheila's alliance with Ronnie was described as dishonest or inauthentic. She was not interested in dealing with Ronnie's complaint, and it was only her envy of Monica which made her side with Ronnie. The fact that Ronnie saw his parents at times made Sheila feel better about depending on her own mother. There was no altruism in her support of Ronnie. Sheila resented Monica's decision to withdraw from methadone maintenance because this made her feel guilty. Her feelings of inadequacy were projected and displaced to Monica and Woodrow.

The concerted efforts of the leaders and the group tempered the fury of the four angry members, and permitted discussion of the real problem raised by Ronnie, which was not insoluble. Ronnie's way of presenting the problem and the unthinking responses of Woodrow, Monica, and Sheila, which originated in anxiety, caused the uproar. Only the firmness of the leaders, the imposition of silence on the disputants, and insistence on reflective thinking averted a worse explosion. The strategy of the leaders was twofold: 1) to return to the practicalities of Ronnie's complaint about conditions in the kitchen while upholding the established rules of the program, and 2) to reflect on the behaviors of the four members and interpret their responses as examples of dysfunctional communication while offering alternative coping methods.

SUMMARY

Acceptance, socialization, and instillation of hope were identified as aspects of common-problem groups which may be either self-led or professionally led. The boundaries of common-problem groups for alcohol and drug abusers were identified. Alcoholics Anonymous programs were contrasted with traditional group therapy for alcoholics, and divergent views on abstinence as a group goal for alcoholics were presented. Problematic issues such as dependency, denial, and anger in alcoholism groups were discussed, along with appropriate intervention strategy. Selecting alcoholics for Alcoholics Anonymous or for traditional group treatment is a difficult issue for professionals. Available data indicate that the cognitive orientation of an alcoholic entering treatment may be a significant variable in making a referral either to an Alcoholics Anonymous chapter or to traditional group treatment for the alcoholic.

The disparate characteristics of abusers of specific categories of drugs were compared. Identifying personality types among drug abusers was considered to be less important than relating to drug abusers as individuals who should learn new ways of living and coping. Problematic issues such as unclear motivation and the dissembling behaviors of drug abusers were presented, and possible interventions were suggested. Finally, adjunct forms of group treatment for drug abusers, such as family and therapeutic community meetings, were described briefly. The unique role of the nurse in comprehensive drug-abuse programs was also discussed.

REFERENCES

Anderson, R.E., and I. Carter. *Human Behavior in the Social Environment.* Chicago: Aldine, 1978.

Battegay, R. "Different Kinds of Group Psychotherapy with Patients with Different Diagnoses." *Acta Psychiatry* (Scandinavia), 1977, pages 345–354.

Brown, S., and I.D. Yalom. "Interactional Group Therapy with Alcoholics." *Journal for Studies on Alcohol* 38, 1977, pages 426–456.

Burkhalter, P.K. *Nursing Care of the Alcoholic and Drug Abuser.* New York: McGraw-Hill, 1975.

Feeney, D.J., and P. Dranger. "Alcoholics View Group Therapy." *Journal for Studies on Alcohol* 37, 1976, pages 611–618.

Fontana, A.F.; B.N. Dowds; and M.H. Bethel. "A.A. and Group Therapy for Alcoholics." *Journal for Studies on Alcohol* 37, No. 5, 1976, pages 675–682.

Glasser, W. *Reality Therapy.* New York: Harper & Row, 1966.

Gilmour, V. "How Nurses Feel About Alcoholics," *New Zealand Nursing Journal*, September 1973, pages 31–32.

Goldstein, A., and J. Wolpe. "Behavior Therapy in Groups." In *Comprehensive Group Psychotherapy*, H.I. Kaplan and B.J. Sadock, Eds. Baltimore: Williams and Wilkins, 1971.

Gust, D. *Face to Face with Alcoholism.* Center City, ME.: Hazelden Literature, 1979.

Hyde, A. "The Alcoholic Personality." *Medical Counterpoint* 5, 1971, pages 10–12.

Heyman, M.M. *Alcoholism Programs in Industry: The Patient's View.* Monographs of Rutgers Center of Alcohol Studies Vol. 14, no. 12. New Brunswick, N.J.: Rutgers Center of Alcohol Studies, 1978.

Janosik, E.H. "Reachable and Teachable: Report on a Prison Alcoholism Group." *Journal of Psychiatric Nursing and Mental Health Services,* April 1977, pages 24–28.

————.; S. Trimborn; and E. Milanese. *Cognitive Orientation, Curative Factors, Treatment Outcomes in Alcoholism Group Programs.* Research Report CNA Grant ONR-N0014-76-0001, 1978.

Janzen, C. "Family Treatment for Alcoholism: A Review." *Social Work* Vol. 23, No. 2, 1978, pages 134–141.

King, A.S. "Experimenter Expectancy Effects on Organizational Change." *Administration Science Quarterly* Vol. 19, No. 2, 1974, pages 221–230.

Lachar, D.; C.L. Gdowski; and J.F. Keegan. "MMPI Profiles of Men Alcoholics, Drug Addicts, and Psychiatric Patients." *Journal for Studies on Alcohol* 40, 1979, pages 45–56.

Leake, G.J., and N.S. King. "Effect of Counselor Expectations on Alcohol Recovery." *Alcohol Health and Research World* 3, 1977, pages 16–22.

Lowinson, J., and I. Zwerling. "Group Therapy with Narcotic Addicts." In *Comprehensive Group Psychotherapy,* H.I. Kaplan and B.J. Sadock, Eds. Baltimore: Williams and Wilkins, 1971.

Mills, T.M. *Sociology of Small Groups.* Englewood Cliffs, N.J.: Prentice-Hall, 1967.

Moody, P.M. "Attitudes of Nurses and Nursing Students toward Alcoholism Treatment." *Journal for Studies on Alcohol* 32, 1971, pages 172–175.

Mullan, H., and I. Sanguilano. *Alcoholism Group Psychotherapy and Rehabilitation.* Springfield, IL.: Charles C Thomas, 1960.

Pepper, S.C. *World Hypothesis.* Berkeley, CA.: University of California Press, 1942.

Rosenbaum, M., and M. Berger. *Group Psychotherapy and Group Function.* New York: Basic Books, 1963.

Scott, E.M. "The Alcoholic Group: Formation and Beginnings." *Group Process* 7, 1976, pages 95–116.

Seelye, E.E. "Relationship of Socioeconomic Status, Psychiatric Diagnosis and Sex to Outcome of Alcoholism Treatment." *Journal for Studies on Alcohol* 40, 1979, pages 57–62.

Thompson, R.W. *Road to Recovery: Cognitive and Behavioral Styles of Recovering Alcoholics.* Paper, March 1979, Dept. of Anthropology, University of Illinois.

Weil, A. *The Natural Mind.* Boston: Houghton Mifflin, 1972.

Wurmser, L. "Drug Abuse: Nemesis of Psychiatry." *The American Scholar* Vol. 41, No. 3, 1972. Reprinted by New York Narcotic Addiction Control Commission.

Yowell, S., and C. Brose. "Working with Drug Abuse Patients in the Emergency Room." In *Psychiatric-Mental Health Nursing: Contemporary Readings*, B. Backer, P.M. Dubbert, and E.J.P. Eisenmann, Eds. New York: D. Van Nostrand, 1978.

16

Psychotherapeutic Group Work

Ellen Hastings Janosik

Group psychotherapy represents a trend which began during the 1930s and 1940s and was, in part, a pragmatic response to the psychosocial pressures of the depression and war-time years. This was a period when psychoanalytic theory was in ascendance, but the demand for psychiatric treatment far exceeded the supply of therapists. Over time, many persons who were neither psychiatrists nor psychoanalysts became active in the group therapy movement and made impressive contributions to group theory and practice. At present, group work, including group psychotherapy, is the most widely used treatment in the United States (Morgan and Moreno, 1973).

Psychotherapists are notoriously individualistic in their methods, and group psychotherapy reflects the diverse preferences of the group leader. Spotnitz (1971) observed that a literature review gave the impression that there were as many forms of group psychotherapy as there were group therapists. Slavson (1964) made a nice distinction between group counseling, group guidance, and group psychotherapy. Group guidance and group counseling were considered aspects of psychosocial nursing; only groups organized to induce intrapsychic change were regarded as psychotherapy.

The continuum presented in Chapter 3 shows psychotherapeutic methods which range from repressive-inspirational to regressive-reconstructive (Rosenbaum, 1965). Each pole of the continuum represents the extent of personality change being sought, with repressive-inspirational groups seeking the least change and regressive-reconstructive groups seeking the most. Supportive, adaptational, and reparative groups fall at less extreme points on the continuum.

Yalom (1975) found so much diversity in the field of group therapy that he preferred to classify groups according to operative curative factors rather than the orientation of the group leader or the nature of group goals. Yalom differentiated the *front* and the *core* of various group psychotherapies. The front consisted of the form, techniques, and language surrounding individual schools of psychotherapy. The core included only the mechanisms of change or curative factors present in the group. When the front of group psychotherapy was disregarded, various therapeutic approaches were found to be quite similar across groups.

DEFINITION OF GROUP PSYCHOTHERAPY

Group psychotherapy may be viewed as a treatment modality which seeks any number of diversified goals. Usually the goals involve psychological change of one kind or another. Sometimes psychological change is clearly addressed; at other times psychological change is pursued by means of behavioral or social adaptation.

The role of the psychotherapeutic group leader includes various directorial or managerial responsibilities. In order for a therapy group to be successful, its organization, leadership, and goals must meet the needs of group members. The contract of a psychotherapeutic group is a mutually negotiated, explicit agreement which outlines the conditions under which the group operates. Thus the contract shapes and is shaped by the expectations of members and the interventions of group leaders (Klein and Gould, 1973; Levinson and Astrachan, 1974).

Many groups manage to achieve therapeutic ends without actually venturing into psychotherapy. Unlike therapeutic groups, group psychotherapy is rooted in psychiatry and psychology, although its scope and depth vary. The broad prerequisites for group psychotherapy include regular meetings of three or more persons held at specific times and places for the purpose of improving psychosocial health. A narrower definition of group psychotherapy is that it is the use of group methods to treat the psychopathology of members. The shortcoming of this definition is that it omits an explanation of what really constitutes psychopathology. For purposes of this chapter, group psychotherapy is considered to be a treatment whose chief purpose is to produce social and psychological change through monitored interactions in a group setting. Psychological change includes interpersonal and intrapersonal modifications produced through exploration of the past, the present, and the anticipated future (Marram, 1978).

The term *group therapy* was first used by Jacob Moreno, who opposed the rigid tenets of psychoanalysis by treating groups rather than individuals, and by emphasizing the therapeutic aspects of the group experience (Morgan and Moreno, 1973). Even though many psychoanalytic concepts are used in group work, Moreno conceptualized group psychotherapy as a departure from traditional psychoanalytic dogma.

BASIC CONCEPTS IN GROUP PSYCHOTHERAPY

Group members bring to the experience residual feelings and behaviors which have been influenced by early familial experience. In psychoanalytic terms, the group becomes a replication of the first primary group, with leaders seen as surrogate parents and members as siblings, although this perception is seldom conscious. The corrective reenactment of the original primary group experience may be used to alter emotional conflicts and maladaptive defenses which are the legacy of early life.

In group psychotherapy, which deals with interpersonal rather than intrapersonal factors, the group is perceived not so much as a family but as a microcosm of society. The appraisals and responses of group members counteract feelings of social isolation, and encourage the discovery and testing of alternative behaviors. Within interpersonal groups, shared communication moves from inchoate to articulate expression. The increased dignity and understanding which ensue constitute the group equivalent to exploring the unconscious.

Most group therapists subscribe to a particular theoretical framework, although some are more consistent than others in adhering to a singular approach. Although they may be used in different ways, depending on group variables such as goals, composition, and contracts, six concepts are intrinsic to group psychotherapy (Lego, 1979). These concepts were designated as: 1) transference, 2) countertransference, 3) resistance, 4) acting out, 5) insight, and 6) working through.

Transference This is an unconscious process in which individuals transfer to others the conflicted wishes and fears which were experienced with significant persons in early life. For instance, a group member who filled the role of "Daddy's little girl" in the original family configuration may try to relive that role with the male leader. Recognition by group members of the dynamics beneath this behavioral pattern may ultimately permit "Daddy's little girl" to grow up and behave more like an adult. Transference, then, is an unconscious idiosyncratic distortion which the group has the potential to correct.

Countertransference   This is the transference by the group leader, to one or several members, of conflicted fears and wishes which originated in the leader's primary group. A group leader who is incited to anger by a member may be responding to internal distortion rather than the reality of the group situation. Countertransference which is realized may be consciously controlled. Like all other mortals, group leaders do not always examine their own reactions objectively and may engage in denial and rationalization. Because it is the leader who must be challenged, only a mature group will be able to deal with this. Supervision and observation of group sessions are important for all group leaders, but they are crucial for leaders of psychotherapeutic groups. In addition, the leader must engage in introspection for the purpose of raising his or her own self-awareness. A lengthy discussion of transference issues is found in Chapter 3.

Resistance   An unwillingness on the part of the members to relinquish distortions and accept consensually validated interpretations is known as resistance. It may be individual or collective, overt or covert, conscious or unconscious. Some manifestations of resistance are anger, inattention, sarcasm, flippancy, lateness, or erratic attendance. Like transference and countertransference, resistance in groups can be exceedingly complex, being directed toward the leader or toward group members in ways not immediately apparent.

Acting Out   Often confused with acting-up behavior, which is usually a form of resistance, acting out is deeper and more profound. Acting out means that an individual expresses old conflicts symbolically or behaviorally instead of talking about them. Acting-out behavior is usually unconscious and merits interpretation by the leader and, if possible, by group members. Many times the interpretation is not accepted initially, but evenutally the acting-out members may recognize the accuracy of the interpretations, thus taking a step toward insight.

Insight This is the conscious connection made between behavior and underlying motives. The acquisition of insight may be a tedious process, since intellectual understanding is only the beginning. Like the recognition of one's acting out behavior, progress toward insight is a time consuming journey which requires a state of readiness on the part of the individual. Without readiness, the connection between behavior and motivation will not be made. This is among the reasons that group psychotherapy, which has insight as a goal, is of relatively long duration.

Working Through This is another process in group and individual psychotherapy which requires time. In order to change and grow, group members must repeatedly face their infantile conflicts. During individual psychoanalysis, regression is allowed so that ineffective defenses and coping mechanisms may be eradicated and reconstructed. A group functions, however, to prevent excessive regression by upholding a social order. The multiplicity of relationships and interrelationships in groups is thought to weaken transference phenomena. These limitations have caused some theorists to question the value of group psychotherapy in producing genuine personality change.

Even the advocates of group psychotherapy question how much intrapsychic change occurs, compared to individual psychotherapy. Slavson (1964) straddled both sides of the question by asserting that the depth and thoroughness of group work cannot compare to individual work, and that the therapeutic process is hastened in groups because of the increased productivity of group members. Without venturing into further comparisons, it is safe to state that neither transference nor regression are as extreme in group psychotherapy as in individual work. In the absence of extreme transference and regression, the psychotherapy groups offer such curative factors as: identification, universality, imitativeness, hopefulness, cohesion, altruism, interpersonal learning, and catharsis (Yalom, 1975).

CATEGORIES OF PSYCHOTHERAPEUTIC GROUPS

A triadic classification of group psychotherapy transcends the dichotomy of intrapersonal and interpersonal groups, and incorporates the polarities of repressive-inspirational groups and regressive-reconstructive groups. These categories may be identified as: 1) nondirective, 2) directive, and 3) didactic.

In nondirective group therapy a climate of nonjudgmental acceptance is maintained which encourages members to express positive and negative feelings without fear of rejection or censure. Member to member, or member to group interactions are promoted rather than leader-centered interactions. The leader assumes some responsibility for preserving an atmosphere of safety, but does not become an authority figure. One interesting distinction made between nondirective and directive group therapy is that the directive leader sets limits upon the group members, whereas nondirective leaders set limits on themselves. In nondirective groups decision making remains within the purview of group responsibility, and autonomous functioning is permitted (Spotnitz, 1971; Swanson, 1978). Among the many nondirective forms of group therapy are sensitivity groups, encounter groups, gestalt-existential groups, music and art therapy, analytic group therapy, and psychodrama. Two of these, analytic group therapy and psychodrama, will be used as illustrations of nondirective groups.

Analytic Group Psychotherapy

As in individual analytic therapy, these groups adhere to major psychoanalytic principles. The leader is passive and reflective; transference is prominent and, like resistance, is analyzed and interpreted. To intensify transference the leader does not engage in self-disclosure or status denial to any extent (Yalom, 1975). Anthony (1971) stated that the goal of individual and group analytic work is to help individuals become their own therapists. For this reason the analytic group leader fosters the notion that help is forthcoming not from the leader but from the group, and that the growing insight and awareness of each member is a resource to be tapped.

The early stage of analytic work tends to be leader-centered. Unrealistic expectations of the leader are entertained; members at first regard one another as intruders who prevent a one-to-one relationship with the leader. At this time members may leave the group without much attention being paid to their departure. Newcomers are not warmly welcomed, since every new member is thought to reduce the attention available from the leader. Eventually the jealousies of the early phase are replaced by positive factors of identification, mutuality, imitation, and cohesiveness (Yalom, 1975). Transference and other irrational phenomena subside as the group begins to mature.

There are many adaptations and modifications of traditional analytic approaches in group work. The nondirectiveness of group leaders is not absolute but may be plotted on a continuum. Relatively few group leaders are purists who preserve a totally neutral position. Most group leaders, even those with a psychoanalytic bias, deviate from a noninterventionist position. In general, no indication is made by nondirective group leaders that attitudes and feelings are right or wrong in and of themselves. What is sought by this type of leader is chiefly an honest expression of feelings.

During the preparatory period the nondirective group leader may present rules regarding *how* feelings may be expressed, but does not set restrictions on *what* may be expressed. In some nondirective groups a contract is established that only verbalization of feelings will be allowed. In other groups feelings may be expressed nonverbally through actions and gestures. During the preparatory period, permissible means of expression must be clearly delineated. For example, touching may be used to show emotion, but members should know what is allowable in a group session. Even though the nondirective leaders are not authority figures, they may not forgo responsibility for the group atmosphere or the safety of individual members. If rules are understood before the group commences, the nondirective leader need not become a disciplinarian.

Psychodrama Groups

Psychodrama is considered a nondirective group even though this form of group therapy is overlaid with rules and structure. What makes psychodrama nondirective is the fact that no content areas are forbidden, nor are any feelings or actions of members considered inherently good or evil. This is a form of psychotherapy in which verbalization is subservient to action. When first introduced, psychodrama was considered revolutionary in its denigration of verbal communication, the activity on which psychoanalysis was based (Moreno, 1971). In conceptualizing psychodrama, Moreno insisted man's need to integrate the past, present, and future. This was another digression from psychoanalytic theory, which is preoccupied with antecedent events and the past.

What psychodrama attempts is an enactment of events, real or fantasized, which have produced emotional discomfort in a group member. As formulated by Moreno, psychodrama is an elaborate procedure requiring a definitive format and an adequate number of staff members who may be actors or observers. Modified versions of psychodrama are possible, and these modifications enable smaller psychiatric facilities to engage in the psychodramatization of significant events (Fried, 1971).

In psychodrama the content and roles of the scenario are prearranged. The group member who has outlined the script to be enacted may play his or her own role, or select another group member to do this. Other actors are chosen for roles by the protagonist member who has devised the script. According to Spotnitz (1971) five components are required for psychodrama: 1) a group whose members function as audience and actors; 2) the protagonist or group member who has supplied the script; 3) a "therapeutic space" or stage on which the drama is enacted; 4) "auxiliary egos" or group members playing assigned roles; and 5) the leader-director who orchestrates the drama. The spontaneity, catharsis, and reality testing which accompany psychodrama are thought to contribute to its effectiveness as a therapeutic tool.

Psychodrama can be an excellent source of information about group members, and can also be used for assessments. Feelings of group members toward one another and toward significant persons in their lives are revealed through the drama. The experience is also beneficial for members who are not in touch with their feelings because of repression or denial. Internal experiences which seem overwhelming may be reviewed and tolerated by means of dramatization. The simple act of dramatizing a sequence helps to decrease inhibited expressiveness concerning it.

The Value of Psychodrama   There are those who question the value of psychodrama on the grounds that it is stressful for members and fosters gratification rather than growth. Other critics decry the ritualization demanded by Moreno, who cautioned leaders of psychodrama on the need for restraint. At the same time failure to allow random behavior during psychodrama may prevent it from having an impact (Anthony, 1971). It must be remembered, however, that the cartharsis and free expression offered by psychodrama contain certain hazards. Techniques such as role exchange, role reversal, and cognitive directorial interventions offer a measure of caution and safety. Occasionally a protagonist who is overcome by the drama may be asked to direct the scene instead of acting it or to become an observer for a time. Identifying with the protagonist or extrapolating themes of the drama are other stratagems aimed at restraint. A post-session in which the drama is discussed and generalized to the group is essential for achieving therapeutic closure.

Moreno (1971) indicated certain conditions or procedures which are advisable when psychodrama is attempted:

- Conflicts should be enacted, not merely described.
- Enactment takes place in the here-and-now, regardless of whether events occurred in the past, will occur in the future, or are fantasies.

- Auxiliary egos should be used; the function of auxiliary egos is to represent absent persons and internalized objects, ideals, or distortions of the protagonist.
- The protagonist has the right to discard the script or choose another scene. The director-leader may return to the script at a later time, or may discuss with the protagonist and the group the reasons for abandoning the script.

ORGANIZING NONDIRECTIVE GROUPS

Because of the nondirective posture of the leader, certain precautions must be taken when organizing this form of group. The optimal number of members is six or seven, with nine members considered maximal. In psychodrama groups membership may appear larger because of the presence of staff members who augment the ranks of audience and cast. The composition of the group is another important consideration; prospective members of nondirective groups should be assessed and prepared very carefully. Group members should have the ability to engage in reality testing and to withstand heightened levels of anxiety. Ego strengths such as judgment and rationality must be evident and integrated into the behavioral patterns of members. Persons who are extremely hysterical, blatantly psychotic, or suicidal should be excluded. The last exclusion does not extend to somewhat depressed patients unless they are unable to interact with others. Suitable for admission to nondirective groups are persons with moderate neurotic symptoms, persons who suffer psychophysiological disturbances, and persons who exhibit interpersonal difficulties (Solomon and Patch, 1974).

The following psychological or social problems are considered responsive to interventions in nondirective groups.

- *Shyness and loneliness:* When such persons express fear of joining a group they may be told that this is exactly why they should join. Reassurance may be given that shyness and loneliness are universal feelings.
- *Dependency conflicts:* Multiple interactions in the group cause dependency needs to be distributed rather than concentrated on one person.
- *Role and identity confusion:* Clarification is offered and adaptive change is reinforced by the group.
- *Self-defeating behaviors:* Maladaptive behavior is identified and confronted by the group.

Table 16-1   TYPES OF GROUP PSYCHOTHERAPY

Nondirective	Directive	Didactic (Cognitive)
Leader may be active or inactive, but is always permissive	Leader is active; guides, directs, and regulates	Leader is active; instructs, teaches, and guides
Transferences and resistance analyzed	Interpersonal behavior stressed; transference acknowledged	Learning and adaptive behavior stressed
Concern with the unconscious to promote insight	Concern with covert and manifest content	Concern with overt and manifest content
Affective issues explored; cognitive understanding sought	Affective issues explored; cognitive understanding sought; operant conditioning used	Cognitive understanding stressed; affective issues secondary; behavioral modification used
Past is explored in order to understand and alter the present	Here-and-now reality of the group is explored	Present and future events are explored

DIRECTIVE GROUP PSYCHOTHERAPY

A basic premise of directive group psychotherapy is that the success of the group experience can be assured by an active, directive leader (see Table 16-1). The leaders of directive groups reject the proposal that problems can be resolved through spontaneous group interaction, contending that a group which is not regulated by the leader may be malignant rather than benign in its effects (Kaplan and Sadock, 1971). Catharsis and ventilation of affect are not considered therapeutic unless followed by learning and growth, which are promoted by directive leadership.

In nondirective groups (Table 16-1) some persons become active, contributing members while others continue to be uncommunicative for extended periods or throughout the life of the group. In directive groups leaders exert the power invested in their position in order to mobilize the members. The directive leader wants to provoke cognitive understanding rather than affective responses, not only to regulate the emotional level of the group but to provide guidance and maintain order. Some directive group leaders may be compared to behavioralists who use operant conditioning, since in both cases a leader's interventions are used to reinforce adaptive and inhibit maladaptive behaviors (Yates, 1975). When a directive leader praises the behavior of a withdrawn member who has just spoken, the act of involvement is rewarded or reinforced. Witnessing the reinforcing activity of the leader causes group members either to join the leader in promoting the involvement of the withdrawn member or to engage in similar behavior in order to win the same approbation for themselves.

Goal specificity is another way of differentiating between directive and nondirective group therapy. Berne (1966) made a distinction between diffuse or "soft" therapeutic goals and clearly defined or "hard" therapeutic goals. The overall goal of group psychotherapy is to help individual members to change in some way. This is true of directive and nondirective groups, even though their specific goals differ. In general the goals of directive groups tend to be more clearly defined, but the differences between the two types of groups are methodological rather than substantive. Repressive-inspirational groups usually require directive leadership; socialization, transactional analysis, and behavior modification are among the group experiences which rely upon a leader who is both active and directive. Chapters 12 and 13 of this book contain descriptions of various directive groups designed for children, adolescents, and the elderly.

Behavioral Group Psychotherapy

The behavioral therapist is a health professional who is not concerned with psychodynamics or interpersonal processes except as they directly affect behavior. Therefore a behavioral group leader carefully selects members who have similar, localized dysfunctions, rather than global symptomatology. Desensitization, relaxation, and assertiveness training are among the behavioral modifications which may be attempted in groups. Obesity groups, stop-smoking groups, and aversive therapy for alcoholics are other examples of behavior modification programs.

The nature of behavioral therapy necessitates a homogeneous selection of members. Therapy occurs during the group sessions but is not directed by members or the collective group. Instead, the interaction is leader-centered, and group activities include explanations, discussions, simulations, and role modeling, all conducted under the guidance of the leader. Verbalization is used to implement the modification program, but is minimally used for the expression of feelings.

Group behavioral therapy may be used advantageously with many neurotic persons, especially those with fears or phobias. Relaxation exercises may be used to reduce the distress of persons who are very anxious. Psychotic or delusional persons are rarely helped by behavioral approaches because of the idiosyncratic nature of their responses.   Some individuals with impulse control problems may decompensate unless they are permitted to engage in behaviors which offer an outlet for their impulses. A rigid behavioral modification program may change their behavior, but the unexpressed impluses may then take the form of more severe neurotic symptoms or of psychophysiological disorders. For these reasons it is important that the behavioral modification group not become a punitive agency, and that the members be carefully screened and prepared (Spotnitz, 1971).

Assertiveness training is a form of behavior modification which can proceed expeditiously in groups. Members are selected who have expressed a wish to be more assertive in their dealings with others.   Initial meetings might include explanations of assertive responses, and reassurance that assertiveness does not necessarily denote aggression or hostility. The leader might ask group members to describe everyday situations in which they have difficulty being assertive. An agreement might then be made that members try to show assertive behavior whenever a similar situation arises. They would be expected to report to the group any progress or lack of progress made in being assertive. During group sessions any display of appropriate assertiveness would be commented on favorably by the leader. Asking members to keep an assertiveness journal or log is an excellent daily reminder of the group task. A majority of the members involved in behavioral group psychotherapy have reported that the altered behaviors generated in the group can be transferred to daily life (Spotnitz, 1971).

Membership Limitations

Directive groups may safely accommodate slightly more members than nondirective groups, but ten to twelve members is probably the optimal size (Kaplan and Sadock, 1971). When the group is too large, fragmentary interactions arise between subgroups while the leader is occupied in dealing with the main body of the group. Control resides in the leader, whose directiveness sometimes arouses the resentment of the group. As is customary, the composition of the group and the dimensions of the common problem determine the group goals; these are usually circumscribed and specific in behavioral group therapy.

Special Techniques in Directive Groups

In directive groups the corrective re-enactment of the early family experience is not emphasized. Affective responses, intellectual understanding, and behavioral conditioning; may be included in the scope of directive groups. In addition, there are certain techniques favored by directive leaders to accelerate group progress. The following are some of the techniques which may be used selectively.

Go-Around The go-around is a technique in which each member is sequentially given an opportunity to contribute to group discussion. Perhaps one member is facing a crisis with which the group is trying to deal, and the go-around is being used to solicit suggestions from group members as to how the crisis might be handled. At other times the go-around may be used to allow every member to report personal accomplishments or failures in the interval between sessions. The presence and interventions of the leader are directed toward keeping the go-around orderly and rational. At the end of the go-around, when every member has had a turn, the leader may summarize the proceedings, assess the current status of the group, and suggest areas for future discussion.

Subject Session The topics suggested by the leader may include issues the leader deems important, but suggestions from the members are acceptable. Whatever the topic, the subject session is another way of structuring the group. Some subjects which might be chosen for discussion include: infidelity; loneliness; and problems with parents, spouses, peers, or "bosses."

The proponents of directive group psychotherapy present empirical evidence of the value of the method. Kaplan and Sadock (1971) reported that during a period of eighteen years no patient in a structured interactional therapy group committed or attempted suicide, even though numbers of depressed patients were included. The same source also pointed out an extremely low drop-out rate of less than five percent.

Membership Criteria

In selecting members for directive groups the criteria for inclusion far outweigh exclusionary criteria. Except for persons suffering severe organic defects or extreme regression, directive group psychotherapy may be attempted with virtually every type of interpersonal, neurotic, or personality disorder. Because the directive leader uses interventions which help all members to participate, depressed and withdrawn patients are especially suitable. Even persons who suffer latent, borderline, or residual psychosis may be considered appropriate members because of the protection afforded the group by the directive leader. In the directive group the amount of stimulation, anxiety, and tension in the group are regulated to avoid emotional overload.

Composition of directive groups should be heterogeneous with respect to sex, age, clinical diagnosis, personality patterns, and interactional styles. Heterogeneity operates to prevent the strengthening of maladaptive behavior through reinforcement or imitativeness. There are two types of patients who seem to do better in homogeneous groups: adolescents, and very regressed persons, whose needs generate resentment among heterogeneous members because of the time and attention required to deal with them.

As a regulatory agent, the leader preserves order in the group. At the same time the individual needs of members must be met. Monopolizing members may need to be confronted, even when the confrontation is seen as rejection. Withdrawn members may have to be encouraged to participate either through techniques like the go-around or the subject session. When a new member enters the directive group that person is introduced by name and may be asked to tell something about the reason for coming. This strengthens the group norm that participation is an expectation. At the same time members are expected to orient the new member to the group and to introduce themselves, all under the protective presence of the directive leader.

DIDACTIC GROUP PSYCHOTHERAPY

Didactic group psychotherapy (Table 16-1, p. 332) has as its purpose the transmitting of factual information about the problems of group members and of using a cognitive rather than an affective approach. In discussing didactic groups one is aware of the blurred distinctions between directive and didactic group therapy. It may be stated that a nondirective group leader seeks to inculcate, a directive group leader seeks to indoctrinate, and a didactic group leader seeks to educate the members (Solomon and Patch, 1974) by facilitating cognitive understanding.

Some didactic groups do not constitute group therapy but there are many appropriate utilizations for didactic group therapy. An education group organized for alcoholics which deals with the debilitating psychological, physical, and social effects of problem drinking is an example of didactic group therapy (Janosik, 1977). Sex education groups for young people, reality orientation groups for the elderly, and discharge groups for chronic schizophrenics are other forms of didactic group therapy. In addition to the didactic material presented in these groups, there is an implicit hope that increased knowledge will lead to psychological and behavioral change. In other words, cognitive understanding is not an end in itself but a mechanism of change.

Didactic group work takes place in many settings; the depth of psychotherapeutic intervention ranges from superficial to moderate. Members of didactic groups are taught about the dimensions and implications of their shared interests or problems. Cognitive material is emphasized in didactic groups, based on the assumption that cooperation and acceptance follow an intellectual comprehension of facts (Solomon and Patch, 1974). Factual knowledge transmitted in didactic groups may relate to physical, psychological, or social issues. The cognitive approach which characterizes these groups is reassuring for persons incapable of or reluctant to make a commitment to more stressful groups.

Many psychiatric facilities offer programs which use nondirective, directive, and didactic group therapy. A therapeutic community in a day treatment center is a form of milieu therapy which includes didactic groups. Orientation groups, vocational rehabilitation groups, and discharge groups are aspects of a therapeutic community which uses didacticism to improve the psychological status and social functioning of members (Davis, 1978).

Organizing Didactic Groups

Primary, secondary, and tertiary levels of prevention may be accomplished through the medium of didactic group work. There is probably no form of group intervention more consistent with nursing process than this form. Because many didactic groups are offered in settings which are not psychiatric, generalist nurses, community health nurses, school nurses, and gerontological nurses are apt to be involved. The list of patients suitable for didactic group work is extensive. The following is only a partial list of appropriate candidates.

- Preoperative and postoperative patients.
- Patients with chronic medical or psychiatric problems requiring long-term aftercare.
- Persons facing a developmental crisis such as prospective parenthood or retirement.
- Persons facing situational crises such as disasters or catastrophic illness.

- Persons with organic brain damage.
- Persons suffering addictive disorders.
- Persons experiencing loss of body image or body functions because of illness.

Some individuals who might be considered suitable for a didactic group experience may refuse to participate. In some instances the refusal must be accepted, but reassurance and persuasion may be used if it is thought that the group will prove beneficial. The interaction in didactic groups is facilitated if the members possess commonalities which induce motivation and promote cohesiveness. Although their responses to the shared experience will be heterogeneous, the members will be drawn together by their homogeneous concerns.

The leader of a didactic group may use formal lecture methods or informal presentations. Unless a lecture is followed by a group discussion, the leader is not using group process to promote learning and change. Teaching is an interpersonal endeavor which consists of a series of related interactions. The success of the learning experience depends partly on the expertise of the leader, but is greatly affected by the use or misuse of group dynamics.

The leader of a didactic group may be the expert, but acceptance of the leader's expertise may be conferred or withheld by the group. Acceptance of the leader's expertise is a crucial matter if the group is to achieve the goal of cognitive learning, followed by psychological or behavioral change. Three possible modes of accepting the expertise offered by the leader may be identified: *compliance, identification,* and *internalization* (Sampson and Marthas, 1977) (Table 16-2).

Compliance This is acceptance which depends on fear of the consequences of noncompliance. This mode of acceptance is relatively unsatisfactory, since it depends upon the presence or vigilance of the leader who is therefore considered an agent of retribution or surveillance. Leaders who use warnings which provoke alarm in the group may obtain compliance based on feelings of dependency and powerlessness. The compliance which results from severe or authoritarian leadership allows little room for autonomy or initiative among group members.

Identification This causes the group to accept what the leader has to give, motivated by a wish to be more like the leader. For instance, identification may be present in a nutrition group where a slim, attractive leader is a person whom overweight members wish

Table 16-2   ACCEPTANCE MODE IN DIDACTIC GROUPS

Mode	Tactics	Leadership Strategy
Compliance	Rewards and Punishments	Coercion Unilateral Control
Identification	Emulation and Imitation	Role Modeling Unilateral Persuasion
Internalization	Credibility and Mutuality	Reciprocal Compromise Bilateral Persuasion

Source: After Sampson and Marthas, 1977

to emulate. Emulation or imitation persists whether the leader is present or absent, since a positive image of the leader has been internalized by the group. Acceptance based on identification develops when the leader is admired by the group or has convinced the group that certain values are important. Acceptance through identification is possible even when a leader is somewhat authoritarian, as long as members are convinced of the leader's integrity and of their own capabilities. Thus, any derogation of the group's potential reduces the inclination of members to identify with the leader.

Internalization   This goes a step beyond identification. Here, acceptance by the group of the leader's offerings is based upon mutual negotiation. The leader must show willingness to adapt to the values, beliefs, and capacities of the members. Credibility of the leader and reciprocal trust are prerequisites for this mode of accepting the leader's message. Usually it is a democratic leader who induces internalization, since reciprocity is needed, and persuasive rather than coercive tactics are employed. In some respects the didactic group leader is a teacher embarked on an educational journey which is propelled or impeded by forces within the group, some of which are controlled by the leader.

CLINICAL EXAMPLE: CONTRASTS IN NONDIRECTIVE, DIRECTIVE, AND DIDACTIC GROUP THERAPY

Bernice was a psychiatric patient attending a day treatment center which offered an extensive group program. She was referred to the day treatment center after discharge from a state psychiatric hospital, had been attending the center for six weeks, and was involved in the group program of the therapeutic community. Her medication was Prolixin Enanthate 25 mgm, which was administered by injection every two weeks. Although her affect was flat, there were no indications of psychosis or impaired reality testing.

She was a young black woman, nineteen years old, whose diagnosis was chronic, undifferentiated schizophrenia. Brought up in a rural southern state, Bernice had migrated to a northern city with her mother, sister, and maternal grandmother and they had lived in the North about five years.   Until her breakdown and psychiatric hospitalization eighteen months earlier, she had lived with her family.   When Bernice was discharged from the hospital she returned home and, to her dismay, found many changes.   Her mother had married a widower and moved into his home.   Her older sister was living with a male friend. This meant that only the grandmother was still in the home, but she, too, was greatly changed.   During Bernice's stay in the hospital the grandmother had suffered a series of strokes and had become quite incapacitated.

The staff of the day treatment center realized that Bernice was very unhappy with her living arrangement, even though she talked little about it.   Her withdrawn manner and listlessness had been noted by the staff, and they were working together to avert the pattern of apathy and chronicity which Bernice seemed to be developing. Helping Bernice cope with her living situation became a high priority for the staff.   Certain characteristics were identified which caused Bernice to be unable to handle her current situation — poor problem-solving skills, poor communication skills, low self-esteem, and high anxiety levels (Finkelman, 1977).

It had been assumed by Bernice's mother and sister that responsibility for the grandmother could be delegated to Bernice. Even though the girl was unable to verbalize her resentment of this, there were indications that the care of the grandmother was extremely burdensome. With this background data, the staff began addressing the issue of Bernice's problematic lifestyle. Since the family members were unwilling to become involved with the day treatment center, the staff decided to deal with Bernice's problems through integrated group experiences which incorporated nondirective, directive, and didactic approaches.

Nondirective Group Therapy: Psychodrama

At the suggestion of the leader-director, Bernice devised a script which revealed the demanding behaviors of the elderly grandmother, the girl's reluctant care of her grandmother, her rage at her whole family, and her violent impulses toward her grandmother.   When Bernice tried to deny resentment and to feign affection for her grandmother, the leader encouraged her to examine her real feelings. As the drama was enacted, auxiliary egos gave voice to Bernice's anger, which constantly threatened to erupt as she bathed, fed, and dressed her grandmother.   Gradually Bernice lost her apathetic manner and began to talk to her grandmother in a hostile way. Her fear of losing control and of striking her grandmother came to dramatic life when the director-leader handed the girl a pillow, instructing her to treat the pillow as if it were her grandmother. The audience watched as Bernice began to tear at the pillow, ripping and punching it savagely. Finally she threw the pillow across the room, yelling that she wanted to be left alone. At the end of the scene Bernice was sobbing loudly.

Several of the patients who had been watching the drama began to comfort Bernice. The leader-director allowed time for the girl to become more composed and then began a discussion period. Many persons in the audience, staff members and patients, identified with Bernice and were able to say this to her. The leader used interventions which reassured Bernice that her feelings of entrapment were human, universal, and understandable. A staff member spent considerable time with Bernice on a one-to-one basis for the remainder of the day. The same staff member promised to be available that evening if Bernice needed to talk to someone by phone.

Directive Group Therapy

In the directive social learning group the predicament of Bernice became the focus of a subject session. With the help of the leader the group began to examine the contribution of Bernice's passivity to the problem. The group was supportive about the drastic changes which had occurred while she was in the hospital, but she was advised not to take responsibility for the turn of events. Anticipatory guidance was provided at the instigation of the leader. Bernice was confronted with her lack of self-assertiveness. She was given opportunities in the subject session and in subsequent meetings to practice making reasonable demands of other people. She was encouraged to ask for more help from her mother and sister, and to set some limits for her grandmother, who was a cantankerous old lady. Between the group sessions Bernice was asked to record interactions with her mother, sister, and grandmother, and to bring these accounts to the group. Any examples of assertive behavior from Bernice, either during meetings or between meetings, were rewarded with praise; examples of passivity or timidity received little attention and no approval from the leader of the group.

Didactic Group Therapy

The adolescent group held in the day treatment center used part of a session to help Bernice with her problem, but the approach was generalized to all the group members. The leader began by discussing developmental tasks at different periods during the life cycle. The developmental issues of individuation and separation were attributed to the adolescent and young adult stage of life. Then the developmental tasks of parents and grandparents were introduced. Bernice, along with others in the group, was encouraged to examine the developmental tasks of the elderly, especially after a serious illness. The question of who takes care of elderly relatives was raised by the leader. Dividing responsibility for the elderly was suggested as a way of reducing the burden laid upon one family member. Limit-setting, simplification of housekeeping tasks, and recourse to community support systems were discussed as aids for the elderly. As the session continued, Bernice became more willing to reveal her special problems. Practical methods of helping her grandmother were discussed. The group leader placed the discussion within the context of developmental tasks, indicating to Bernice that her own growth would be promoted if she won more freedom for herself. The cognitive assistance available in the group made the care of her grandmother begin to seem more manageable to Bernice. The emotional effects of the interventions caused her anxiety level to decline, and the support of the leader and members alleviated her sense of worthlessness. Placing Bernice's dilemma in a developmental framework enabled the leader to keep to the group contract, which was to consider the problem of adolescence. The leader also extended the message that the excessive demands being made on Bernice had counterparts in the lives of many individuals, including the leader and the group members. This form of intervention increased group cohesion and mobilized the members on Bernice's behalf. The mode of acceptance which developed in the group was identification rather than compliance.

SUMMARY

The difficulty of defining group psychotherapy was acknowledged and several alternative definitions were presented. In this chapter group therapy was defined as a treatment modality whose purpose is to produce psychological and social change through monitored group interactions. The difficulty of classifying types of group psychotherapy was discussed, and a triadic scheme was adopted. Psychotherapeutic groups were broadly categorized as nondirective, directive, and didactic; distinctions were based on the leadership perspective being used. Analytic group psychotherapy and psychodrama were given as examples of nondirective group therapy. Behavioral group therapy was discussed as representative of a directive group approach. Several special techniques suitable for directive group work were presented; these included the go-around and the subject session. Didactic group therapy was conceptualized as an educational experience which utilizes group forces and group dynamics. The didactic group leader was described as the group expert whose message may be accepted in different ways by the group. Three modes of acceptance displayed by group members were contrasted. Acceptance modes were differentiated along the lines of compliance, identification, or internalization by group members. The organizational procedures, selection, and preparation of members for each of the three categories of group psychotherapy were included.

REFERENCES

Anthony, E.J. "Comparison between Individual and Group Psychotherapy." In *Comprehensive Group Therapy*, H.I. Kaplan and B.J. Sadock, Eds. Baltimore: Williams and Wilkins, 1971.

Berne, E. *Principles of Group Treatment.* New York: Oxford University Press, 1966.

Davis, H.R. "Management of Innovation and Change in Mental Health Services." *Hospital and Community Psychiatry* 29, 1978, pages 649–658.

Finkelman, A.W. "The Nurse Therapist: Outpatient Crisis Intervention with the Chronic Psychiatric Patient." *Journal of Psychiatric Nursing and Mental Health Services* August 1977, pages 27–32.

Fried, E. "Basic Concepts in Group Psychotherapy." In *Comprehensive Group Psychotherapy*, H.I. Kaplan and B.J. Sadock, Eds. Baltimore: Williams and Wilkins, 1971.

Janosik, E.H. "Reachable and Teachable: Report on a Prison Alcoholism Group." *Journal of Psychiatric Nursing and Mental Health Services* 15, 1977, pages 24–28.

Kaplan, H.I., and B.J. Sadock. "Structured Interactional Group Psychotherapy." In *Comprehensive Group Therapy*, H.I. Kaplan and B.J. Sadock, Eds. Baltimore: Williams and Wilkins, 1971.

Klein, E., and Gould, L. "Boundary Management and Organizational Dynamics: A Case Study." *Social Psychiatry* 8, 1973, pages 204–211.

Lego, S. "Group Dynamic Theory and Application." In *Comprehensive Psychiatric Nursing*, J. Haber, A.M. Leach, S.M. Schudy, and B.F. Sideleau, Eds. New York: McGraw-Hill, 1979.

Levinson, D.J., and B. Astrachan. "Organizational Boundaries: Entry into the Mental Health Center." *Administration in Mental Health* Summer 1974, pages 3–12.

Marram, G.D. *The Group Approach in Nursing Practice.* St. Louis: C.V. Mosby, 1978.

Moreno, J.L. "Psychodrama." In *Comprehensive Group Therapy*, H.I. Kaplan and B.J. Sadock, Eds. Baltimore: Williams and Wilkins, 1971.

Morgan, A.J., and J.L. Moreno. *The Practice of Mental Health Nursing: A Community Approach.* Philadelphia: J.B. Lippincott, 1973.

Rosenbaum, M. "Group Psychotherapy and Psychodrama." In *Handbook of Clinical Psychology,* B.B. Wolman, Ed. New York: McGraw-Hill, 1965.

Sampson, E.E., and M.S. Marthas. *Group Process for the Health Professions.* New York: Wiley, 1977.

Slavson, S.R. *A Textbook in Analytic Group Psychotherapy.* New York: International Universities Press, 1964.

Solomon, P., and V.D. Patch. *Handbook of Psychiatry.* Palo Alto, CA.: Lange Medical Publications, 1974.

Spotnitz, H. "Comparison of Different Types of Group Psychotherapy." In *Comprehensive Group Psychotherapy,* H.I. Kaplan and B.J. Sadock, Eds. Baltimore: Williams and Wilkins, 1971.

Swanson, M.G. "A Check List for Group Leaders." In *Psychiatric Mental Health Nursing: Contemporary Readings,* B.A. Backer, P.M. Dubbert, and E.J.P. Eisenman, Eds. New York: D. Van Nostrand, 1978.

Yalom, I.D. *The Theory and Practice of Group Psychotherapy.* New York: Basic Books, 1975.

Yates, A.J. *Theory and Practice in Behavior Therapy.* New York: Wiley, 1975.

PART FOUR

Evaluation and Analysis of Group Work

17

Empirical Investigation: Research Strategy

Thomas R. Zastowny

Richard S. DeFrank

Evaluation of group work is endorsed by responsible clinicians seeking to judge the effectiveness of the group experience.

THEORETICAL PERSPECTIVES

In the absence of systematic evaluation of the group, interventions sometimes tend to be intuitive rather than deliberative and to be based on expedience rather than clinically sound concepts. Competent leadership based on a suitable theoretical framework, behaviorally defined objectives, and baseline or pregroup assessment of members are among the conditions that contribute to systematic evaluation of group effectiveness. General evaluative guidance was offered by Loomis (1979), who listed five sources of information pertaining to group effectiveness: 1) individual group members; 2) group leaders; 3) group as a whole; 4) significant persons outside the group; 5) group observers and supervisors.

Listing sources of information about group effectiveness does not guarantee the accuracy of data collected. Subjective data from any source, although quantified before collection, may be distorted. Even when carefully designed, pre- and post-group questionnaires filled out by leaders or members may not always reflect the changes which have occurred. Group members may be unaware of the extent to which they have changed, or leaders and members may attribute to the group more change than actually occurred. Reports of progress by significant others or by representatives of the external system, although generally more objective, may also be affected by unadmitted bias. Only through careful research — which minimizes subjectivity, quantifies change, and permits replication — can the effectiveness of the group experience be fairly evaluated.

When attempting to evaluate the group experience the investigator must decide what aspects of the group are to be explored. In addition, Loomis (1979) identified major perspectives of group experience which merit investigation. These are: 1) Group Structure, 2) Group Process, and 3) Group Outcomes. Having determined available sources of the data to be collected, and the major areas of investigation, the clinician engaged in evaluation must then turn to the complex issue of research design and strategy.

Rationale for Group Research

Group research is a problematic and challenging endeavor, and few research projects are more fraught with methodological difficulties (Frank, 1979; Hartman, 1979). The difficulties of the investigator are compounded by the widespread application of diverse forms of group treatment to different problems and by growing attention to such issues as leadership behaviors (Lieberman, Yalom, and Miles, 1973), group environment (Moos, 1974, 1973; Moos, Insel, and Humphrey, 1974), and patient perceptions (Peteroy, 1979). Despite methodological problems and variability in group outcome studies, some advances have been made in group research. Systematic research of group experience is currently being conducted in both clinical and laboratory settings (Parloff and Dies, 1977).

A critique of progress by Hartman (1979) revealed many remaining problems in group research. Much needs to be done in clarifying theory and refining methodology (Bednar and Kaul, 1978; Lewis and McCants, 1973). Since emphasis in this chapter is on general evaluative strategies in group research, a complete discussion of methodology and previous research findings is not attempted. For a thorough review of methodology, the reader is referred to Dunphy (1972). Excellent reviews of substantive findings in group research are available in Hare (1976), Gibbard, Hartman, and Mann (1974), and Ofshe (1973).

Conceptual Orientation

It is impossible to overstate the importance of lucid, concise hypotheses and objectives in any research project. To avert preliminary problems in group research the investigator must first consider alternative dichotomies such as: group versus individual approaches; clinical versus statistical methods; and process versus outcome variables. It is also important to appreciate the intimate relationship among conceptual frameworks, methodology, and research adequacy, and to recognize that groups are not merely aggregates of separate individuals (Lewis and McCants, 1973).

How well hypotheses and objectives have been defined by the investigator may be ascertained by asking certain questions (Maher, 1978). If these questions are answered affirmatively, alternative experimental methods may be considered, and their strengths and weaknesses compared.

- Is there an explicit hypothesis?
- Has the origin of the hypothesis been made explicit?
- Was the hypothesis correctly derived from the theory cited?
- Are other opposing hypotheses compatible with the same theory?
- Is there an explicit rationale for the measures chosen, and was the rationale for the measures derived logically from the hypothesis?

STRATEGIES FOR RESEARCH AND EVALUATION

Experimental Designs

Experimental designs appropriate for group research may be divided into two categories: 1) single subject/single group designs, and 2) within subject-within group/between subject-between group designs. Each of these experimental designs has its own strengths and weaknesses.

Single Subject/Single Group Designs

Single organism or single case experimental designs represent, in their most basic form, an extensive study of the individual. Such designs, employed in many early investigations, suffered a temporary setback with the advent of group comparison methodologies and inferential statistics. Single case research designs, however, have been revitalized, especially in the behavioral sciences (Hersen and Barlow, 1976). Recent progress in single subject methodology and statistics, the detailed information obtainable, and the resurgence of single case designs warrant their inclusion here.

Single case experiments within a group and case study research using a single group as subject are both viable, and afford undeniable advantages. In single case research there is more control over experimental conditions related to subject variability. When single subject or single group experiments are used, influences such as subject/environment, subject/setting, or subject/experimental manipulation are constant, because only a single subject is being studied. In using subjects as self-experts or self-reporters with regard to intrasubject conditions and variation, the subject pool is small ($n = 1$). More time can then be invested in differentiating change due to personal characteristics from change due to experimental manipulation. An assumption of the single case experiment (in which subjects monitor themselves) is that individuals can record self-change accurately and that their perceptions of change can be reported meaningfully.

Savings relative to investigative resources constitutes another advantage of single case research. Essential here is the notion of statistical power, or how able the experiment is to detect expected differences in proportion to the time and effort the investigator is willing to expend in order to achieve the statistical power. Single case experiments can also sometimes avoid ethical issues which accompany control groups. Frequently in single subject or single group studies, the same treatments are administered to all subjects, thereby avoiding the ethical dilemma of placing some subjects in a situation of receiving no treatment, particularly when this might constitute a violation of their rights.

Developmentalists long ago recognized the value of longitudinal studies in which single subjects or single group observations are made over time. Since single case designs emphasize intrasubject and intragroup variability, they are practical for isolating relatively small effects and differences (Shontz, 1976). Between group comparisons, which pool subject changes to obtain group means, may overlook important individual differences of small magnitude.

Within Subject-Within Group Designs and Between Subject-Between Group Designs

The methodological issues relevant to within-group designs have been described extensively by Hersen and Barlow (1976). Methodological issues relevant to between group designs have been presented by Campbell and Stanley (1963). In this chapter, guidelines for using these designs are summarized and possible threats to experimental adequacy are discussed briefly.

Given the differences in within subject designs and between subject designs, there are situations in which one type of design is more appropriate than the other. Between subject designs may be used to evaluate treatment packages, to compare treatment strategies, and to modify group behavior. Within subject designs may be used to evaluate changes in the individual member; to study certain areas, such as obesity research, which show great intersubject and intrasubject variability; and to conduct research where defined clinical reversals are possible (Wilson, 1978).

Problems with between subject designs include possible ethical issues, practicality, averaging of results, generality of the findings, and intersubject variability. Difficulties with within subject designs, especially the single subject approach, include large variations in the individual baseline, intrasubject variability, and auto-correlation.

Under what conditions are group designs more appropriate than single case study designs? According to Kazdin (1978) and Shontz (1976), group designs rather than single subject designs should be adopted when the group rather than the individual is the focus of interest, when the research study attempts to isolate effects of member/leader or member/treatment variables, and when the relative efficacy of treatment packages or treatment components is being evaluated.

In contemporary research, emphasis is on flexibility and on rather complicated interactionist designs. In constructing a research design, some experienced investigators advocate combinations of within subject and between subject strategies. It has also been suggested that because of high intersubject variability in group treatment outcomes, single subject data should be reported in the context of between group designs (Wilson, 1978). Another recommendation is to use single case designs to isolate therapeutic factors and then to use a group design to further evaluate the identified therapeutic factors. Suggestions for a comprehensive design sequence include the following steps:

1) Use of intensive single subject designs to isolate salient treatment factors (Hersen and Barlow, 1976).
2) Extrapolation of salient treatment factors to group settings.
3) Replication on a small scale of studies which combine finalized treatment factors with multiple assessments for evaluation (Hartman, 1979).

4) More comprehensive study of the identified factors in multivariate experiments.
5) Replications on a larger scale, using different sites and different populations.

Methodological Refinements

Solutions to many problems of group research may be refined initially through attention to the following concerns. Consideration should be given to background and demographic characteristics of subjects (Garfield, 1978), to subject selection and attrition (Frank, 1979; Wilson, 1978), and to follow-up after termination of the group (Hartman, 1979; Malan, Balfour, Hood, and Shooter, 1976). Follow-up procedures can help answer questions about the maintenance and generalization of change (Ashby and Wilson, 1977; Lieberman, Yalom, and Miles, 1973).

Consideration should be given to the leaders' characteristics, experience, and effectiveness regarding the treatment in question (Frank, 1979; Wilson, 1978). Inclusion of both member and leader attributes allows evaluation of optimal treatment combinations such as member/leader and leader/treatment interactions along relevant dimensions (Zastowny and Janosik, 1981; Posthuma and Carr, 1975; Best, 1975; McLachlan, 1972).

Some common threats to experimental adequacy include the use of nonspecific hypotheses and unrepresentative samples; absence of random assignment; poor definition, inadequate assessment, and implementation of experimental factors; uncontrolled variables, inaccurate replication of causal relationships; inappropriate data presentation and interpretation, and faulty conclusions. Recognition of these potential hazards may serve to improve the effectiveness of the experimental design.

EVALUATION PERSPECTIVES

Previous research dealt with structure, process, or outcomes in group settings; rarely have investigators combined these areas, even though many studies indicate their interrelatedness. In discussing group process and group outcomes it may be stated that comprehending one enhances understanding of the other. In outcome studies one often fails to specify process; in process studies one often fails to consider outcomes (Hartman, 1979). Furthermore, considerations related to group structure are frequently ignored (Yalom and Rand, 1966). Therefore the evaluation perspectives of group structure, process, and outcome are discussed in some detail, with attention to their interrelatedness.

Definitions

For purposes of discussion, group structure is defined as the pattern of interrelationships among the members of a group at a particular point in time. Process is conceptualized as the dynamic interplay occurring within the group over time. A reasonable research question might consist of asking how group structure or interrelationships have altered over time. Outcome is defined as change resulting from the experimental intervention, from group structure and process, and from subject variables. Without an understanding of relationships between individual members (structure), changes in the group over time (process), and eventual effects (outcomes), exploration of group phenomena remains limited in scope. Simultaneous assessment and ongoing measurement of structure, process, and outcomes provide a wide vantage point from which to study groups (Piper, Doan, Edwards, and Jones, 1979).

Structure

There are a number of ways in which group structure or patterned interrelationships may be assessed. One set of techniques is called *sociometrics*. When sociometric techniques are used, group members may be asked to select from their ranks those members who are most liked, most respected, most powerful, and so on. These choices, denoted by directional arrows, may be charted on a figure or sociogram which shows the extent of selection, mutual selection, the presence of stellar members who are selected most often, and the existence of group isolates. The sociogram can generate data about intragroup attraction, status, power, and cohesiveness. This last factor can be estimated by identifying the influence, size, number, and composition of subgroups as shown in the sociogram.

Figures 17-1 and 17-2 illustrate sociograms of a hypothetical obesity therapy group at the beginning and at the end of treatment. At the start of therapy there is little cohesiveness and only two mutual selections (1:5 and 3:4). Some people (X_6) are isolated and do not make or receive any selections. It may also be stated that person X_5 appears to be the relative "star" of the group, attracting three selections. The end of treatment (Figure 17-2) shows a very different configuration, with some people ($X_2 : X_3 : X_4$ and X_7) forming a fairly close-knit group while others still remain relatively isolated.(X_6). Notice also that subgroup ($X_1 : X_5$) can be identified. This type of analysis yields considerable information about groups with regard to power, likes and dislikes, and deference than can help investigators more fully conceptualize group structure and dynamics.

Figure 17–1   SOCIOGRAM OF OBESITY THERAPY GROUP AT THE START
OF TREATMENT

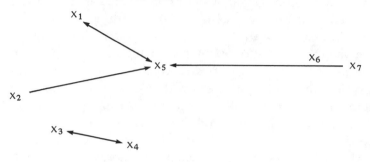

Figure 17–2   SOCIOGRAM OF THE SAME OBESITY THERAPY GROUP
PRESENTED IN FIGURE 1 AT THE END OF TREATMENT

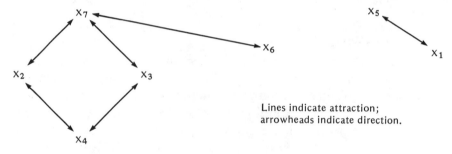

Lines indicate attraction;
arrowheads indicate direction.

The procedure of asking members about their peers can be used to
delineate group roles as well. Hare (1976) reviewed a body of research
which suggested that differentiation of group roles leads to the development of a task leader and a socioemotional leader, and that these
leaders may or may not be the same person. Using a sociogram or
other sociometric procedure helps differentiate such leaders and show
their emergence over time.

Communication Network   Another aspect of group structure
is the communication network or the pattern of who talks to whom.
The structure of a communication network can be distinguished from
the actual act of communicating, since observing a communication
network deals with communication channels evident among members.
Observation of group interactions through sociometric procedures
helps the investigator to recognize the modes of communication usually employed, whether communication is verbal or nonverbal, and

the frequency of communication attempts made in the group. The data are comparable to information obtained by using a sociogram.

Process

There is considerable overlap between group structure and process as the terms are applied here. This is shown by the observational techniques used to assess both these aspects of group experience. Process may be evaluated through observational methods employed in several ways. First, measured observations may be made of naturally occurring group interactions, either in the laboratory or in a natural setting. Some investigators choose to develop their own rating scales with which to measure interactional variables. It is true that individualized scales have the advantage of dealing with the group dimensions of greatest interest to the investigator. At the same time such scales may not be as reliable as more standardized observational measures. One of the latter is Bales's Interaction Process Analysis (IPA) (Bales, 1950). This measurement uses twelve categories of behavior, three of which relate to positive reactions within the group, three to negative reactions, three to problem-solving attempts, and three to conformation-seeking behavior. The extent to which these categories of behavior are demonstrated is partly a function of the group task. Some groups are engaged in a task which demands high amounts of information-giving activity while other groups, which are oriented to process, may show little frequency of informational communication (Hare, 1960, 1976). Categories for Bales's Interaction Process Analysis (adapted from Bales, 1950, and Hare, 1976) follow below.

I. Social-Emotional Behavior

    A. Positive reactions:
        1. Shows solidarity: jokes, raises others' status, gives help
        2. Shows tension release: laughs, shows satisfaction
        3. Shows agreement: passive acceptance, understands, complies

    B. Negative reactions:
        4. Shows disagreement: passive rejection, formality, withholds help
        5. Shows tension: asks for help, withdraws from field
        6. Shows antagonism: deflates others' status, defends or asserts self

II. Task Behavior

    A. Problem-solving:

        7. Gives suggestions: direction, implying autonomy for others

        8. Gives opinion: evaluation, analysis, expresses feeling, wish

        9. Gives information: orientation, repeats, clarifies, confirms

    B. Questioning:

        10. Asks for information: orientation, repetition, confirmation

        11. Asks for opinion: evaluation, analysis, expression of feelings

        12. Asks for suggestions: direction, possible ways of action

The Bales interaction scoring method conceptualizes the group as an ordered system and helps the scorer attend to each transaction as it occurs. Problem-solving activities are extracted from the total proceedings and are scored, but other dimensions of the group experience are not. Some deficiencies of the scoring method have been acknowledged by Mills (1967) as follows:

1. Substantive aspect of interaction is not recorded either in detail or thematically. (Content)
2. Intent, purpose, or aim of the actors are not recorded. (Motivation)
3. Affective content of actors is not recorded. (Feelings)
4. Cognitive experiences which stimulate or are stimulated by the interactions are not recorded. (Thoughts)

Consensus Rorschach A second method of making observations is to give the group a specific task to accomplish and to examine members' interactions while thus engaged. One advantage of this is that it improves comparisons among groups by standardizing the task situation. Some of the research using IPA has involved groups working on assigned problem-solving. The analyses of such activities may be used to determine qualities of intragroup functioning and to note intergroup differences. A further example of this type of procedure is the *consensus Rorschach*, which asks a group to agree on the perceived contents or meaning of an inkblot. This technique has been used extensively with families, especially with respect to research on schizophrenia (Herman and Jones, 1976; Wynne, 1968). The consensus Rorschach can generate information about how group members acknowledge one another's ideas, about positive and negative relationships, and about the development of consensus. Observations of naturally occurring group behavior and observations of group behavior around specified tasks provide valuable insights into the nature of group process.

Procedures described so far have dealt with observations of interactions expressed mostly through verbal language. Other aspects of group behavior around specific tasks can provide valuable insights into the nature of group process.

Many investigators have studied the ways in which people maintain, increase, or decrease distance from one another, and have commented on the implications of space as a variable in interpersonal transactions (Shaw, 1976, 1964; Altman, 1975; Evans and Howard, 1973). Intentional and unintentional messages may be transmitted through nonverbal channels such as facial expressions, eye contact, and body positioning.

Outcome

The evaluation of outcomes in group research reflects the complexity of group research in general. Deciding what to measure and obtaining a measurement tool are only the beginning of an often difficult process. Evaluation of outcomes in group settings may be one of the most difficult challenges faced by an investigator (Hartman, 1979; Parloff and Dies, 1977; Abramowitz, 1976; Smith, 1975). Without theoretical and methodological clarity, the researcher may encounter baffling results and become entangled in a web of diffuse outcome considerations. The state of outcome research suggests that single perspective evaluations are usually limited and that multiple assessments (repeated measures) in different domains (physiological, psychological, and behavioral), collected from leaders, members, and observers will yield more robust findings (Strupp and Hadley, 1977).

Because of the foregoing considerations, the premise that adequate outcome evaluation involves several levels of functioning and requires various evaluation perspectives seems reasonable. Previously the use of different outcome criteria across studies made it virtually impossible to compare findings. What is now essential is that investigators include in group studies behavioral, interpersonal, and intrapersonal outcome measurements which can be quantified and compared (Hartman, 1979).

Environmental Influences

A relatively neglected area of group reserach is the interaction between groups and their environment. Characteristics of the environment in which the group operates can affect group structure, process,
and outcomes. One approach to the study of these relationships is
found in *ecological psychology*. Ecological psychology or behavioral
ecology is the study of naturally occurring behavior, showing how
behavior is enacted over various environmental locations designated
as behavior settings. Such studies offer information about how
different groups use different environments, and how group patterns
of use, influenced by the environment, may affect group outcomes.
One investigator who examined patient activities in a rehabilitation
unit found that patterns of involvement in various hospital settings
such as the ward, the occupational unit, and physical therapy facilities
affected the length of a patient's stay in the rehabilitation unit
(Willems, 1976).

The architectural plan of a care facility may affect the behaviors
of hospital staff and of patients (Holahan and Saegert, 1973; Ronco,
1972). Attractiveness of the group setting (Mintz, 1956), seating
arrangements (Strodtbeck and Hooks, 1961), and room temperature
are among the environmental variables which affect group interaction
(Griffitt and Veitch, 1971). These and similar studies attest to the
value of observing group behavior from an ecological viewpoint.

As an outgrowth of concern for environmental effects, attempts
have been made to develop tools which measure the social and emotional climate of the environment. A Ward Atmosphere Scale was
developed by Moos (1974) to measure treatment programs in relation to environmental involvement, support, autonomy, clarity,
and other factors. The Group Atmosphere Scale (Silbergeld, Manderscheid, and Koenig, 1977) assessed patient-environmental effects
by means of the "perceived psychosocial atmosphere" within the
group. Although these scales were devised for psychotherapy groups,
they might well be adapted for use with less specialized groups.

SUMMARY

This chapter discussed general strategies, experimental designs, and
relevant issues for group research. A recommendation was made that
comprehensive group research include simultaneous consideration of
structure, process, and outcome perspectives using a multiple assessment viewpoint. Longitudinal studies with repeated measurements
and follow-up were described as having potential for yielding com-

plete and accurate data. Systematic and carefully designed research was suggested to improve comparability of data across studies, to permit understanding of causation, and to make cumulative contributions to theory. Various experimental designs for group research were compared and contrasted. Sociometric observations and interactional process analysis were described, along with methods of assessing the effects of environmental factors on group process and outcomes. Literature cited in the chapter was selective because of the abundance of material available, but the selected references offer perspectives from which to study groups.

REFERENCES

Abramowitz, C.V. "The Effectiveness of Group Psychotherapy with Children." *Archives of General Psychiatry* 33, 1976, pages 320–326.

Altman, I. *The Environment and Social Behaviors.* Monterey, CA.: Brooks/Cole, 1975.

Ashby, W.A., and T. Wilson. "Behavior Therapy for Obesity: Booster Sessions and Long-Term Maintenance of Weight Loss." *Behavior Research and Therapy* 15, 1977, pages 451–463.

Bales, R.F. *Interaction Process Analysis: A Method for the Study of Small Groups.* Cambridge, MA.: Addison-Wesley, 1950.

Bednar, R.L., and T.J. Kaul. "Experimental Group Research: Current Perspectives." In *Handbook of Psychotherapy and Behavior Change*, S.L. Garfield and A.E. Bergin, Eds. New York: Wiley, 1971.

Best, J.A. "Tailoring Smoking Withdrawal Procedures to Personality and Motivational Differences." *Journal of Consulting and Clinical Psychology* 43, 1975, pages 1–8.

Campbell, D.T., and J.C. Stanley. *Experimental and Quasi-Experimental Designs for Research.* Chicago: Rand McNally, 1963.

Carr, J.E. "Differentiation Similarity of Patient and Therapist and the Outcome of Psychotherapy." *Journal of Abnormal Psychology* 76, 1970, pages 361–369.

Dunphy, D.C. *The Primary Group: A Handbook for Analysis and Field Research.* New York: Appleton-Century-Crofts, 1972.

Evans, G.W., and R.B. Howard. "Personal Space." *Psychological Bulletin* 80, 1973, pages 334–344.

Frank, J.D. "The Present Status of Outcome Studies." *Journal of Consulting and Clinical Psychology* 47, 1979, pages 310–316.

Garfield, S.L. "Research on Client Variables in Psychotherapy." In *Handbook of Psychotherapy and Behavior Change*, S.L. Garfield and A.E. Bergin, Eds. New York: Wiley, 1978, pages 191–232.

Gibbard, G.S.; J.J. Hartman; and R.D. Mann, Eds. *Analysis of Groups.* San Francisco: Jossey-Bass, 1974.

Griffitt, W., and R. Veitch. "Hot and Crowded: Influences of Population Density and Temperature on Interpersonal Affective Behavior." *Journal of Personality and Social Psychology* 17, 1971, pages 92–98.

Hare, A.P.; E.F. Borgatta; and R.F. Bales. *Small Groups, Studies in Social Interaction.* New York: Knopf, 1965.

Hare, A.P. *Handbook of Small Group Research.* 2nd ed. New York: Free Press, 1976.

Hartman, J.J. "Small Group Methods of Personal Change." *Annual Review in Psychology* 30, 1979, pages 453–476.

Herman, B.F., and J.E. Jones. "Lack of Acknowledgment in the Family Rorschachs of Families with a Child at Risk for Schizophrenia." *Family Press* 15, 1976, pages 289–302.

Hersen, M., and D.H. Barlow. *Single Case Experimental Designs.* New York: Pergamon Press, 1976.

Holahan, C.J., and S. Saegert. "Behavioral and Attitudinal Effects of Large-Scale Variation in the Physical Environment of Psychiatric Wards." *Journal of Abnormal Psychology* 82, 1973, pages 454–462.

Kazdin, A.E. "Methodological and Interpretive Problems of Single-Case Experimental Designs." *Journal of Consulting and Clinical Psychology* 46, 1978, pages 629–642.

Lewis, P., and J. McCants. "Some Current Issues in Group Psychotherapy Research." *The International Journal of Group Psychotherapy* 23, 1973, pages 268–278.

Lieberman, M.A.; I.D. Yalom; and M.B. Miles. *Encounter Groups: First Facts.* New York: Basic Books, 1973.

Lindzey, G., and E. Aronson, Eds. *Handbook of Social Psychology.* 2nd ed. Menlo Park, CA.: Addison-Wesley, 1969.

Loomis, M. *Group Process for Nurses.* St. Louis: C.V. Mosby, 1979.

Maher, B.A. "A Reader's, Writer's, and Reviewer's Guide to Assessing Research Reports in Clinical Psychology." *Journal of Consulting and Clinical Psychology* 46, 1978, pages 835–838.

———. "Stimulus Sampling in Clinical Research; Representative Design Reveiwed." *Journal of Consulting and Clinical Psychology* 46, 1978, pages 643–647.

Malan, D.H.; H.G. Balfour; V.G. Hood; and A.M.N. Shooter. "Group Therapy: A Long-Term Follow-Up Study." *Archives of General Psychiatry* 33, 1976, pages 1303–1315.

McLachlan, J.F.C. "Benefit from Group Therapy as a Function of Patient-Therapist Match on Conceptual Level." *Psychotherapy: Theory, Research, Practice* 9, 1972, pages 317–323.

Mills, T.M. *The Sociology of Small Groups.* Englewood Cliffs, N.J.: Prentice-Hall, 1967.

Mintz, N. "Effects of Esthetic Surroundings: II. Prolonged and Repeated Experience in a 'Beautiful' and an 'Ugly' Room." *Journal of Psychology* 41, 1956, pages 459–466.

Moos, R.H. *The Social Climate Scales: An Overview.* Palo Alto, CA.: Consulting Psychologist Press, 1974.

———. *Evaluating Treatment Environment: A Social Ecological Approach.* New York: Wiley, 1974.

———. Conceptualization of Human Environments. *American Psychologist* 28, 1973, pages 652–665.

——— ; P.M. Insel; and B. Humphrey. *Preliminary Manual for the Family, Work, and Group Environment Scales.* Palo Alto, CA.: Consulting Psychologist Press, 1974.

Ofshe, R.J., Ed. *Interpersonal Behaviors in Small Groups*. Englewood Cliffs, N.J.: Prentice-Hall, 1973.

Parloff, M.B., and R.R. Dies. "Group Psychotherapy Outcome Research 1966–1975." *The International Journal of Group Psychotherapy* 27, 1977, pages 321–341.

Peteroy, E.T. "Effects of Member and Leader Expectations on Group Outcome." *Journal of Counseling Psychology* 26, 1979, pages 534–537.

Piper, W.E.; B.D. Doan; E.M. Edwards; and B.D. Jones. "Cotherapy Behavior, Group Therapy Process, and Treatment Outcome." *Journal of Consulting and Clinical Psychology* 47, 1979, pages 1081–1089.

Posthuma, A.B., and J.E. Carr. "Differentiation Matching in Psychotherapy." *Canadian Psychological Review* 16, 1975, pages 35–43.

Ronco, P.G., "Human Factors Applied to Hospital Patient Care." *Human Factors* 14, 1972, pages 461–470.

Sellitiz, C.; M. Johoda; M. Deutsch; and S.W. Cook. *Research Methods in Social Relations*. New York: Holt Rinehart & Winston, 1959.

Shaw, M.E. *Group Dynamics: The Psychology of Small Group Behavior*. New York: McGraw-Hill, 1976.

——————. "Communication Networks." In *Advances in Experimental Social Psychology*, L. Bakowitz, Ed. Vol. 1. New York: Academic Press, 1964.

Shontz, F.C. "Single-Organism Designs." In *Data Analysis Strategies and Designs for Substance Abuse Research*. P.M. Bentler, D.J. Lettieri, and G.A. Austin, Eds. Research Issues 13. MD.: National Institute on Drug Abuse, 1976.

Silbergeld, S.; R.W. Manderscheid; and G.R. Koenig. "The Psychosocial Environment in Group Therapy Evaluation." *The International Journal of Group Psychotherapy* 27, 1977, pages 153–163.

Smith, P.B. "Controlled Studies of the Outcome of Sensitivity Training." *Psychological Bulletin* 82, 1975, pages 597–622.

Strodtbeck, F.L., and L.H. Hooks. "The Social Dimensions of a Twelve Man Jury Table." *Sociometry* 24, 1961, pages 397–415.

Strupp, H.H., and S.W. Hadley. "A Tripartite Model of Mental Health and Therapeutic Outcomes with Special Reference to Negative Effects in Psychotherapy." *American Psychologist* 32, 1977, pages 187–196.

Willems, E.P. "Behavioral Ecology, Health Status, and Health Care: Applications to the Rehabilitation Setting." In *Human Behavior and Environment: Advances in Theory and Research*, I. Altman and J. Wohlurill, Eds. New York: Plenum Press, 1976.

Wilson, G.T. "Methodological Considerations in Treatment Outcome Research on Obesity." *Journal of Consulting and Clinical Psychology* 46, 1978, pages 687–702.

Wynne, L.C. "Consensus Rorschachs and Related Procedures for Studying Interpersonal Patterns." *Journal of Projective Techniques and Personality Assessment* 32, 1968, pages 352–356.

Yalom, I.D., and K. Rand. "Compatibility and Cohesiveness in Therapy Groups." *Archives of General Psychiatry* 15, 1966, pages 267–275.

Zastowny, T.R., and E.H. Janosik. *Alcohol Treatment Planning and Evaluation: A Brief Report on Cognitive Orientation, Identified Curative Factors* and *Depression as Predictors for Treatment Outcomes in Alcoholism Group Therapy Programs.* Publication in progress, 1981. Center for Naval Analysis Grant, Office of Naval Research-Grant #N0014-76-0001.

18

Empirical Investigations: Data Analysis

Richard S. DeFrank

Thomas R. Zastowny

When assessing group structure, process, or outcome, it is essential that the variables of interest be measured as specifically as possible, and that these variables be analyzed, theoretically and empirically, in appropriate fashion. This chapter surveys some of the concerns and options available in selecting and using analytic techniques.

RELIABILITY

Whether the investigator develops measurement tools expressly for the project at hand or adopts standardized measurements, several major issues should be routinely raised about the measures used. Initially, it should be determined if the measure is reliable; that is, whether the instrument produces consistent results for the same subject over a number of administrations (multiple measurements), or whether it is influenced by extraneous factors which may increase its variability. Reliability also refers to the degree of agreement among different raters using the same instrument with the same sample.

Highly reliable measures are valuable because they indicate that changes across time are due to experimental manipulations and, therefore, are not attributable to random fluctuations in the data.

VALIDITY

Another important concept in this area is validity, which has several components which must be considered: an initial question is whether the measure has *content* validity; that is, does it measure the variable it was intended to measure? Second, does it have *face* validity, or the appearance of being a valid test? Third, does the measure have *criterion-related* validity; that is, does it predict behavior adequately? Validity becomes a problem when the measurement tool used to rate a behavior or attribute does not measure what it purports to measure.

OBJECTIVITY AND PRACTICALITY

Objectivity, related to intra-rater and inter-rater reliability, asks whether the measurement procedure relies on simple, overt behaviors or attributes, or depends on more complicated inferences made by the observer. Objectivity may be questionable when scores assigned by one rater differ from scores assigned by a second rater using the same measurement tool with the same subjects. In addition, objectivity might be questioned whenever the same rater assessing the same persons fails to obtain consistent scores. Practicality of an instrument relates to its cost in terms of time, work, and money, and to the availability of appropriate analytic procedures. The reliability, validity, objectivity, and practicality of an instrument tool should be carefully considered prior to its use in an investigation.

GENERALIZABILITY

Besides evaluating various aspects of a group experience, clinicians are also interested in generalization of the findings. Generalizability refers to the application of the data to other populations or, in this instance, to other groups. An investigator who found that drop-out rates in a group were significantly related to the number of preparatory sessions might choose to generalize this finding to future group undertakings. At the same time the investigator might well continue to replicate the first small-scale study in order to validate the findings.

In group research a single causal factor can seldom be isolated. In general there are two theoretical ways of thinking about causation in research. *Deterministic* causes are those which are necessary and sufficient to produce a certain effect. *Probabilistic* causes are necessary, but are not in and of themselves sufficient to produce a certain effect. An example of a deterministic cause is the fact that one must first join a group in order to be a group member. Joining determines membership in the group. A *probabilistic* cause is that joining a group will produce beneficial effects on the members. The probability of beneficial effects cannot be tested unless an individual joins the group, but group membership cannot of itself produce beneficial results unless other conditions are also present. Research endeavors to identify variables of the group experience, isolate those variables, and demonstrate relationships among them. Analysis shows the strength and direction of relationships among two or more variables, but causality is often not proven.

CLASSIFICATION OF VARIABLES

Another important consideration in the selection of measurement techniques is the type of variable being investigated. One approach is to use the experimental design, in which some factors are treated as independent variables under the control of the experimenter and are assumed to have some effect on the subjects. Examples of independent variables include group composition or leader intervention techniques. Other criteria are viewed as dependent variables. Dependent variables indicate in some way the impact of the independent variables on the subjects. Examples of dependent variables are group performance, length of hospitalization, or rates of recidivism.

Variables are described as intervening when they operate between independent and dependent variables. Group interaction may be considered an intervening variable which may or may not influence dependent variables. Antecedent variables predate the implementation of independent variables and are not under experimental control, unless included as selection criteria. Prior acquaintance of group members or their previous health history are examples of antecedent variables; classification of variables has implications for the selection and application of data analytic procedures.

MEASUREMENT

Physiological Measurement

A distinction has been made between physiological, psychological, and behavioral measurements (McGrath, 1970). While these categories overlap somewhat, they are useful in illustrating the dimensions of various measurements. Physiological measures are often used in group settings to assess such variables as obesity (skin-fold measures) or hypertension (blood pressure levels). Stress measurements include galvanic skin responses (Lazarus et al., 1963; Lazarus, 1966), heart and pulse rates (Selye, 1976), trace measurements of corticosteroids (Mason et al., 1976), and catecholamines (Frankenhaeuser, 1975). The exact nature of the physiological measures used depends on the research questions, subject population, and resources available to the researcher. Frequency and intrusiveness of data collection are other considerations in the selection of measurement procedures.

Psychological Measurement

Although self-report scales have limitations, they are the most popular method of psychological assessment. Examples of specific measures are the Taylor Manifest Anxiety Scale (Taylor, 1953) and the Minnesota Multiphasic Personality Inventory (Hathaway and McKinley, 1967), which assess such variables as anxiety and personality composition. Other scales have been designed to evaluate responses to potentially stressful situations such as hospitalization, one of which is the Hospital Rating Scale (Volicer, Isenberg, and Burns, 1977). Additional psychological data may be obtained from external indicators of intrapsychic functioning, such as nonverbal behaviors (Mehrabian, 1970, 1972), or from projective tests, such as the Thematic Apperception Test (Murray, 1943) or the Rorschach Inkblot Test (Rorschach, 1942). References to a wide range of psychological scales are made by Chun, Cobb, and French (1975) and Andrulis (1977). Other works focus on specific areas such as personality (Sundberg, 1977; Cattell, 1973; Buros, 1970) or attitudes (Robinson and Shaver, 1973). Thus there is an impressive range of measurement scales available to ascertain the psychological characteristics and reactions of group members.

Behavioral Measurement

Measurement tools are also available for examining behavioral variables, among which is the Interaction Process Analysis of Bales (1950), which was discussed in Chapter 17. Behavior checklists may be used to assess the occurrence of specific activities in a group (Walls et al., 1977). Straus and Brown (1978) reviewed a variety of measurement tools for the investigation of family groups. An innovative method of evaluating behavior using goal attainment scaling (GAS) was devised by Kiresuk and Sherman (1968). This evaluative procedure asks staff members to rate clients on expected outcomes. Actual results and deviations of expected outcomes from actual outcomes give an indication of the effectiveness of the program.

This brief review directs investigators to consideration of relevant measures for research studies, and to selection of several different evaluative tools which measure the same theoretical construct. After the administration of measurement tools, the collected data must be analyzed. Discussion of the analytic phase of the investigative process follows.

ANALYSIS OF DATA

Analytic Techniques

As research in group structure, process, and outcome has increased in quantity and become qualitatively more complex, the number of analytic procedures available to researchers has expanded correspondingly. A few of the more common methods of data analysis are presented here and additional reference sources are recommended. For general information on statistical procedure, Blalock (1979) and Hays (1963) are suggested. Researchers are also reminded of nonparametric statistics (Siegel, 1956), which may be used under certain conditions and offer alternatives to the techniques described here. Nonparametric designs are appropriate when certain assumptions cannot be made. No matter which statistical approach is taken (parametric or nonparametric) generalizability may be limited in small group research. Replication of studies and intergroup comparisons are also strongly recommended in this research area.

Factor Analysis

This procedure is primarily used for its data reduction capabilities. Factor analysis determines the existence of a small set of factors or components which may underlie a larger data set. It is used primarily in an exploratory way or to test hypotheses about the presence or characteristics of the factors. Factor analysis may also be used when constructing measurement tools, since it shows major groupings in a large pool of items. It also notes redundant and irrelevant items, and the significance of these to the obtained factors. The researcher who is concerned with the construction of scales should be cognizant of factor analytic techniques. Further information is available in Comrey (1973, 1978), Gorsuch (1974), and Mulaik (1972).

Cluster Analysis

This is another set of important data description/data reduction techniques useful for identifying clusters of entities, generating schemes for classification, and uncovering structure inherent in data. A common procedure involves first considering each observation as a cluster, then combining the two closest observations into a single cluster, merging the closest clusters of the new set, and so on until one is left with a cluster containing all observations. The intermediate clusters are then examined to determine the best solution for the data at hand. This is an especially valuable technique when attempting to identify groups of individuals who are similar on a number of characteristics.   For example, clustering individuals on a number of shared variables may help predict behavior in different group settings, an approach with applications to clinical research in nursing. Additional explanations of cluster analysis are available in Anderberg (1973), Everitt (1974), Hartigan (1975), and Wolfe (1970).

Cluster sampling is sometimes used instead of random sampling when the resources of the investigator are limited. An investigator might wish to study curative group factors emphasized by alcoholism group leaders throughout the state, but find it too difficult to reach every group leader. A reasonable alternative might be to include ten leaders from every county in the state. In this way the entire state is represented with considerable economy of time and work. The clusters of group leaders might be considered as one unit, thus reducing the number of subjects for data collection and analysis. A degree of randomness or representativeness may be sacrificed, but sometimes practical considerations prevail.

Analysis of Variance

This procedure estimates the differences among group means and is appropriate for the comparison of groups in an experimental design. For example, the effects of different leadership styles on member satisfaction among comparable groups may be examined by using analysis of variance techniques. Analysis of variances estimates whether differences between group means are greater than mean differences within groups. The impact of a number of variables may be viewed simultaneously, which allows for the inclusion of covariates and specification of independent effects. Detailed information is available in the work of Wilkinson (1975) and Woodward and Overall (1975).

Multivariate Analysis

When an investigator looks into relationships between variables, what is being sought is the extent to which one variable is associated with another. An investigator considering attrition in a psychotherapy group might want to learn whether age, sex, education, or preparation for the group experience are variables associated with high drop-out rates. When the investigator compares an independent variable (sex) to a dependent variable (premature termination), the hypothesis is that the first causes the latter. However, the cause of premature termination may not necessarily be related to the sex of the member. More women than men may drop out of the group, not because they are women but for other reasons. The question which must be confronted is: What factors other than female gender cause more women than men to drop out of the group?

One way of comparing more than one variable is to engage in multivariate analysis, which discovers correlations between multiple variables. *Univariate analysis* takes a single independent variable, such as sex of group members, and attempts to discover its relation to premature termination. *Bivariate analysis* uses two independent variables, such as age and sex, and attempts to analyze simultaneously their relation to a dependent variable, such as premature termination. The researcher might want to investigate why some members left the group while others of the same age and sex continued. Data might be collected which included marital status, employment, and residence, since these are variables which might affect group attendance. Cross tabulation or multivariate analysis is limited only by the resources of the investigator. Obviously, the more variables considered, the greater probability of establishing causal relationships. While cross tabulation may be done by hand, large amounts of data are usually tabulated and analyzed by computer (Overall and Klett, 1972).

Multiple Regression and Correlation

Complete experimental control over independent variables is difficult to attain, especially in natural settings. Recognition of this has expanded interest in multivariate techniques which employ various methods of dealing with the complexities existing in clinical settings. A popular form of multivariate analysis is multiple regression and correlation. This statistical procedure attempts to identify and classify relationships between one dependent (*criterion*) variable and a number of independent (*predictor*) variables. Correlational techniques measure the association among independent variables and their effect on the dependent variable. Regression procedures use these analyses to derive the line or curve which best fits the data so that future behavior may be adequately predicted.   Further discussion of these techniques are to be found in Cohen and Cohen (1975), Kerlinger and Pedhazur (1973), and Overall and Spiegel (1969).

Evaluating Analyses

Researchers may find the following inquiries, as outlined by Maher (1978), to be helpful in reviewing a completed data analysis:

- Were the statistics used with appropriate assumptions?
- Were appropriate tests of significance used and recorded?
- Have statistical significance levels been defined in practical terms?
- Has consideration been given to limited and abnormal distributions?
- Was the statistical strategy in line with the experimental design and measurement procedures?
- Was the number of significant findings compared with the total number of comparisons made?
- Were theoretical expectations in line with outcomes?

Questions and issues regarding effective and promising directions for research and evaluation strategies are numerous. The answers to these methodological concerns will not arrive easily, but are best sought through systematic replications of past research and careful planning of future studies. The following guidelines are important in the pursuit of meaningful group research.

1. Hypotheses should be stated clearly, particularly with regard to substantive intent. Groups should be defined according to the perspectives of structure, process, and outcome, as well as other dimensions that are of consequence to the research design.
2. Experimental designs should be considered in terms of their relative costs and benefits, and various approaches should be considered. These include combinations of within subject and between subject designs, along with individual and multiple group procedures.
3. There should be greater reliance on multitrait/multimethod paradigms, which allow simultaneous consideration of the same phenomena, utilizing measurements in behavioral, physiological, and psychological domains. Distinct evaluation perspectives of leaders, members, observers, and significant others should be noted.

4. There should be more emphasis on examination of structure, process, and outcome within the same study.
5. More in-depth, multidimensional measurement procedures should be utilized from individual and group perspectives, with greater acceptance of the combined use of proven measurements and newly developed tools. This should maximize the comparability of disparate group studies, allow for easier replications, and generate new research techniques.
6. Analytic techniques should be selected judiciously, with consideration given to assumptions of the procedures and hypotheses of the study.
7. More use should be made of multivariate statistics and stochastic models to examine group structure, process, and outcome.

SUMMARY

This chapter sketched briefly some approaches to the complexities and challenges of group research, approaches which must be continually refined and made complementary to theoretical viewpoints. Basic research terminology was defined and a few analytic techniques were outlined. Need for care in the selection and use of measurement tools and in data analysis was stressed. Through the research process, group phenomena may be explored systematically in order to understand group dynamics more fully.

REFERENCES

Anderberg, M.R. *Cluster Analysis for Application.* New York: Academic Press, 1973.

Andrulis, R.S. *Adult Assessment: A Source Book of Tests and Measures of Human Behavior.* Springfield, IL.: Charles C Thomas, 1977.

Bales, R.F. *Interaction Process Analysis: A Method for the Study of Small Groups.* Menlo Park, CA.: Addison-Wesley, 1950.

Blalock, H.M. *Social Statistics.* New York: McGraw-Hill, 1979.

Buros, O.K., Ed. *Personality: Tests and Reviews.* Highland Park, N.J.: Gryphan Press, 1970.

Cattell, R.B. *Personality and Mood by Questionnaire.* San Francisco: Jossey-Bass, 1973.

Chun, K.; S. Cobb; and J.R.P. French, Jr. *Measures for Psychological Assessment: A Guide to 3000 Original Sources and Their Applications.* Ann Arbor, MI.: Survey Research Center, Institute for Social Research, 1975.

Cohen, J., and P. Cohen. *Applied Multiple Regression/Correlation Analysis for the Behavioral Sciences.* New York: Wiley, 1975.

Comrey, A.L. *A First Course in Factor Analysis.* New York: Academic Press, 1973.

————— . "Common Methodological Problems in Factor Analytic Studies." *Journal of Consulting and Clinical Psychology* 46, 1978, pages 648–659.

Everitt, B. *Cluster Analysis.* London: Heinemann Educational Books, 1974.

Frankenhaeuser, M. "Experimental Approaches to the Study of Catecholamines and Emotion." In *Emotions — Their Parameters and Measurement*, L. Levi, Ed. New York: Ravin Press, 1975.

Gorsuch, R.L. *Factor Analysis.* Philadelphia: Saunders, 1974.

Hartigan, J.A. *Clustering Algorithms.* New York: Wiley, 1975.

Hathaway, S.R., and J.C. McKinley. *Minnesota Multiphasic Personality Inventory: Manual for Administration and Scoring.* New York: Psychological Corporation, 1967.

Hays, W.L. *Statistics.* New York: Holt Rinehart & Winston, 1963.

Kerlinger, R.N., and E.J. Pedhazur. *Multiple Regression in Behavioral Research.* New York: Holt Rinehart & Winston, 1973.

Kiresuk, T.J., and R.E. Sherman. "Goal Attainment Scaling: A General Method for Evaluating Comprehensive Community Mental Health Programs." *Community Mental Health Journal* 4, 1968, pages 443–453.

Lazarus, R.S. *Psychological Stress and the Coping Process.* New York: McGraw-Hill, 1966.

—————; J.C. Speisman; and A.M. Mordkoff. "The Relationship between Autonomic Indicators of Psychological Stress: Heart Rate and Skin Conductance." *Psychosomatic Medicine* 25, 1963, pages 19–30.

Maher, B. "Stimulus Sampling in Clinical Research: Representative Design Reviewed," *Journal of Consulting and Clinical Psychology* 46, 1978, pages 643–647.

Mason, J.W.; J.R. Maher; L.H. Hartely; E. Mongey; M.J. Perlow; and L.G. Jones. "Selectivity of Corticosteroid and Catecholamine Responses to Various Natural Stimuli." In *Psychopathology of Human Adaptation*, G. Serban, Ed. New York: Plenum, 1976.

McGrath, J.E. "Settings, Measures, and Themes: An Integrative Review of Some Research on Social-Psychological Factors in Stress." In *Social and Psychological Factors in Stress*, J.E. McGrath, Ed. New York: Holt Rinehart & Winston, 1970.

Mehrabian, A. "A Semantic Space for Nonverbal Behavior." *Journal of Consulting and Clinical Psychology*, 35, 1970, pages 248–257.

————— . *Nonverbal Communication.* Chicago: Aldine-Atherton, 1972.

Mulaik, S.A. *The Foundations of Factor Analysis.* New York: McGraw-Hill, 1972.

Murray, H.A. *Thematic Apperception Test.* Cambridge, MA.: Harvard University Press, 1943.

Overall, J.E. "Note on Multivariate Methods for Profile Analysis." *Psychological Bulletin* 61, 1964, pages 195–198.

————— , and C.J. Klett. *Applied Multivariate Analysis.* New York: McGraw-Hill, 1972.

————, and D.K. Spiegel. "Concerning Least Squares Analysis of Experimental Data." *Psychological Bulletin* 72, 1969, pages 311–322.

Robinson, J.P., and R.P. Shaver. *Measures of Social Psychological Attitudes.* Rev. ed. Ann Arbor, MI.: Survey Research Center, Institute for Social Research, 1973.

Rorschach, H. *Psychodiagnostics: A Diagnostic Test Based on Perception.* Berne, Switzerland: Huber, 1942.

Selye, H. *The Stress of Life.* New York: McGraw-Hill, 1976.

Siegel, S. *Nonparametric Statistics for the Behavioral Sciences.* New York: McGraw-Hill, 1956.

Straus, M.A., and B.W. Brown. *Family Measurement Techniques: Abstracts of Published Instruments, 1035–1074.* Rev. ed. Minneapolis, MN: University of Minnesota Press, 1978.

Sundberg, N.D. *Assessment of Persons.* Englewood Cliffs, N.J.: Prentice-Hall, 1977.

Taylor, J.A. "A Personality Scale of Manifest Anxiety." *Journal of Abnormal and Social Psychology* 48, 1953, pages 285–290.

Volicer, B.J.; M.A. Isenberg; and M.W. Burns. "Medical-Surgical Differences in Hospital Stress Factors." *Journal of Human Stress* 3, 1977, pages 3–13.

Walls, R.T.; T.J. Werner; A. Bacon; and T. Zane. "Behavior Checklists." In *Behavioral Assessment: New Directions in Clinical Psychology*, J.D. Cone and R.P. Hawkins, Eds. New York: Brunner/Mazel, 1977.

Wilkinson, L. "Response Variable Hypothesis in the Multivariate Analysis of Variance." *Psychological Bulletin* 82, 1975, pages 408–412.

Woodward, J.A., and J.E. Overall. "Multivariate Analysis of Variance by Multiple Regression Methods." *Psychological Bulletin* 82, 1975, pages 21–32.

Wolfe, J.H. "Pattern Clustering by Multivariate Mixture Analysis." *Multivariate Behavioral Research* 5, 1970, pages 329–350.

GLOSSARY

abstinence The state of being without a substance on which an individual depends for gratification.

acting out Behaviors or actions which express unconscious emotional conflicts.

adaptive Functional adjustment to changes in the environment by an individual, family, or group.

addiction Use of a chemical substance to the extent of physiological or psychological dependence.

affect Any mood, emotion, or feeling experienced or expressed by an individual.

affective Emotional experiential states such as anger, grief, joy, and anxiety.

aftercare Follow-up care after episodes of acute illness or hospitalization.

aggression Forceful actions which may be appropriate or inappropriate, are directed against other persons or objects, and do not necessarily respect the rights of others.

Alcoholics Anonymous A group program whose membership is composed of acknowledged alcoholics receiving and extending help through collective work which stresses sobriety and recourse to a "higher power."

altruism Commitment to the well-being and improvement of others.

ambivalence Coexistence of opposing thoughts or feelings toward the same person, object, or situation.

anxiety Intrapsychic discomfort arising from anticipation of danger or threat, usually of nonspecific origin.

apathy   Absence of affect or feeling, often manifested by withdrawal or disinterest.

assertiveness   Forceful but appropriate actions which make demands of others but respect their rights.

authentic   Awareness or recognition of the self as genuine and valid.

autism   Excessive preoccupation with self which is usually accompanied by interpersonal and situational distortions.

aversive therapy   Reduction or removal of undesirable behavior by associating unpleasant experiences with the behavior.

basic assumption   Conceptualization by Bion of prevailing group behaviors which are alternatives to productive work and which take the form of dependency, flight–fight, and pairing activities.

behavior therapy   A treatment modality which modifies behavior without exploring intrapsychic or interpersonal factors.

blocking   Interruption or interference with the flow of thought or speech due to the intrusion of anxiety or other unconscious factors.

boundaries   Psychological limits surrounding groups which help determine group membership, in addition to individual boundaries which surround each group member and maintain separateness despite pressure to merge with the group.

catharsis   Therapeutic release of repressed material achieved through affective verbalization of unconscious material.

change agent   A catalytic force or person which operates to produce adaptive change.

cognition   An ego function which includes such mental processes as learning, knowledge, and judgment.

cohesion   Feelings of belonging experienced by group members, generated by a common purpose or need.

compulsion   Persistent desire to perform a repetitive act in order to reduce or control anxiety.

confabulation   Defensive fabrication of forgotten details in order to conceal memory lapses or informational gaps.

confrontation   Technique used to help others become self-directive and self-aware.

consensual validation   Correction of idiosyncratic distortion by feedback from others in the same group or setting.

content   Substantive or factual material brought up in the group.

corrective reenactment   Reenactment in a favorable group setting of distressing psychological experiences of the past.

cotherapy   A form of therapy in which more than one person treats an individual or a group.

crisis   A hazardous event which is unresponsive to usual coping behaviors, resulting in confusion and disorganization.

crisis intervention   Brief treatment of a circumscribed, immediate problem by directive, active therapeutic means.

curative factors   Aspects of group life which facilitate therapeutic change or a positive group experience.

defense mechanism   An unconscious, protective mental process used to relieve conflict and anxiety which threaten the ego.

denial   Refusal, expressed verbally or behaviorally, to accept the reality of a disturbing fact or event.

depersonalization   A sense that one's person, existence, or surroundings are unreal.

detoxification Gradual or abrupt removal of the toxic effects of a drug.

deviance Behavior which does not conform to accepted standards of the group.

displacement Substitution of one target for another toward which negative feelings may be safely expressed.

eclecticism Selection of concepts and principles from various theoretical frameworks according to their suitability in a particular situation.

ego A major component of personality described by Freud whose major function is mediation between demands of the id and prohibitions of the superego; includes such material processes as perception, memory, thinking, and reasoning.

ego alien Thoughts, feelings, or actions which are not acceptable to the individual and therefore increase anxiety levels.

ego ideal The aspect of personality which includes identifications and values defining the self as one would like to be.

ego syntonic Thoughts, feelings, or actions, which are acceptable to the individual and do not increase anxiety levels.

egocentric A form of self-involvement which is characterized by self-absorption and relative indifference to the needs of others.

emotion The affective climate of a group resulting from positive and negative feelings between individual members, and from shared feelings toward the group.

empathy Objective awareness of the feelings and behavior of others, in contrast to sympathy which is subjective.

enabling solutions Group behaviors which explore essential issues, maintain open communication, and avoid superficiality and evasion.

encounter group A group whose major purposes include self-awareness and emotional expressiveness.

existentialism A school of thought which stresses self-determination and responsibility for one's choices and which discounts biological and cultural determinants as major factors of existence.

feedback Response of a group or individual to the behavior or communication of another.

focal conflict Shared feelings of group members concerning such issues as dependency, authority, and inclusion.

gestaltism A school of thought which emphasizes a total configuration of perception and experience based upon needs which become dominant, are met, and give way to other urgent needs.

goals Major purposes or objectives for which groups are organized.

grief work Active mourning which loosens bonds between survivors and lost objects or persons.

group An interaction between two or more persons occurring within boundaries which contain the interaction and define the membership.

group conflict A psychological struggle in the group arising from opposing drives, needs, and impulses.

group pressure Overt and covert demands by group members that others submit to group rules, goals, and norms.

group process Covert acts and feelings in the group, including the emotional nuances, unconscious goals, and latent forces which impel the group toward or away from its goals.

herd behavior Desire to belong to a group and to engage in behavior like that of other group members.

id Aspect of the personality which is present from birth and is the repository of instinctual needs and drives.

identification An unconscious psychological process by which one individual adopts or assumes the values, behaviors or attributes of another.

insight Understanding the meaning of behavior and making connections between behavior and underlying causes.

instincts Innate drives or needs which include, among others, sexuality and aggression.

interpersonal Forces or transactions operating between individuals.

interpretation Examination of the meaning or motivation underlying behavior of the group or an individual member.

intellectualization Converting a strong urge or impulse into an intellectual concept, thus reducing its strength and impact.

interaction analysis A quantified analytic technique used to score and evaluate group interaction.

intrapsychic Feelings, drives, or motives arising within the self.

intrapsychic conflict Conflict arising from opposing feelings or drives within oneself.

kinesics Study of body movement and nonverbal expressiveness.

libido Energy associated with instinctual drives and goals.

life cycle group Conceptualization of group development as an evolutionary movement from immaturity through maturity to eventual decline and demise.

linear progressive group Conceptualization of group development as a forward movement from immaturity to mature productivity.

metacommunication Communication about communication, which conveys information about the relationships among the participants.

milieu therapy Treatment which emphasizes environmental influences, interpersonal experience, and a sense of community.

motivation Impetus or incentive to behave in ways which satisfy needs and desires.

narcissism Self-love or egocentricity which is not necessarily likened to genital expression.

National Training Laboratory (NTL) for Applied Behavioral Science A program established in 1947 to teach group dynamics to government and industrial executives in which member to member relationships are emphasized.

network therapy Group work involving the nuclear family, extended family, relatives, and friends involved in life of the client.

neurosis Mental disorder characterized by excessive anxiety which may be discharged through somatic channels, converted, displaced, or projected.

nondirective A leadership style in which the therapist follows the direction indicated by the client or clients.

norms Pressures toward conformity established over time through collaborative actions and shared expectations of the group.

nuclear conflict Behavior of an individual which reflects conflicts and problem-solving behaviors originating in childhood.

obsession Recurrent idea, thought, or feeling which cannot be dispelled.

oedipal Conflict related to erotic attachment to the parent of the opposite sex and the need to identify with the parent of the same sex.

orientation Awareness of the relation of self to space, time, and other persons.

panic Severe anxiety accompanied by confusion, disorganization, and a tendency to engage in herd behavior.

pendular or recurrent groups Conceptualization of group development as recurrent movement between poles representing either success or failure in accomplishing stage critical tasks.

personality disorder Mental disorder characterized by maladaptive behaviors which are motivated by self-interest and accompanied by little subjective anxiety.

phobia Intense fear associated with an external stimulus, object, or situation.

prevention Primary: a concept of health care which is directed toward reducing the incidence of illness. Secondary: a concept of health care which is directed toward treating illness which has developed. Tertiary: a concept of health care which is directed toward alleviation and rehabilitation of the disabling effects of illness.

primary groups Significant groups which confirm identity, inculcate social values, and provide emotional support for the members. The family is an example of a primary group.

projection Defense mechanism in which the unacceptable thoughts and feelings of one person are attributed by that person to another.

protagonist A term used in psychodrama for the person who is the center of the scenario or script being enacted.

proxemics Study of space maintained between individuals involved in interpersonal transactions.

psychodrama A technique of group psychotherapy in which individuals enact their psychological conflicts and problems in order to achieve therapeutic effects.

psychoanalysis Application of Freudian concepts to bring unconscious conflicts to awareness, to explore their origin through free association and interpretation in order to reduce maladaptive defenses and coping mechanisms.

psychosexual Psychoanalytic theory in which personality develops through oral, anal, phallic, and latent periods, culminating with the genital stage in which mature, sexual intimacy is achieved.

psychosis Mental disorder in which the capacity to recognize and relate to reality is impaired.

psychosocial Life cycle theory of Erikson, characterized by eight stages of human life, with a developmental task specific to each stage.

psychotherapeutic groups A treatment modality which endeavors to produce psychological and social change through monitored interactions in a group setting.

rapport A state of responsive relatedness between two or more persons.

rationalization A defense mechanism which transforms irrational behaviors and motives into rational, logical ones.

reaction formation A defense mechanism in which behaviors are the antithesis or opposite of actual thoughts and impulses.

reference groups Groups which influence the attitudes, values, and behaviors of members but are less pervasive than primary groups.

regression Defense mechanism in which the individual returns to behaviors appropriate to earlier development stages.

repression   Defense mechanism in which unacceptable thoughts and feelings are removed from conscious awareness.

resistance   Conscious or unconscious opposition to bringing repressed materials into conscious awareness.

restrictive solutions   Group behaviors which relieve anxiety and maintain interpersonal comfort but avoid dealing with essential issues.

reversal   Change of a strong wish or impulse into its opposite after gratification of the wish or prolonged frustration of the wish.

role   A set of behavioral expectations shared by group members concerning the occupant of a position in the group.

role enactment   Observable verbal and nonverbal behavior of a role occupant.

rules   Stipulated standards of group conduct agreed to by leaders and members.

scapegoat   Group member who expresses shared feelings which others disavow, thereby becoming the target of negative feelings.

secondary groups   Groups limited to a specific task and time frame, less influential and more specialized than primary groups.

self-actualization   An attempt to make maximal use of one's potential.

self-analytic groups   Activities in which members function as participant observers while sharing subjective and objective data relevant to the group experience in which all are involved.

self-esteem   The degree to which an individual feels competent and valued.

sociogram   A schematic method of generating data about intragroup attraction, status, power, and cohesion.

sublimation   Defense mechanism in which unacceptable drives and impulses are expressed through socially approved behaviors.

superego   The aspect of personality which censors the instinctual demands of the id and which is formed by identification with the standards and values of parents and other significant figures in early life.

suppression   Defense mechanism in which an unacceptable impulse or feeling is consciously controlled.

symbiosis   A close and mutually dependent relationship between two persons, often maintained at the cost of individuation.

systems theory   Conceptualization of groups as social systems in which members are units or components which are interdependent and interrelated.

T-Group (Training Group)   A form of group which emphasizes self-awareness and understanding of group process.

tabula rosa   An empty page or screen symbolized by the psychoanalyst who utilizes free association and transference as integral parts of the therapeutic relationship.

Tavistock groups   A model used to study intragroup phenomena by emphasizing the importance of relationships between the leader and members.

termination   The orderly conclusion of the therapeutic relationship whether individual or group.

therapeutic groups   A group experience which offers the possibility of interpersonal adaptation or support.

transsexual   An individual dissatisfied with the socially assigned gender; dissatisfaction may be psychological only, but may also involve physiological ambiguity.

transference   Unconscious transfer to others of feelings and responses originally attached to significant persons in early life. Counter-transference is a subjective response to transference phenomena experienced by a therapist or group leader.

undoing   Defense mechanism in which an individual attempts to reverse an unacceptable action.

values   Shared ideas of what the group should become.

working through   Process of increasing insight through frequent exploration of a problem or conflict.

INDEX